VYĀYĀMA-YOGA

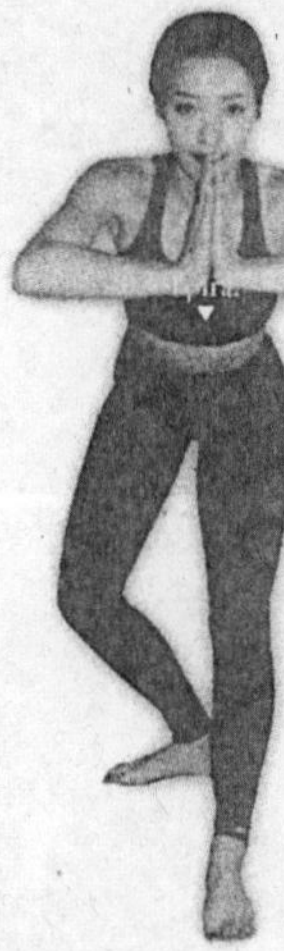

Vyāyāma Yoga

The Art of Dynamic Breathing

Javier Plazas

New Age Books

ISBN: 978-81-7822-174-8

First Edition: Delhi, 2008

Published by
NEW AGE BOOKS
A-44, Naraina Industrial Area, Phase I
New Delhi-110 028 (INDIA)
Email: nab@vsnl.in
Website: www.newagebooksindia.com

Printed in India
at Shri Jainendra Press
A-45, Naraina Phase-I, New Delhi-110 028

Contents

Dedication

tvaṁ bhāskaraścet kamalaṁ tato 'ham
tvaṁ sāgaraścet kaṇikā tato 'ham !
tvaṁ pāvakaścet śalabhas tato 'ham
chāyā tavāhaṁ nahi saṁśayo 'tra !!

"If you are the Sun, I am a lotus flower;
if you are the ocean, I am a drop;
if you are the fire, I am a moth.
There is no doubt that I am nothing more
than your shadow"
SWAMI TILAK

This work sheds light on the Vyāyāma practice and its basic fundamental knowledge. It is dedicated to the memory of my beloved Master Shri Swami Tilak, who gave me the inspiration I needed to integrate the 'curative art' and to share it with those near to me.

The *Vyāyāma Yoga* saved me from certain death when malaria was threatening my life in Western Bengal and the doctors had given up hope on my recovery. The last resource of my will to live came back from within myself from the same source I had learned when I met Swami Tilak, at the age of sixteen.

The medicine of the Vyāyāma Yoga practice miraculously gave me healthy energy, gave me strength and showed me what the Master told me so many times: "The secret of life and death is very near, in your breath."

I love Vyāyāma Yoga as much as I love life, thus I love to teach it to share this very love to show my constant gratitude.

I started to learn Vyāyāma Yoga in 1976 in the traditional manner being by the Master, watching the Master, without limits of time, without anxiety, as an apprentice, becoming impregnated with the knowledge. A few years later I started teaching to my monastic pupils in a simple method through the use of 18 positions of *Sukha Vyāyāma* or 'Happy Vyāyāma', but it was not until 1994 that I structured the teaching and shaped it in an accessible way, so that it could be learned by men and women who have many needs and little time.

The book in your hands is a historic event in itself, it is the first methodological Vyāyām book ever published, not only in Spain, but in the entire world. I shall honour the New Delhi's Vishvāyatan Yogāshram Master Dhirendra Brahmachārī, disciple of Shrī Kārtikeya Mahāriṣi, who taught a basic form of energetic Vyāyām and showed it in his book titled 'Yogic Sūkshma Vyāyāma', published in 1975.

"To my students and friends, I say thank you for the collaboration and enthusiasm, who helped to compile this book. I would also like to make a special mention to my students who are presently teachers who posed for the pictures: Satomi Miyagoshi, David Beriain and Eva Maral. Thanks to Ulises Miranda who collected and shaped this book. Thanks to Cristina Morencos who revised, corrected and styled the text and honoured me by writing the prologue. Thanks to Lisardo Sanchez for his ability in photography. Thanks to Edaf publishing for being enthusiastically involved in the realization of the Spanish edition of this book, especially Sebastian Vazquez, my patient editor in Spain. To Fay Williams and Ondine Savage for their collaboration in checking the English text. To New Age Books and especially Mr. Rajeev Jain for his interest in publishing the English translation of the book."

I will never forget what Swami Tilak advised when I was taking my first steps in Yoga and what I see as the essence of Vyāyāma. "My son! We do not need more wise men and saints in this world. We only lack men. Try to become one."

November 1st, 2002 JAVIER PLAZAS

Prologue

What I carried out moved by rage,
vigorously grew from dusk to dawn,
but did not survive the fight with elements.

What I sowed moved by love,
sprang firmly and matured slowly,
and enjoyed blessings from heaven.

PETER ROSEGGER

Rosegger's verses reveal that serenity provides us with love and love with blessings. In the same way, this book reveals long-time jealously-kept secrets that lead us to deep calmness, showing a path, towards well being, thus far unknown to most people.

The author of this book, Javier Plazas, is what Lawrence would call "an aristocrat of spirit", a man whose thinking and conduct are in perfect agreement.

He chose the hard way, not the easy one and in this way he forged himself into a man who could be flattered or seduced, but never intimidated.

He tirelessly helps us and reminds us that we should not become victims of time, looking back into the past with melancholy and sadness, that it is never too late to change, while at the same time protecting us with his wisdom, love and courage in the same way he protects life itself. We can think of him as an essential person in our invisible path ahead, for the power and depth of his thoughts, a guide, a protector, a friend, a master.

The word "Virtue" regains its meaning when linked to his name. It is of great consolation to know that wise men always come back to the Earth. And with the humility that only the *knowledge about how to live provides,* he encourages us not only to be led by him, but to surpass him. This book is an irrefutable proof of his interest for anyone willing to approach the hard path of knowing oneself.

This work has been bred by the selfless love of a great master and his ancient lineage to teach us a highly perfected route, which helps us to achieve the calmness and inner peace necessary for us to obtain our own happiness.

It is a complete and straightforward tract on Vyāyāma Yoga, a discipline unknown not only in the Western world, but also in the majority of India, its country of origin. During its lecture, we should not forget that complete lines of masters-disciples have been preserving this knowledge allowing it to remain intact to the present day.

Vyāyāma Yoga is a healing art that keeps our physical body healthy and opens a wide space to spirituality. A tool that unifies, simplifies and structures the principles necessary for introspective relationships at the human level and with the rest of the beings dwelling in the Universe.

There is a genesis process that acts in reciprocity between Vyāyāma Yoga and the person who practises in which the physical body and its energy interact in a beneficial way. It is a self-liberating way, giving the sound back to the inner voice that can be heard at the very core of Being.

In the present day, man lives in constant agony and self-misunderstanding. Science, advanced technology and Reason impose on the westerner an unnatural tension that gets involuntarily incorporated in our daily life. Man keeps looking for something but he does not know exactly what he is looking for. Little by little we have been demolishing myths and values that remind us of the objective of our search and now we are blindly searching desirous of our ideal.

This book, besides being a guide for everyone who wishes to learn this healing practice, is a historical document, because it is the first methodological book of Vyāyāma Yoga that has been published in the world.

Reading this book opens doors to a universe of possibilities capable of improving and transforming one's quality of life, health and well-being.

Vyāyāma Yoga holds out its hand to us, let us embrace it with strength.

CRISTINA MORENCOS
November 1, 2002

Introduction

The literal translation of the word *Vyāyāma*[1] is "to tame the inner breath." This Sanskrit[2] term is composed of two words: *yāma*, which means "to tame" and *vyā*, which means to stimulate, to incite.

Vyāyāma Yoga is the discipline that teaches you to tame the energy that comes from air through breathing.

Its different meanings show us the depth of the technique:

- Drag and brake down any solid, subtle or mental structure
- Separate essential elements filling the core
- Healthy sport or physical activity
- Fight between bodies
- Struggle to achieve a goal
- Warrior combat
- That which enables you to successfully make efforts
- Effort for self-improvement.

In all of these definitions we find a common denominator: expression of force in combination with breath that gives a character of energetic exercise, providing the possibility to model the body and strengthen it in a notable way.

Breath control causes different amounts of oxygen consumption, combustion and hence different amounts of energy production to apply to body movement.

One of the basic principles of the practice is that all movements must have its origin in breathing. This means that all the movements have to be coordinated by a concrete type of breathing. The importance of this coordination is based, as previously stated, in a better utilization of body energy which comes from nutrients and directly from breathing.

The effective control of breathing is one of the most important capabilities of the human being. We could be forty days without eating, far fewer without water, but we could barely sustain life some minutes

1. Pronounced 'bee-ah-yam' Vyāyāma.
2. Sanskrit is the classic language spoken by the Aryan people and is the root of the classic European languages. The use of Sanskrit words is habitual in Indian teachings, because of its precision, briefness and tradition when it comes to designate techniques, as well as philosophical concepts and elements. The meanings of the Sanskrit terms translated in this text were taken from the *Sir Monier Monier Williams, Oxford University & Benares Hindu University* dictionary. This is the language in which the *Vedas* are written, the most ancient written texts known to humanity.

without breathing. Breathing is the primal source of nourishment in our lives and the basis of all the processes that support life.

Breath control means achieving the capacity to control our vital processes and unveil the key to contain our energy. There is an intimate connection between body, mind and energy, the alteration of one influences the other two. Through Vyāyāma Yoga practice we learn to control breathing and with that, the movement of our mind.

Keeping in mind the previous concepts it is not strange that this ancient practice was being utilised in India (Bharata Varsha)[3] as the essential training for warriors, yogis, practitioners of martial arts, dancers and performers.

3. The city of light. The Ancient Vedic Empire of India. Land of light

Fundamental Knowledge of Vyāyāma Yoga

ORIGINS AND ROOTS OF VYĀYĀMA YOGA

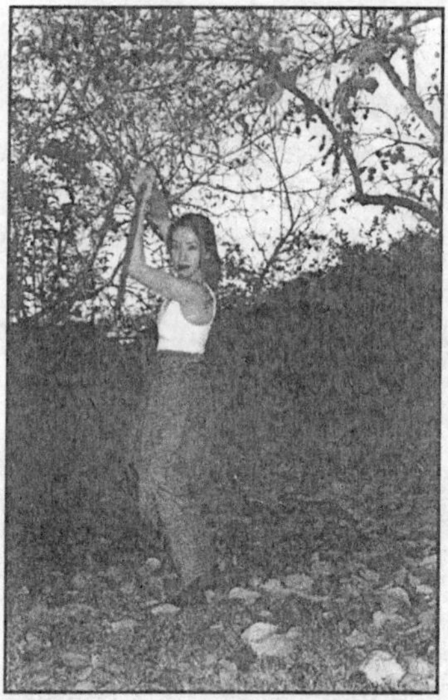

The philosophical principles of Vyāyāma Yoga are contained in the "texts of the tan[1] expansion path" (Tantra Mārga*)*, among which we can highlight the "Mahā Nirvāṇa Tantra" or the "Durlabhvasāra Tantra."

Vyāyāma is the most ancient healing-energetic exercise in the world, which methodologically and culturally inspired other energetic gymnastics and martial arts. Its origins are very ancient and its disciplines were practised in India during the *Vedic* age, before the Buddhist era.

Vyāyāma Yoga was the backbone of the personal training of warriors, for whom a noble spirit and inner knowledge were of great value.

The Vedic art of military science is known in Sanskrit as *Dhanur Vidyā* or *Vīra Vrata Vidyā,* and their meanings in Sanskrit are 'the science of archery' and 'the science of the strong'. Its students were known as *vīravratas,*[2] those who preserved their physical and mental strength, learning to manifest it in a precise way and only when necessary.

1. The singular and inner manifestation of total energy. Its expansion allows oneself to extend far beyond known existential reality and own reality, to a concrete point, a potential and a capacity. It propagates inner energy and extends it beyond one's limits. Its expansion makes the astral body shine through the vital primary energy condensing centres.
2. The concept of the strong (viras) is the same as the one expressed in the tantric texts when they describe the different types of character that people manifest. Only those who show *vira* character, which means strong, self-controlled, and full of physical strength, are able to access tantric knowledge.

Dhanur Vidyā was taught through the knowledge of archery, *Dhanur Veda*,[3] the use of the sword, *Kaṅga Mārga* and *Vyāyāma*. In *Kaṅga Mārga* the basic disciplines were: *Asidhara Vāda* (to clutch the sharp sword), *Kudhana Vāda* (to clutch the wooden sword), *Chicku Vāda* (to clutch the dagger), *Daṇḍa Vāda* (to clutch the cane), and *Hasta Vāda* (to expand the fists) which takes on three basic forms: the monkey with rooted legs, the lion showing its claws, and the man with dense movements, whose mind controls everything.

In *Vyāyāma Yoga* there was a strong emphasis on "*śakti vikāsakas*", practices that provide a great physical preparation of muscular strength and knowledge about the projection of energy in each and every part of the body.

The famous wise kings of the Vedic age, *Rājarṣis*, (among which we can highlight *Janaka-Rājā*) and the Buddhist monks afterwards, stimulated knowledge of the *Dhanur Veda* and introduced the teachings of energetic gymnastics into the monasteries and society in general through physicians, who utilised it as a psycho-energetic gym.

After the age of Janaka-*Rājā*, Bodhidharma, a Buddhist monk, brought Vyāyāma to China in the fifth century, to enable the religious people in the Shaolin temples to defend themselves against bandits and strengthen their bodies, weakened by their ascetic and monastic lifestyle. Afterwards, Chinese energetic gymnastics and martial arts developed, followed by the Japanese martial arts: Tai-chi, Qi-gong, Kung-fu, Shorinji-kempo or Aikido.

Thanks to these past efforts, *Vyāyāma Yoga* can be learned today as a martial training, as a preparation for dramatic art and dance, or as a health therapy.

Although its philosophical and esoteric principles are found in various *Tantra* texts, few vestiges survived time. Some stone and wooden sculptures in many Indian temples representing human and divine figures in *Vyāyāma Yoga* postures are practically the only historic documents in existence.

VYĀYĀMA YOGA TODAY

Nowadays, *Vyāyāma Yoga* is a re-emerging discipline after being

3. This Vedic art of war science is found in the Dhanur Veda, a complementary Vedic text. The bow symbolizes all weapons, because it represents perfect control of the mind and the expression of the energy. In Sanskrit, Dhanur is arch and Veda means knowledge, so Dhanur Veda is translated as 'knowledge of archery'. Two of the legendary warriors known for their prowess were Arjuna (famous for his capacity to hit a bullseye with his eyes closed) and Ekalavya, who surpassed Arjuna's skills.

hidden for centuries due to India's historical circumstances and loss of traditional, spiritual and philosophical values that formerly impregnated these practices. *Vyāyāma Yoga* was not lucky enough to be considered a profane practice as were the Chinese, Japanese or Korean gymnastics and martial arts. It became persecuted by Muslims and afterwards, from the XIX century onwards, by the English during the colonisation period. Its practice was prohibited by law by the British Rāj, so from then on it was clandestinely practised. Through secret transmission by a number of masters, *Vyāyāma Yoga* managed to survive through the years. It is quite unknown in the western world and in India itself. The majority of teachers can be found in the South of India, in Kerala and in Tamil Nāḍu, and are often difficult to access. They are almost exclusively the members of warrior families and princes from old viceroyalties.

In some places, for the most part in South India, we can find the practice of *Maipayat* and *Kalaripayat*. *Vyāyāma Yoga* and *Kalaripayat* are the same, as are *svarodaya* and *maipayat*.[4]

The "Traditional School of *Vyāyāma Yoga*" originated from the venerable Master Swami Tilak, teaches an original and ancestral form of *Vyāyāma Yoga*.

GENERAL BENEFITS

An assiduous Vyāyāma Yoga student is an enthusiastic person, manifesting great vital capacity and mental balance. His/her body, either thickset or thin, appears healthy, strong and compact.

All movements, postures and gestures change, influenced by habitual practice. Incorporating *Vyāyāma Yoga* practice in our lives makes us more conscious of our physical, mental, and energetic movements. Through practising *Vyāyāma* all our movements become energetically more appropriate.

Vyāyāma Yoga brings harmony to the body and mind, strength to muscles and tendons, and the spine is freed from unnecessary tension providing adequate elasticity to the back. It drains the central nervous system, unblocks joints, and prevents diseases such as arthritis, degenerative osteoarthritis and osteoporosis. It gives vitality to the skeletal system, body tissues, and internal organs due to increased oxygenation of the cells.

4. In Ancient India languages were classified in two large blocks: the Aryans, using a Sanskrit form in the Aryan towns, and the Dravidians from the Dravidic towns situated in the South.

FIVE REQUIREMENTS FOR PRACTICE

In every true *Vyāyāma Yoga* practice the following principles should be observed:

Body movement should follow the breath

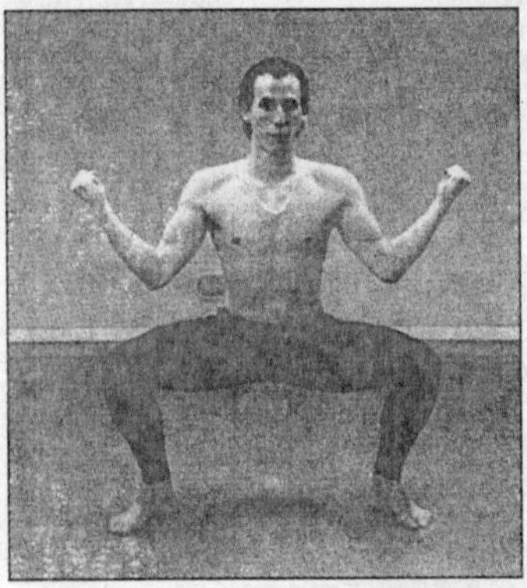

Unlike any other type of gymnastics, *Vyāyāma* is the art and discipline that teaches how to tame the energy that comes from air through breathing. Any movement is preceded by an inhalation or exhalation, and there is always coordination between breathing and body movement.

The mind observes the movement of the body and the breath

To become conscious of our body and of this phenomenon, our mind needs to be focused.

There is always movement in the *Vyāyāma Yoga* practice, either internal or external. The common point between *Vyāyāma Yoga* and meditation is the focus of the mind. While in yogic meditation the mind is concentrated on a fixed point keeping the body still and breathing as calm as possible, in *Vyāyāma Yoga* the mind is focused on the breathing, which is projected through the movement of the body. This is why we call *Vyāyāma Yoga* a meditative and aerobic gymnastic.

The breathing is sonorous and expansive

The sound mixed with breathing allows us to specifically concentrate energy in different parts of the organism, and creates a favourable mental state for practice.

It is expansive because we use all of our lung capacity, alternating between diamphragmatic, thorax and clavicle breathing, and uniting all of them together.

The *haṭha* breath is full of force and provides us with power, vitality and internal heat. This allows for the expansive movements of *Vyāyāma* as well as encouraging correct breathing. This exercise is very beneficial for the lungs because they are exercised to their full capacity.

Every movement is circular and harmonic

After having mastered the preceding principles, the last basic principle in *Vyāyāma Yoga* is the result or consequence of the other four. By linking breathing and body movements, a feeling of 'fluidity' and harmony between the mind, breath and body is produced.

The end of one movement is the beginning of the next movement

If we keep in mind the first principle, which tells us about the link between breathing and movement, we can conclude that in the same way as breathing is composed of a series of inhalations and exhalations, all the movements (*vyāṅgas*) are linked with each other, and are performed without breaking the connection between the breath and body movement.

When we finish a practice session, the final movements consist of taking a few steps back, which represents the will to continue learning and the mental predisposition to do so.

This *Vyāyāma Yoga* principle is actually part of a philosophical premise about the relationship between all that exists and the succession of transformations needed for life to be possible. From this point of view, nothing is destroyed and nothing is created; everything is just transformed.

OTHER IMPORTANT PRINCIPLES

To establish harmony, *Sama*

Sama means to harmonize, to calm down after making an effort. In order to do so, the body needs to remain in a relaxed state, breathing at ease. We look for the natural state in which the mind is in balance with the breath and body.

To become rooted, *Sthānam*

Holding our body still, we draw strength from breath, taking it to the base of the throat, *vāyu kanda*,[5] it is retained. Concentrating on this point and producing a sharp sound with the glottis, we exhale, visualizing the air as a heavy iron ball falling to the *tan*. The mind becomes embodied in a state of concentration, allegorically called "to ground oneself in the sky". On the other hand, the body remains still, "to ground oneself in the earth".

5. The place where Vāyu lives, the wind, is situated at the base of the throat and below the throat.

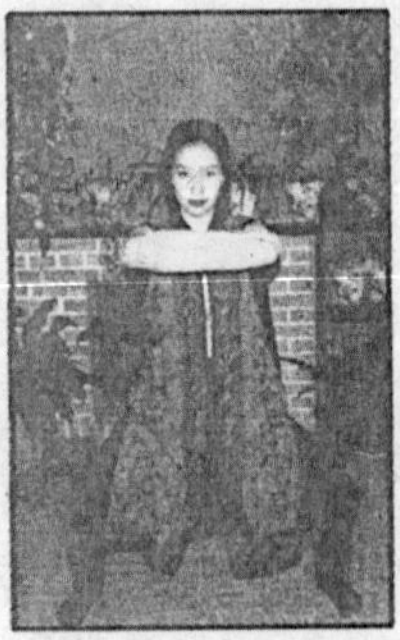

To align the energy distribution centres, *Tālas*

This is achieved by aligning all the *Tālas* situated in the part of the body we use when we perform any *vyaṅga.*

THE TWO ESSENCES OF VYĀYĀMA YOGA

The develpoment of the series of movements in *Vyāyāma Yoga* is called *Krama Abhyāsa* and is basically composed of:

1. Body movements or dynamics, *Vyayakas.*
2. Types of breathing, *Vāyukas.*

THE THREE TYPES OF VYĀYĀMA YOGA

Dense *Vyāyāma, Sthūla Vyāyāma*

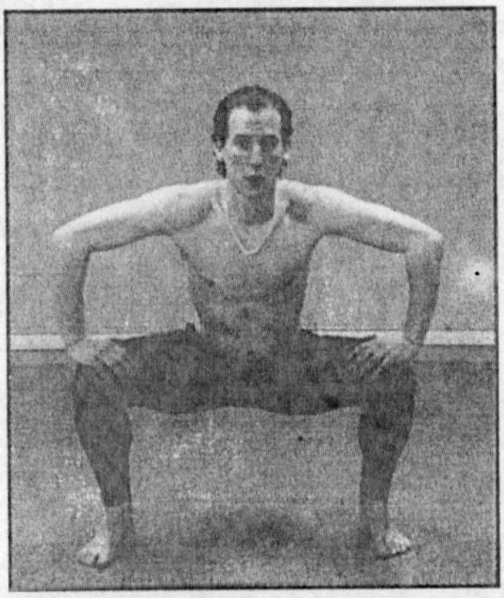

This is the dense or static, internal energetic movement *Vyāyāma Yoga.* It is said to be 'big' because it makes the body glow, 'solid' because it makes the body compact and 'voluminous' because it makes body mass increase. This *Vyāyāma Yoga* constructs the student from the five main elements of *nature.*[6]

In contrast to *Sūkṣma Vyāyāma, Sthūla Vyāyāma* is more internal. Its rule is "with less external movement, there is more internal movement." The body becomes solid, strong and hardened. The person who practises it may have the feeling that his/her body becomes crystalised as if it were a rock. The static *vyaṅgas* provide great physical strength, and can even be held ten minutes or longer in advanced sessions.

Subtle Vyāyāma, *Sūkṣma Vyāyāma*

It is the subtle, external energetic movement Vyāyāma. The meaning of the word *Sūkṣma* in *Sanskrit* is varied, and can be related to the following concepts: 'moment', because the projection of the

6. Earth, water, fire, air and ether. The five elements, named tattvas, are primal states of matter, and to be able to comprehend them in a more precise way we could refer to them as the solidity, the mobility, the heat, the impulse and the vibration.

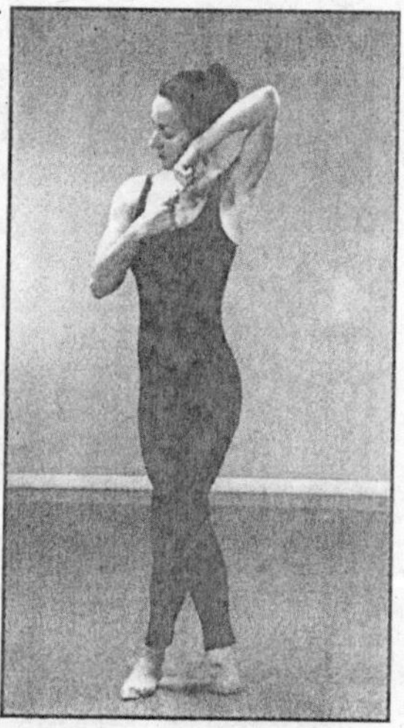

energy is condensed in a very short fraction of time; 'small', because it concentrates all the energy in the *tan*; 'subtle' because it is managed from the vital breath; 'tight', as it stylises the body, and 'tenuous' for being as delicate as silk brocade. It is 'intangible' because its energy extension is only manifested in the sensitivity of the vital centres, cakras. Breathing may be slow, medium or quick paced. It is an energising *Vyāyāma Yoga.*

Mental Vyāyāma

It is the magic mental and psychic energetic movement Vyāyāma. The meanings of the word *kāraṇa* applied to *Vyāyāma Yoga* are the following: 'cause', for being the origin of all dynamics and lying in *the tan*; 'intelligent', because it develops hidden, profound and powerful faculties, like astral travelling, projecting energy through a glance and being able to communicate by shapes and gestures. It is 'expert', because it is a more advanced and complex practice. It is the most subtle and psychic Vyāyāma because it is the thought that transmits energy.

This *Vyāyāma Yoga* teaches us to project energy through the hands, and gives us a basis for understanding the philosophy of the *tan*, which covers the principles of balance. It is the closest to our spirit.

PRACTICE DYNAMICS

The movements and their strength will vary according to the dynamics followed during the practice, and will also depend on the energy we use with them. There are three basic speeds.

Slow, low impact, Adhama kala.
Moderate, medium impact, Madhyama kala.
Decisive, high impact, Uttama kala.

FORMS

The original practice, which is spontaneous and creative, is based on figures and technical movements inspired by phenomena of nature and human tasks, and is called *sahaja krama abhyāsa.*

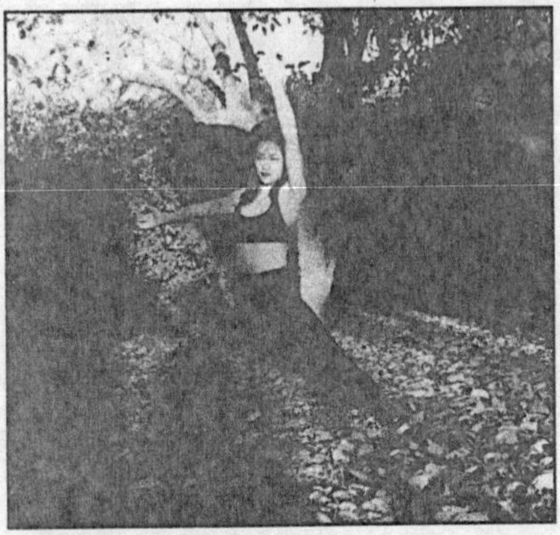

The practice is structured in sets and sub-sets of exercises called *Yoga krama abhyāsa.*

In its basic state, *Vyāyāma Yoga* does not follow any set structure, but is determined by the mobilization of energy by means of breathing and body movement. The objective is to teach it, and in order for the student to learn, teachers have structured a series of exercises.

The structures or *kramas* are divided into a series of positions called *vyaṅgas,* or chains of movements, and can be divided into six classes:

1. Energy strengtheners, or ***śakti vikāsakas.***
2. Energy rejuvenators, or ***śakti vardhakas.***
3. Energy purifiers, or ***śakti śuddhis.***
4. Energy mobilizers, or ***śakti gatis.***
5. Energy pulsation regulators, or ***śakti urdanas.***
6. Energy recoverers, or ***śakti pusṭis.***

Essential Learnings

LEARNING BREATHING

Our quality of life relies on our breathing. Controlled breathing brings more years of life and more resistance, because it provides rich oxygenation to all the body cells.

Prāṇa, vital energy, is present in the whole universe, in solid food, in water, and in air. Just as we need to eat food and drink water, it is absolutely imperative that we breathe air in order to live. When we breathe in air, we inhale positively charged Prāṇa, and when we exhale, we exhale negatively charged Prāṇa. This form of Prāṇa is called Āpāna. Prāṇa manifests itself in the body in five ways, each regulating a different vital function: lungs, Prāṇaprāṇa; excretory organs, Prāṇa-apāna; swallowing organs, Prāṇaudāna; organs that help in the process of assimilation, Prāṇasamāna; and all the processes needed for the circulation of body fluids and nerve currents, Prāṇavyāna.

In our astral body, positive energy, Prāṇa, flows in the form of ha through nāḍī Piṅgalā, which converges in the right nostril. Negative energy, Āpāna, in the form of ṭha, flows through nādī Iḍā, which converges in the left nostril. Throughout the day we breathe approximately 21,000 times. Someone who practises Vyāyāma, a Vyāyāmika, always keeps in mind the following law of nature: "the greater the number of breaths, the shorter the lifespan; the fewer the number of breaths, the longer the lifespan."

Breathing flows through one of the nostrils for approximately one hour, and then alternates and starts flowing through the other. The act of breathing is called svara, and the alternation between each nostril is called udaya. The whole process is called svarodaya. When this alternation in the breath does not occur, an imbalance can arise causing disease and psychological disorders, collapse of vital functions and even death.

There are three main classes of breathing associated with air ingestion, which can be divided according to the area of the lungs to which the air is directed: diaphragmatic, corresponding to the lower area of the lungs; thoracic, in the middle zone of the lungs; and clavicular, in the upper area of the lungs.

Due to the triangular shape of our lungs, diaphragmatic breathing is richer, because of greater lung capacity in the lower area. Clavicular breathing is less efficient, because of the reduced area of the lungs at this level. Each type of breathing produces a different effect:

Diaphragmatic breathing is the natural way of breathing when a human being is born. This type of breathing allows the most air ingestion, and is capable of giving us energy and calming the mind simultaneously. It does not alter the nervous system, but invigorates it. We can use it in **Vyāyāma** yoga, meditation, relaxation, sexuality, and we should also use it spontaneously in our daily lives.

Thoracic breathing is very good in activating our mind and nervous system, but very harmful to our health if practised for long periods of time, as it applies pressure to the organs in a negative way, generating excessive heat and accelerating the destructive mechanisms of the body. It excessively heats our mind, causing states of irritability and mental agitation.

Clavicular breathing provides us with very little air ingestion creating anxious states of mind. It collapses the nervous system and the organs and muscles of our body. It demands a higher number of breathes and increases mental activity.

Complete or yogic breathing is the type of breathing that successively utilizes all these parts.

As we learned in a previous chapter, yogic breathing teaches us the importance of correct air inhalation, exhalation, and air retention. By retaining air in the lungs, the exchange of oxygen and CO_2 is more intense. Under normal conditions, when we exhale without retaining air, an abundant proportion of oxygen is left in the exhaled air. That is why we can, for example, revive another person when we perform mouth-to-mouth breathing.

When practised thoroughly, breath retention stimulates the cells and vital functions and produces rejuvenation.

The centre that controls breathing is located in the medulla oblongata, from where all the data coming from the body is processed. With this information we can consciously assume control of our breathing and help to control the vegetative nervous system, which manages all the vital functions. We are also able to control digestion, body temperature, excretion, and sleep among other functions.

Vital energy, **Prāṇa**,[1] has two basic manifestations: one that produces breathing and the other that moves thought patterns. They are both intimately linked.

1. Prāṇa enters and exits through the nine gates of the body: anus, genitals, nostrils, mouth, eyes and ears. When concentrated on the tip of the nose we obtain control over the elements of air, if we focus it on the manipūra cakra, diseases disappear, and if focused on the toes, the body becomes lighter.

When the breath is in movement, so is the mind; if the breath is under control, then the mind also is. When the vital forces of the body are under the control of the creative mind, a sudden increase in the level of energy and sensitivity can be felt, and the senses are tuned and able to function in a more efficient way.

BREATHING IN VYĀYĀMA YOGA

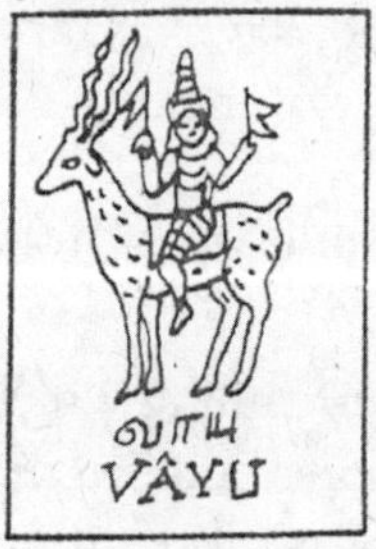

The main objective of Vyāyāma Yoga is to enhance breathing capacity and to master its control.

The ancient yogis knew that the secret to health and mind control was in the breath. This is why they said that breathing is our eternal partner, whom they called Vāyu, the God of Holy Breath; he who gives us our breathing capacity which controls the movement of the mind.

Breath was named Vāyuka, which means 'to have the presence of the God Vayu. This is why the ancient yogis considered the breath as something holy, and believed that men should possess a divine and pure atmosphere.

There is an energetic centre that pumps energy throughout the body. Its physical projection is located four fingers below the navel, called tan in sanskrit, literally "*tan hara śakti*,. The tan is the nerve point of the so-called area of strength, tan hara śakti, and is divided into a frontal region known as tan śakti and a rear region known as tan tala. The tan hara śakti is where the balance of the body is concentrated and where the mind descends for serenity and rest.

In Vyāyāma Yoga, by effectively controlling the breath, we learn the process of projecting vital energy or Prāṇa, and subtle energy or śakti, expanding them from the tan to our body and mind.

We should keep in mind the following objectives in our practice: Phases or timing.

1. Inhalation, Pūraka.
2. Exhalation, Recaka.
3. Internal retention, with the lungs full of air, Kumbhaka antara.
4. External retention, with the lungs empty, Kumbhaka bahira.

Breathing should be expansive and sonorous, and in order to achieve this we partially close the glottis—both the inhalation and exhalation should always pass through both nostrils—emitting a light sound from the base of the throat, vāyu kanda. It is in this area where the breath is transformed into vital energy, Prāṇa, by being polarised at the entrance of the nostrils.

The breathing techniques used in Vyāyāma belong to the science of breathing known as svarodaya. This science includes advanced tantric techniques made up of dynamic breathing consisting of four phases (inhalation, retention, exhalation, retention), svaras; breaths produced by releasing the air suddenly and with sound, vāyukas, and the diverse ways of breathing that polarise our energy meanwhile our body remaining still, Prāṇāyāma.

The breathing used in Vyāyāma is essentially made up of four different types:

1. Sāttvic[2], Bhrāmarī svara, a serene or calm type of breathing which has a soothing effect. It is similar to the buzzing of a bumblebee.
2. Bhastraka svara, a type of stamina, active or rājasic breathing. The thorax contracts and expands quickly and with force, instantly generating body heat and energy. Practising this type of breathing produces expansion of the mind.
3. Ujjayika svara, a whistling, passive or tāmasic type of breath. It is produced in the top part of the lungs and is achieved by emitting a whistling sound, concentrating and focusing the mind.
4. Kapālaka svara, a diaphragmatic, active or rājasic breathing.

Kapālaka breathing is diaphragmatic, and its base is in the energy centre of the solar plexus, Maṇipūra cakra. It gives mental clarity and produces serenity. The vibration that it leaves in the mind reminds us of the cosmic vibration Om.

Breathing and the Body

Good oxygenation occurs with correct breathing, the blood is purified and the organs are cleaned, allowing them to function correctly.

When the blood is rich in oxygen, it allows good functioning of the brain, which has direct influence over the central nervous system and all that is regulated by it. Breathing is oxygenation and prāṇification.

When air loaded with Prāṇa comes in through the nostrils, it is polarized as positive energy, ha, which travels through our organism

2. Matter presents itself in three essential states: Tamas, inertia. Rajas, agitation. Satva, balance. When these terms are applied to the different types of breathing, they indicate the mental and energetic states that are produced in the person who practices it. For example, rājasic breathing will activate energy and the mind, sāttvic breathing will generate calmness, and tāmasic breathing produces inactivity.

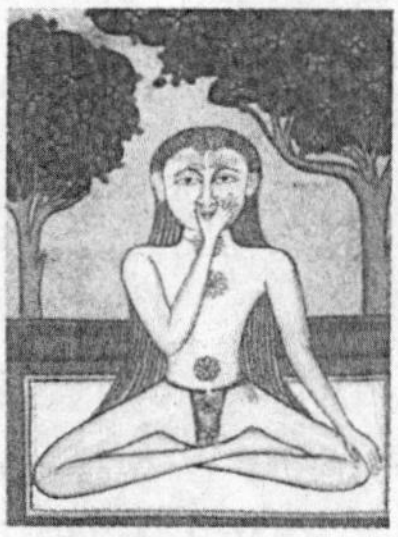

by a subtle energy channel called nāḍī Piṅgalā projecting itself in the right nostril, and as negative energy, ṭha, that travels in our organism through the subtle energy channel known as nāḍī Iḍā, which projects itself through the left nostril. Each one of these energies directly influences the metabolic processes of our organism. Positive energy, ha, acts upon the anabolic processes and negative energy, ṭha, influences the catabolic mechanisms. These facts explain why it is important to breathe through the nostrils and to control air ingestion at will for health and well-being.

Oxygen-enriched breathing allows the delivery of all necessary nutrients to all the parts of the body and helps to eliminate all waste substances. It is fundamental to learn how to breathe ingesting the highest amount of oxygen possible.

Breathing and the Mind

The relationship between thought and breath is established through the movement of the mind.

According to tantra, the mind is known as the organ of inner investigation, antaḥkaraṇa. It is an instrument of knowledge that includes various functions: conscious mind or manas, ego or ahaṁkāra, subconscious mind or citta, and intellect or buddhi. It is located in the subtle body or sūkṣma śarīra, and the dynamics of its existence consist in recognizing and making itself recognized. In order to achieve this it needs to constantly express itelf through the senses, and this is made possible thanks to the energy it receives from breathing.

The states in which the mind manifests itself, wakefulness, sleep, and deep sleep, and the different modifications it can be subjected to depends on the breath, so agitated and uncontrolled breathing will produce dispersed movements of the mind, keeping it from stable and profound thought.

When we think consciously, we are directing thoughts with our force. However, when thoughts are caused by residual force that comes from experiences acquired in the form of desires, they can present themselves with anxiety and in a rebellious way. In some cases, whether wanted or not, this kind of thought appears obsessively and may prevent normal daily routine or activity. In extreme cases it may produce vital function collapse. Exercising control over the mind and the breath that moves it will avoid these kinds of problems.

If you want to move your body in a certain way, you must breathe in a certain way. If you want to think in a certain way, you should breathe in a determined way.

When you want to calm your mind, you should inhale and exhale very little, and very slowly. If you want to activate your mind, you should inhale and exhale quickly and in abundance. If you wish to focus your mind, you should reduce the length of your breathing.

As a result, the relationship that exists between breathing and the mind is identical to the one that exists between breathing and the body. If you breathe properly, the mind receives strength; if you breathe inappropriately, the mind is weakened and so is the body.

Breathing and the Spirit

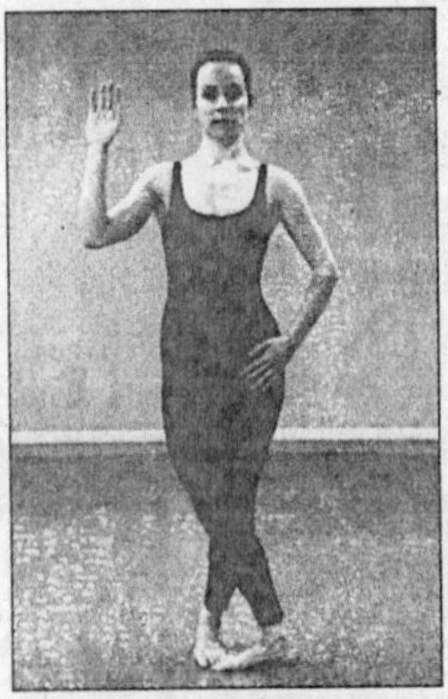

All the processes of knowledge are produced thanks to the mediums available to man, mainly the body and the mind. As previously stated, both body and mind are intimately linked through the breath. It is breathing that drives the body and mind towards spiritual awareness.

In many traditions, especially those of Semitic origin, the soul is considered to be linked to the breath. In accordance with the light of tantra, breath moves the mind and drives it toward the knowledge of the spirit, transcending the mind.

The relationship between the breath and spirit is found, beyond concentration or mental control, in meditation.

To meditate is to allow the mind to become calm through breathing, and through this process it flows towards consciousness.

Meditation teaches us the importance of taking stock of our actions. Man needs to know the course of his life in a determined moment.

We may wonder who we are and what are we doing; these simple questions might give rise to our reconsidering or rethinking every aspect of our lives, but we should face these challenges with courage and determination.

The mind is what gives us an identity and provides us with the realization that we are different from that which we perceive. The mind is an organ that allows us to connect and to disconnect from life each day, providing us with awareness. The mind permits us to constantly keep the idea of 'I am' associated with the body and personality through time and through many transformations. But the Being of 'I am' lies beyond any association to a body or personality. It is that Being that dwells inside us which can be accessed through a door that is common to all Eastern traditions: Meditation.

Thanks to meditation, thoughts become calm and bewilderment and tension due to diverse circumstances is eliminated. One does not become angry or scared, feel hassled or become hostile. A person does not become more emotional than necessary, as the mind is balanced and responds appropriately.

In the Vedas the following saying has existed for thousands of years: "the secret of existence, like the secret of health, is as near to you as the breath itself."

For someone who meditates, meditation becomes a twenty-four hour a day activity, and the source of serenity, harmony, inner power, Siddhi, extra-sensory power, Ṛddhi, and mainly, a state of super-consciousness that answers the most fundamental questions of existence. Meditation is only possible thanks to controlled breathing.

LEARNING BODY ENERGY PURIFICATION

Purification in Vyāyāma Yoga is not based on moral values, but on physical-energetic ones. Purification is necessary to achieve a balanced functioning of our organism and distribution of our energies.

We will start by saying that a poor personal hygiene results in disease and discomfort. An incorrect functioning of our organism prevents us from fully living, as disease and suffering means a state of incapacity. Blockages and absence in the flow of Prāṇa produce physical problems and upset the mind, preventing the possibility of working satisfactorily with the expansion of the tan and the liberation of the mind.

Keeping in mind these principles, we should try to include in our lives those people, animals or things that produce the least amount of waste in the previously stated levels, and in the same way, we should try to eliminate all the physical, energetic, and mentally accumulated waste we hold.

Let's start with personal hygiene, for example, a normal day after waking up. What is the process we should follow?

1. Excretion. If you have difficulty, look for solutions. Constipation is an illness that affects millions of people and unfortunately it is not given the importance it deserves. It is necessary to excrete correctly and in abundance everyday to maintain health; if this doesn't happen then there is a higher risk of attracting infections. We should take the necessary time and dialogue with our intestine. After excretion we should clean the sphincters with water and soap, not with paper, as it is unhygienic.
2. Teeth and tongue cleaning. We should clean the tongue with a small spoon or any other instrument that allows us to smoothly drag the waste that accumulates there.
3. Nostril cleaning. Using a vessel with serum or a solution prepared with lukewarm water, a small amount of salt and bicarbonate of soda.
4. Shower or morning bath. It is highly advisable to repeat this before going to bed. If it is not possible, one should wash the genitals, armpits, feet, hands and face. It is very healthy for men to use cold water on their testicles.
5. Clean clothes. Change them on a daily basis and use natural fibre-made underwear.
6. Food. Vegetables are advised due to their pure energy, sāttvic, in contrast to animal food that contains high amounts of stimulating energy, rājasic and dense energy, tāmasic. The thoughts we have while handling and preparing food are of great importance.

The nature or qualities of the objects or relationships we enjoy, including sexual relationships, are also subject to the interchange of purity, sattva, excitation, rajas and inertia or tamas. Sattva, pure energy, allows Prāṇa to flow in a correct way. On the other hand, this flow is altered and disturbed by agitating or rājasic energies and the dense energies, tāmasic, block the subtle ducts of energy, nāḍīs, preventing their correct flow.

Apart from taking care of hygiene, we should pay special attention in sexual relationships to what type of energy the people we relate to have. Great amounts of energy are exchanged during sexual encounters, and we should observe how these relationships affect us—if they vitalize us, provide us with peace and mental well being, or if, on the contrary, they produce agitation.

In the tan expansion process, all the activities we carry out during our lives have their importance: hygiene, nourishment, sleep, work, sex, satisfaction of our senses, the practices done in order to gain knowledge and develop our inner energy, achieving spiritual awareness, cultural acquisition and other activities. This process globalizes and encompasses the life of human beings.

In order to purify our internal organs and our subtle energy channels, nāḍīs, we can count on a number of practices to help us achieve these objectives in a direct way.

1. Prāṇāyāma: Breathing exercises that are done, in general, sitting cross-legged, which help us to purify the nāḍīs and to regulate the Prāṇa in our vital centres.
2. Kriyās: Internal body cleansing exercises that we should regularly perform.
3. Nyāsas: Touching the body in specific and diverse parts (talas) accompanied by breathing and sounds.
4. Vyaṅgas: Series of movements which are specifically designed to purify the body.
5. Meditation: Absorbing the mind in a point of concentration, to the exclusion of anything else.

This is body energy purification Vyāyāma Yoga.

Body Energy Purification Series

Śarīra śakti Śuddhi Krama Vyāyāma

In each of these movements, vyaṅgas, the energy is carried with your hands from the tan to each part of the body, in order to eliminate the negative, tired, utilized, diseased or inadequate energy and to purify it. It is a highly advisable Vyāyāma for those people with a diseased area of the body, or discomfort in general. During its execution, the whole body is covered resulting in the purification of the physical, mental and psychic body.

For this Vyāyāma Yoga we always move our hands from the tan to the zones of the body we are going to purify. This has the effect of taking energy from the tan to where it is needed.

By working with our legs open and our pelvis positioned in a specific way, the lower back is placed so that the rear tan area energetically recharges itself. This posture is very helpful for people who have lower back problems, and can help to improve problems related to slipped disks, but only if the movements are performed in a correct way, so it is advisable to learn them from a teacher or an expert.

FIRST SERIES OF MOVEMENTS

Vyaṅga pictures: A-1-2-3-4-5-6-7-8

Purifying the tan and the tan Prāṇa area

This movement strengthens and alleviates stiffness in the leg muscles and brings flexibility to the hip, spine and wrist joints. It facilitates deep breathing and purifies the front and rear Prāṇa areas of the tan.

Execution

We start from the initial position in which the body is standing upright with the feet together and the hands placed on the tan. We start by opening the legs, and by taking the hands back to the tan with the index and middle fingers placed together. From here, while inhaling we project the hands toward the kidneys while bending the trunk backwards. Air is retained some seconds and then released while bending the trunk forward, along with our hands. We complete the movement by bringing our hands back to the tan with strength.

SECOND SERIES OF MOVEMENTS

Vyaṅga pictures: A-9-10-11-12-13-14

Purifying the area of the breastplate

This movement has the same effect as the previous one, as well as opening and separating the shoulders, working their talas and their flexibility. It brings flexibility to the wrists and stretches the muscles of the back. When practised correctly it can help lower back pain problems and problems related to the blocking of the so-called 'tiger's eye'. Energetically, it purifies the thorax and the front and rear area of the breastplate.

Execution

Continuing the previous movement with the hands placed on the tan, we raise them up to the chest and from here they are projected to the side and to the front, and then opened and bent backwards to the back and placed at the height of the 'tiger's eye'. From here, we remove them from under the armpits and extend them to the sides to go back to the chest. Afterwards, the movement is performed on the other side and is completed by placing the hands on the tan.

THIRD SERIES OF MOVEMENTS

Vyaṅga pictures: A-15-16-17-18-19-20-21-22

Purifying the right lung and the left lung

This movement allows the purification of both lungs and also balances the talas of the shoulders, strengthens the arms, and opens the shoulder joints. Each time a good breath is taken, more oxygen is brought to the organism and the cells, improving their metabolic functioning. Oxygen takes part in the maintenance of the functions of the organs and improves general health.

Execution

Continuing the previous movement with the hands placed on the tan, both arms and hands are extended towards the ground. From here, one of the arms is raised toward the sky and the other remains downward, as if they wanted to reach the sky and the earth. The arm that is raised comes down passing in front of the face, and both hands meet to go back to the tan. Then the movement is performed changing arms.

FOURTH SERIES OF MOVEMENTS

Vyaṅgas pictures: A-23-24-25-26-27-28-29-30-31-32-33-34-35-36

Purifying the two great rivers, Iḍā and Piṅgalā

The two most important nāḍīs of the body and the energy that flows through them are purified, improving the balance between them. This exercise internally equalizes the energies.

Execution

Continuing the previous movement with the hands placed on the tan, both arms and hands are directed toward the anal sphincter, and from here they move up, crossing each other when they pass the genitals, the solar plexus, heart plexus and the base of the throat. From here, the middle fingers go up, passing the face to the space between the eyebrows, and on through the head, crossing each other behind it and going down again to the base of the throat passing behind the ears. With the fingers of the hands together, the right hand on top of the left, we lower the hands while pressing the sternum until we reach the tan.

FIFTH SERIES OF MOVEMENTS

Vyaṅga pictures: A-37-38-39-40-41-42-43-44-45

Purifying the arms and the 5 Prāṇas in the 5 meridians

The energy of the extended arm is purified, because by moving over the external and internal side of the arm it follows the same route as the meridians. These meridians are on the external side, the large intestine, triple heater and small intestine and on the internal side, the heart, main heart and lung. Āyurvedic traditional medicine teaches that each finger is connected with an organ, from the thumb to the little finger, in the following order: brain, lung, intestine, kidney and heart.

By purifying the energy of each of these meridians, the functioning of the organs they regulate is improved.

It also strengthens the knees and ankles and increases flexibility in the legs.

Execution

Continuing the previous movement with the hands placed on the tan, the hands are moved to the iliac crests, one arm is laterally extended until parallel to the ground and the other hand moves through the trunk reaching the armpit and from there moves along the inner side of the arm and moves back along the outer side reaching the shoulder, descending through the iliac crests. The arm is lowered and both hands meet again at the tan. The same procedure is repeated on the other side.

SIXTH SERIES OF MOVEMENTS

Vyaṅga pictures: A-46-47-48-49

Purifying the nāḍīs, cleansing the lower tan and the knees

In this movement, the hip joint is made more flexible and the internal organs are softly compressed, improving their functioning and the process of peristalsis.

A great benefit is noticeable in the knees.

Execution

Continuing the previous movement with the hands placed on the tan, the arms are turned to one side forming a circle, touching the groin and then dragged down the leg until they reach the knee, inhaling while making the leg vertical and then releasing the force with the hands. Afterwards, the hands return to the tan by moving up the inner side of the leg until the groin and from here the arms turn forming a circle. The same is performed on the other leg.

SEVENTH SERIES OF MOVEMENTS
Vyaṅga pictures: A-50-51-52-53-54-55
Purifying the nāḍīs in the ankles and legs

This movement has a more profound effect on the internal abdominal organs, because besides specifically purifying the ankles a deeper flexion takes pace.

The legs are covered by several meridians; among them we can find the ha meridians in the bladder, stomach and gallbladder, on the outer and rear part of the leg, and the ṭha meridians in the spleen, kidney and liver located on the inner side of the leg.

By executing this leg-purifying Vyaṅga we actively work the circulation of energy in each of the meridians.

Execution

The execution of this exercise is the same as the previous one; the only difference is that the hands go down to the ankles.

EIGHTH SERIES OF MOVEMENTS
Vyaṅga pictures: A-56-57-58-59-50-61-62-63
Purifying the feet and heels

The effects are the same as the previous movements, vyaṅgas, in regard to the purification of the knees and ankles, but this time they are extended to the heels.

Execution

This exercise is executed in the same way as the previous one, but in this case the hands are taken to the ankles without touching the legs. In this way, we drag the energy around them. Then they are crossed at the feet and go up together touching the inner side of the leg.

NINTH SERIES OF MOVEMENTS
Vyaṅga pictures: A-64-65-66-67-68-69-70-71-72-73-74-75-76-77-78-79-80-81-82-83-84-85-86-87-88-89-90-91
Purifying the energetic sphere, taijasa that surrounds the three bodies

This movement activates the circulation of the arms, the neck is mobilized and the cervical joints are made more flexible. The talas of the shoulders and legs are strengthened, improving the functioning of the kidneys.

Execution

We start from the initial position in which the body is standing upright with the feet together and the hands placed on the tan. Next, we open the legs and bring the hands back to the tan with the index and middle fingers together. From here, the hands and arms are projected forward as if we are projecting a sphere of energy out of the tan. We raise the hands to the sky and lower them back to the tan, and then we make it pass through the body towards the back while we lean forward, until the trunk is parallel to the ground. Then we return by bringing the sphere forward and up again and turning the trunk to one side, the arms go down laterally until they meet each other under the legs and then the same is done on the other side. The arms go up and then down and the sphere is brought back to the tan.

Following this, the hands go up from the tan to the chest, then they open to the sides while we turn behind and then they go back to the chest. After this is repeated, the arms form a basket position behind the back while the head is facing the foot. This is repeated in the other direction.

TENTH SERIES OF MOVEMENTS

Vyaṅga pictures: A-92-93-94-95-96-97-98-99-100-101-102-103-104

Balancing the two force poles, Ha and Ṭha

These last movements stimulate and balance the two force poles we have been activating during the previous vyaṅgas, providing great doses of vitality.

They favour the opening and mobility of the lumbar vertebra joints, strengthen the legs, tone the arms increasing their strength from the hands to the shoulders and enhance lung capacity.

Execution

Inhale and exhale turning the arms backwards and forwards from the ground to the tan. Inhale and hold the breath while raising the hands to the shoulders (A-94), and then exhale quickly pronouncing Ha in an expansive way (A-95).

Again, inhale and exhale turning the arms backwards and forwards from the ground to the tan. Inhale and hold the breath while raising the hands to the shoulders and then exhale fast pronouncing Ṭha sharply.

Inhale and exhale turning the arms backwards and forwards from the ground to the tan. Inhale and hold the breath and then exhale quickly, moving the hands to the ground, pronouncing Ha in aṇ expansive way (A-101). Afterwards, inhale and exhale, directing the breath to the sky by pronouncing Ṭha in a sharp way (A-102).

From A-103 to A-107 the movement closes to the initial position.

These exercises strengthen the legs, tone the muscles of the arms from the hands to the shoulders, and allow the opening and mobility of the lower back vertebra joints. It enhances lung capacity and revitalizes the body.

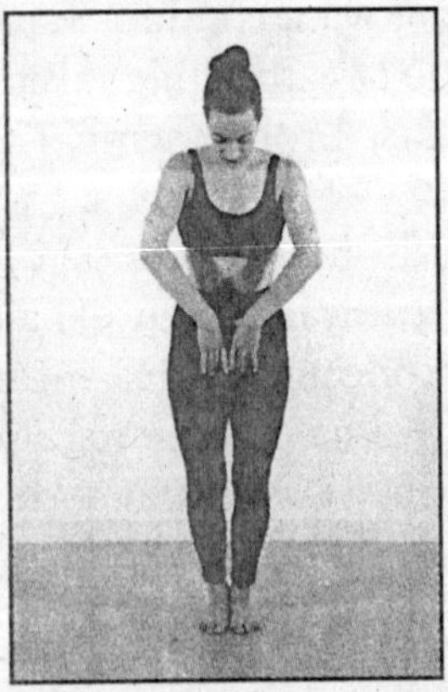

A-1

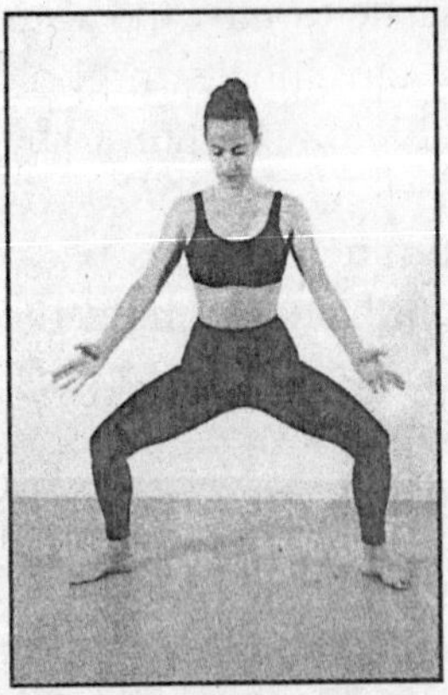

A-2

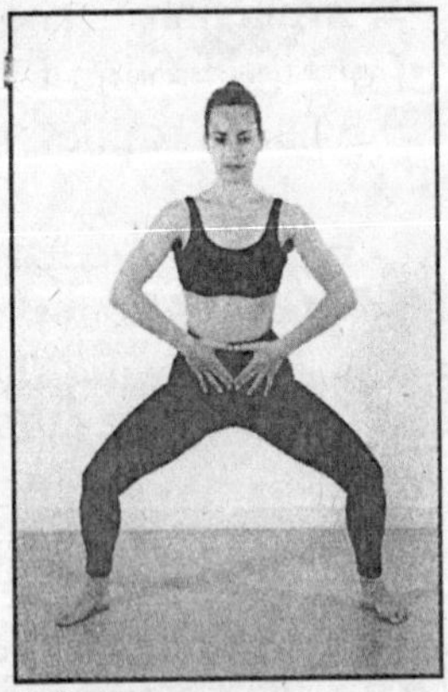

A-3

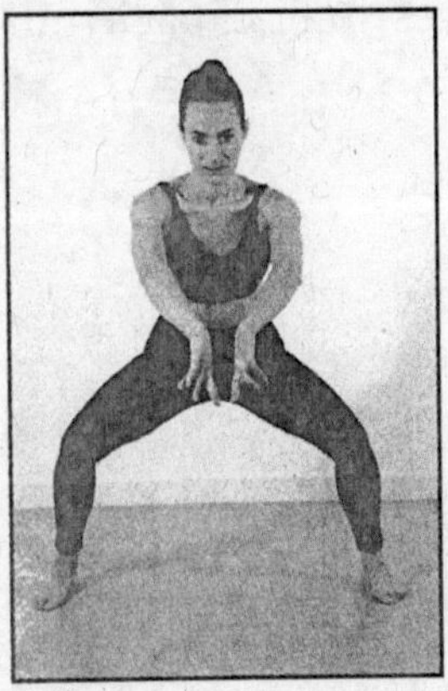

A-4

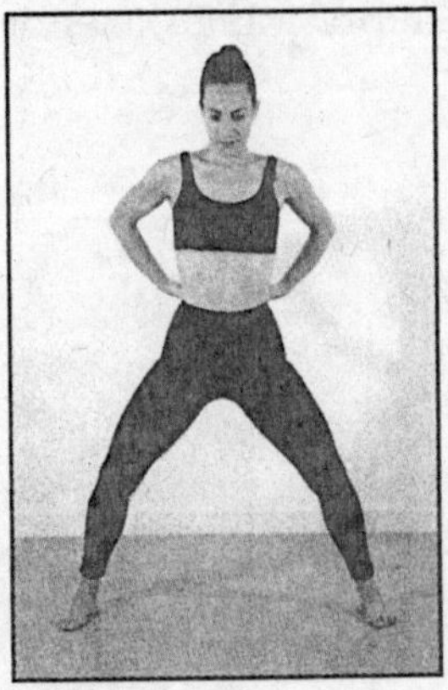

A-5

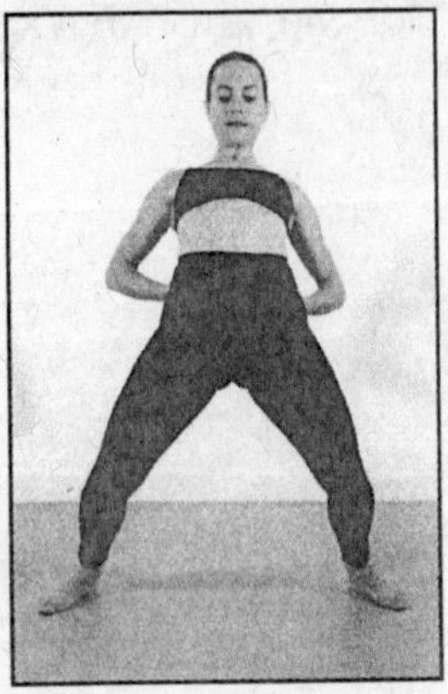

A-6

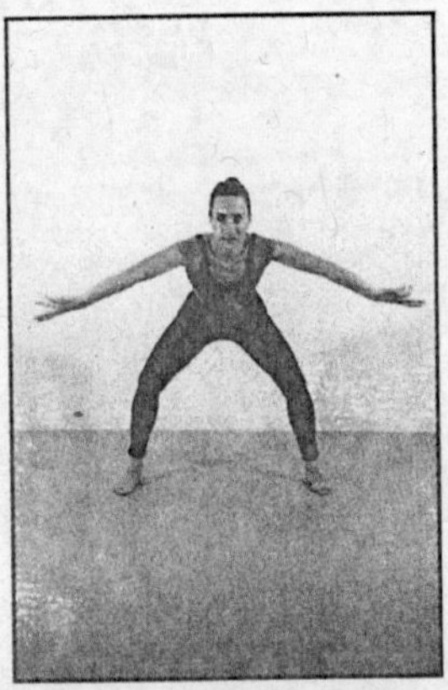

A-7

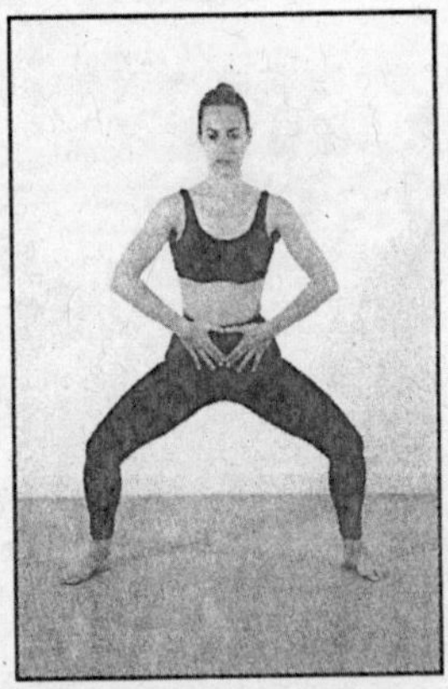

A-8

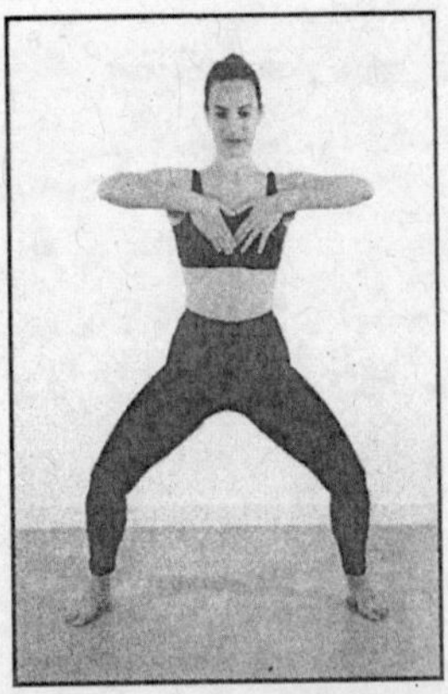

A-9

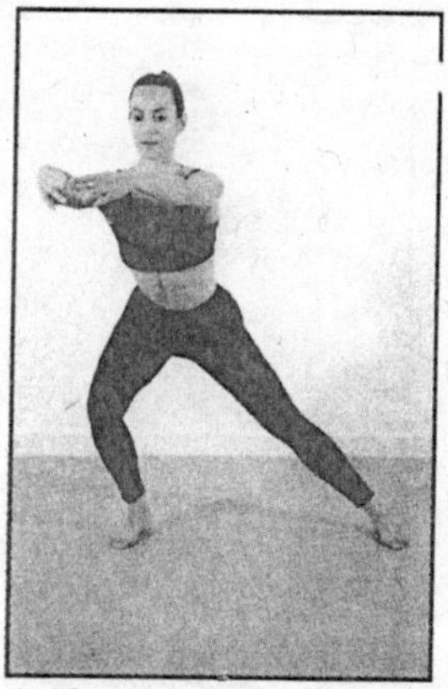
A-10

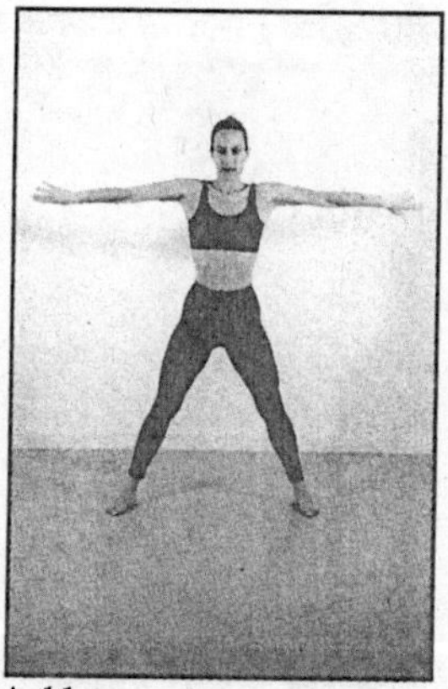
A-11

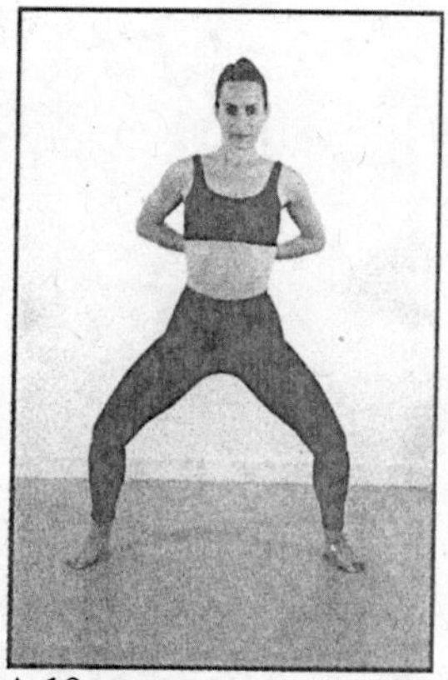
A-12

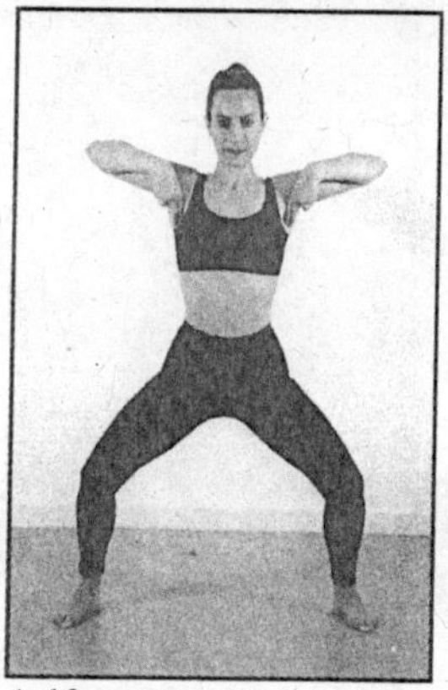
A-13

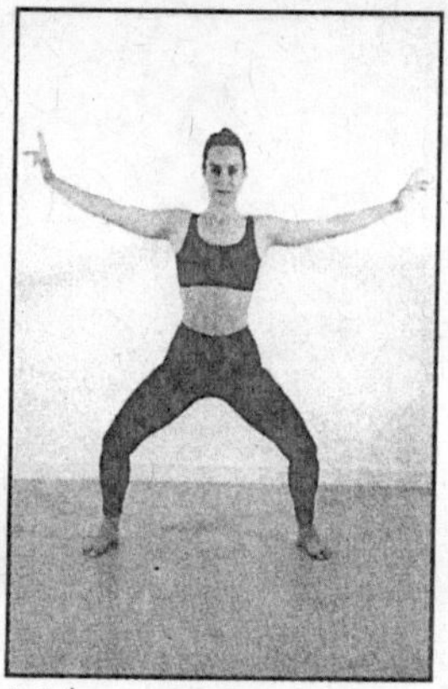
A-14

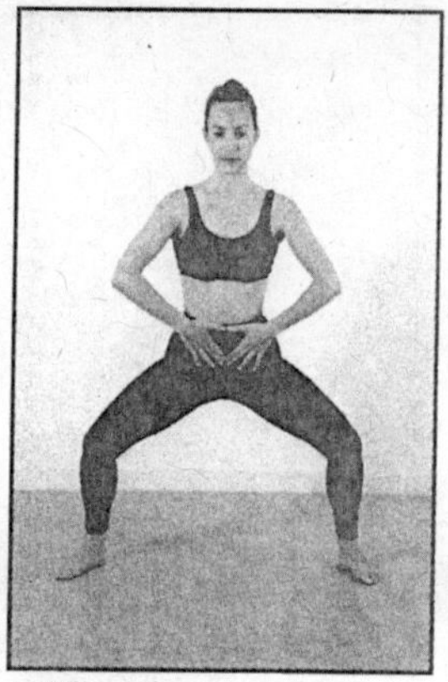
A-15

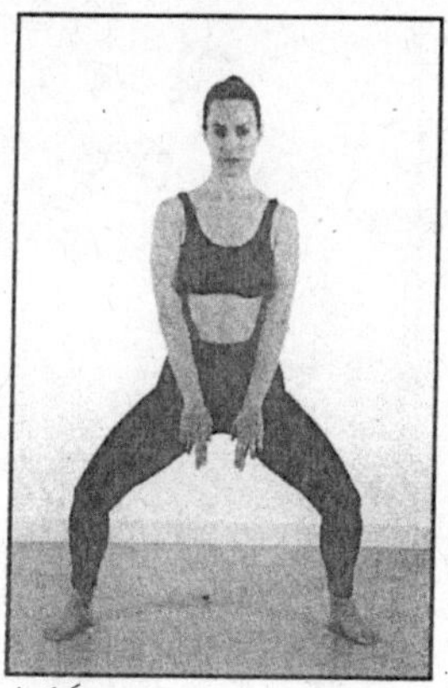
A-16

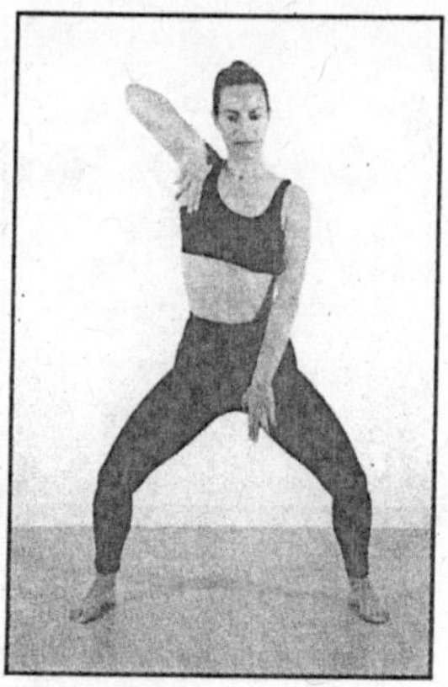
A-17

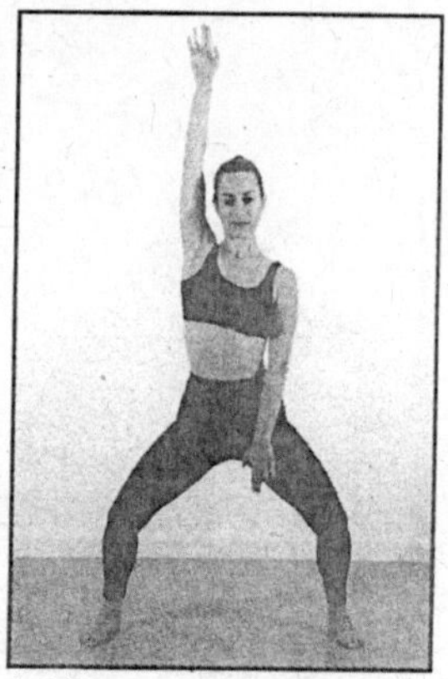
A-18

Repeat movements A-9 to A-14, projecting the arms to the opposite as demonstrated in A-10

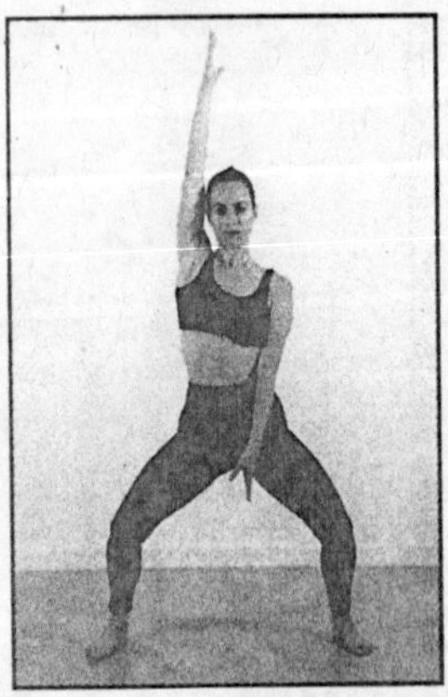
A-19

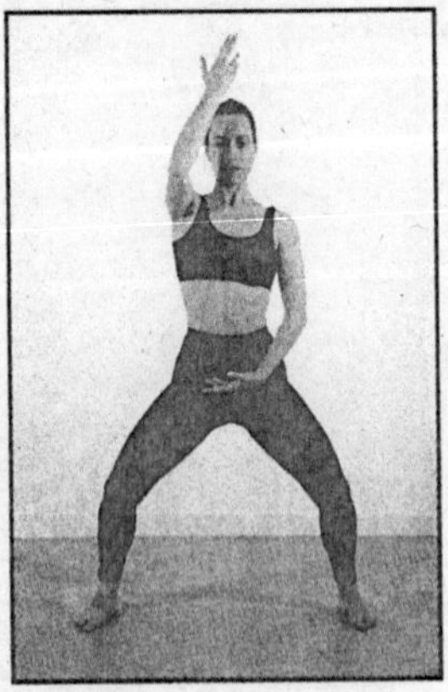
A-20

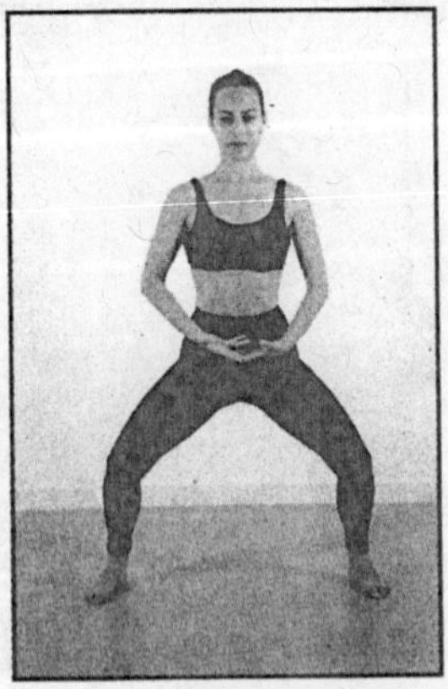
A-21

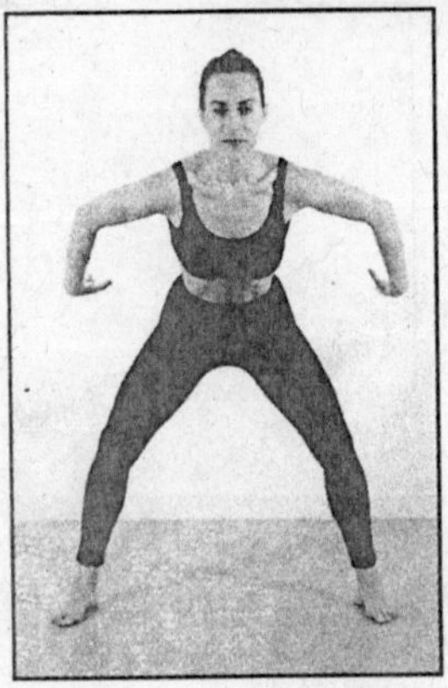
A-22

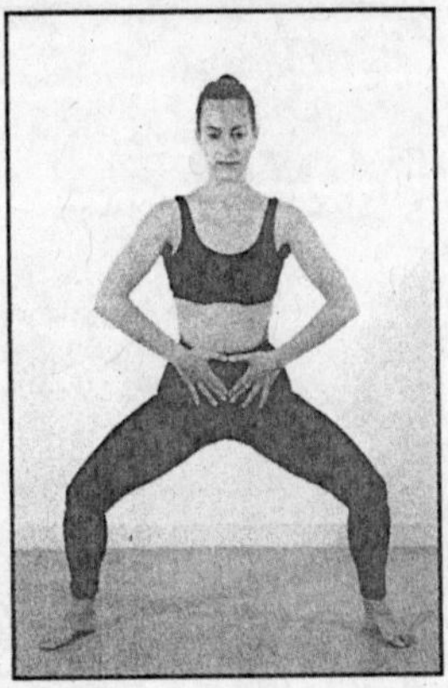
A-23

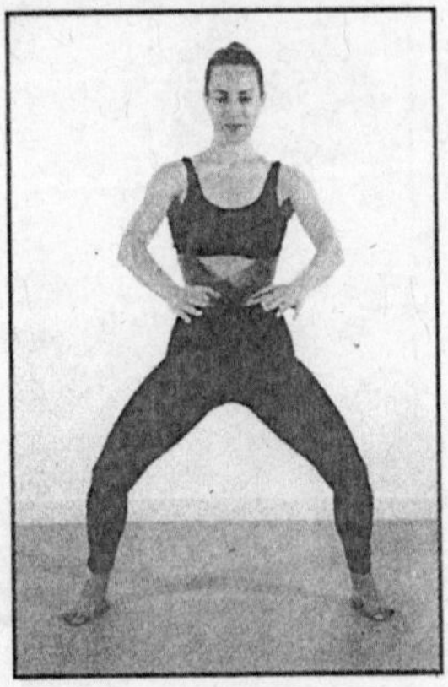
A-24

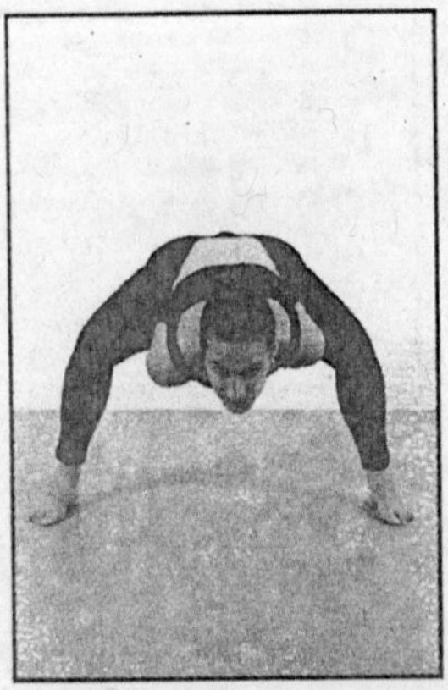
A-25

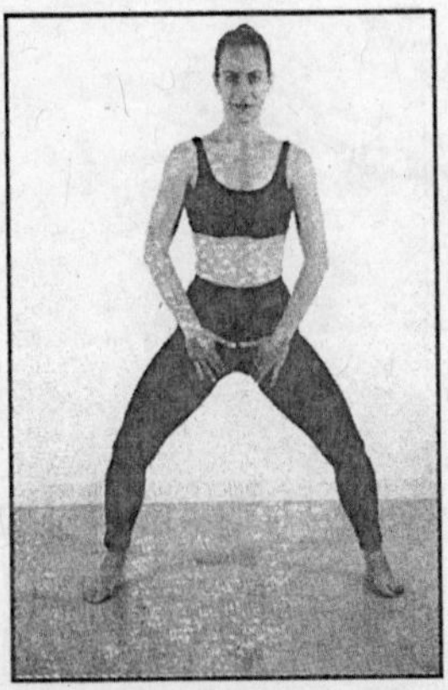
A-26

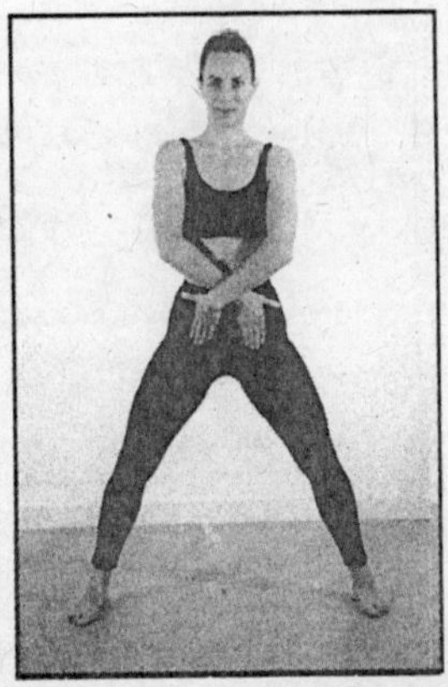
A-27

Repeat movements A-15 to A-22, projecting the opposite arm as demonstrated in A-17,18,19 and 20

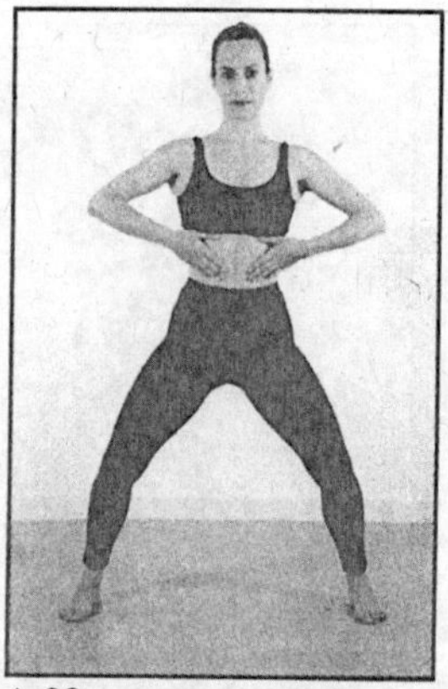
A-28

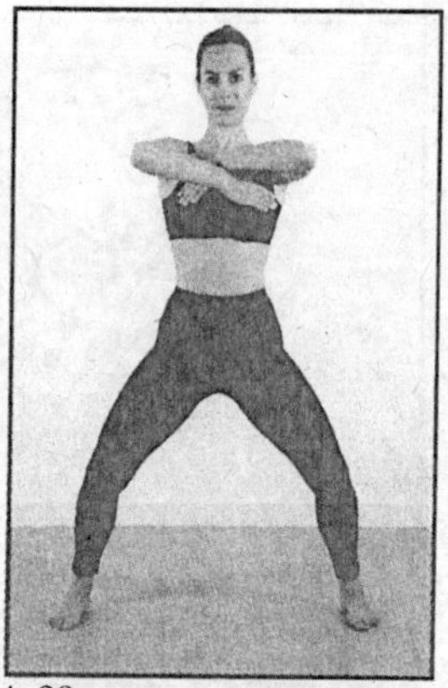
A-29

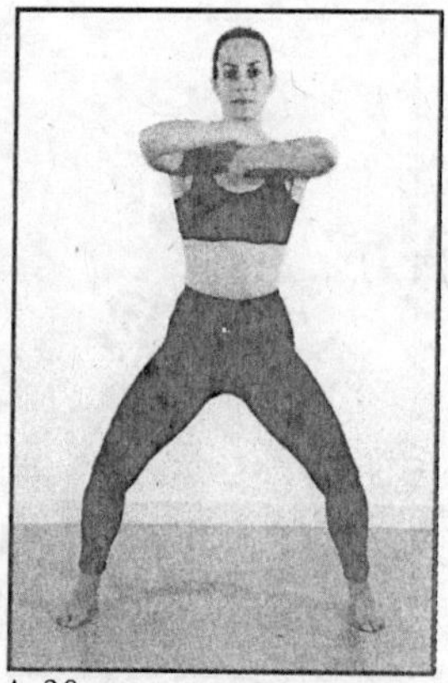
A-30

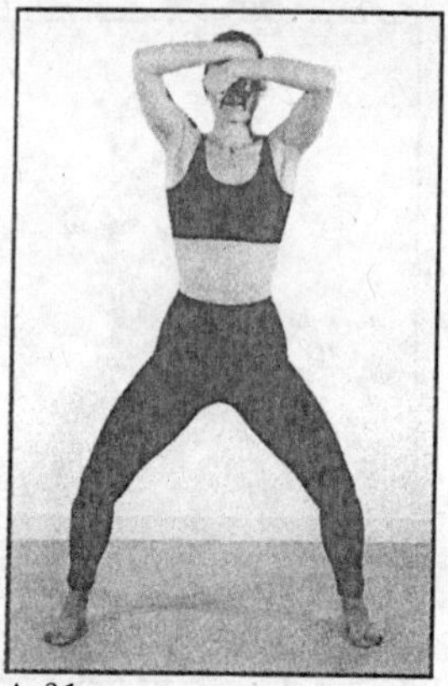
A-31

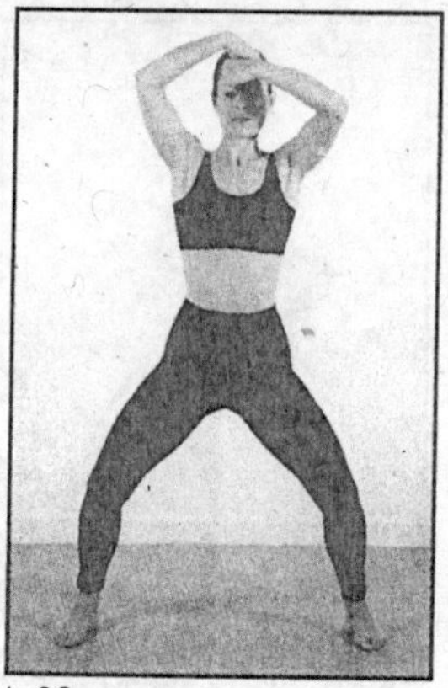
A-32

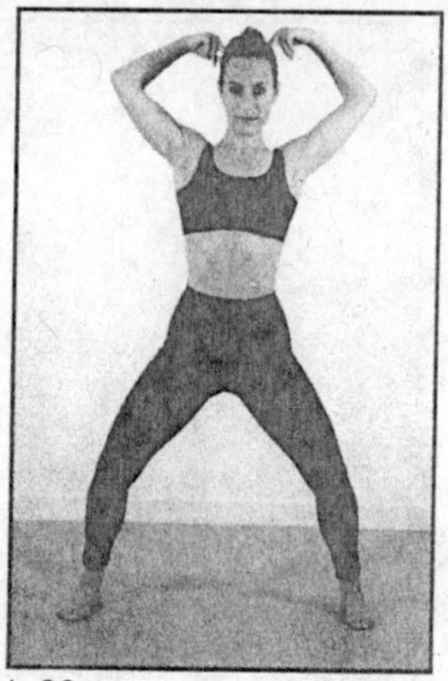
A-33

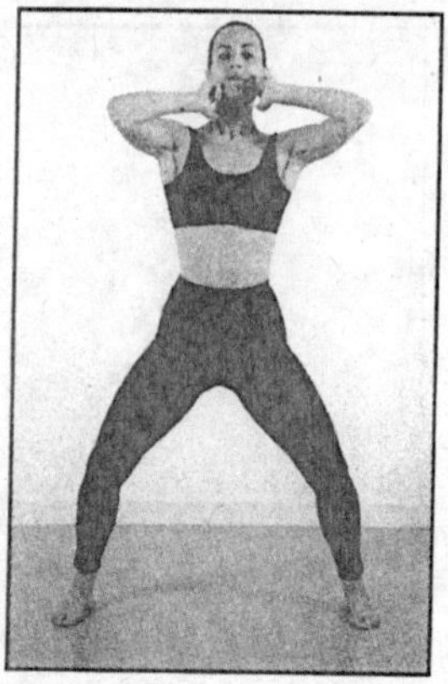
A-34

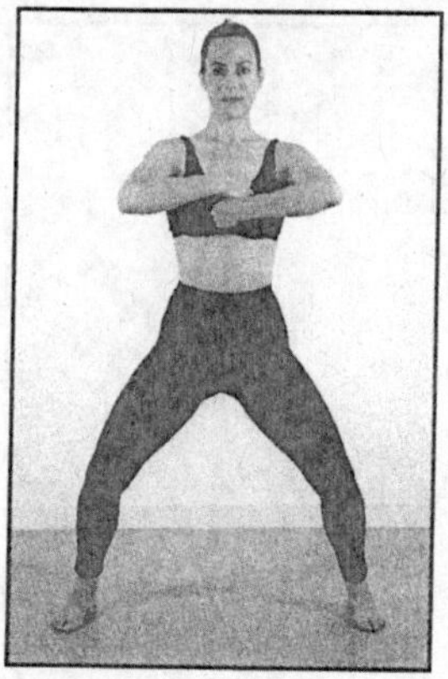
A-35

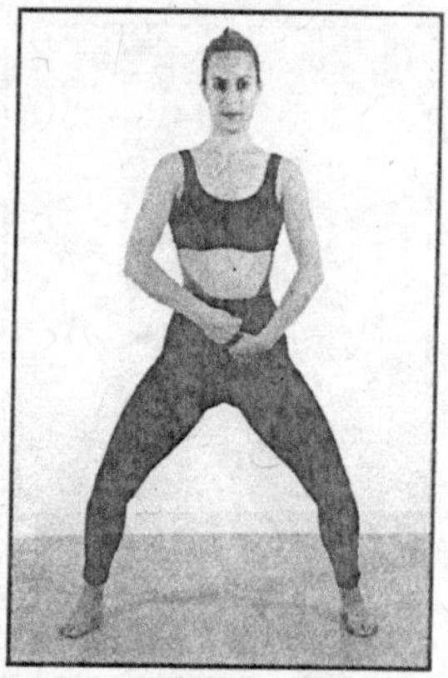
A-36

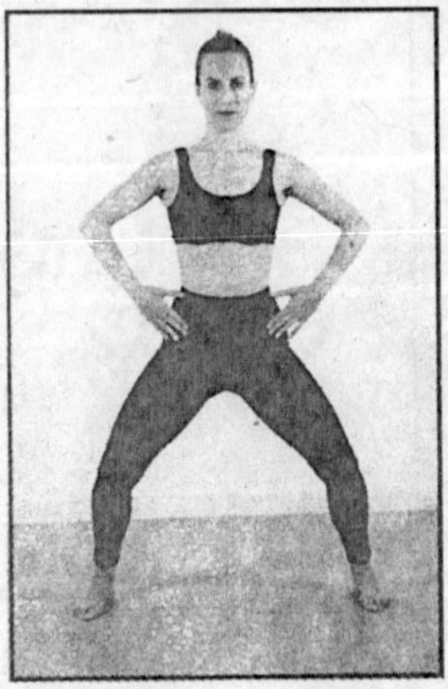
A-37

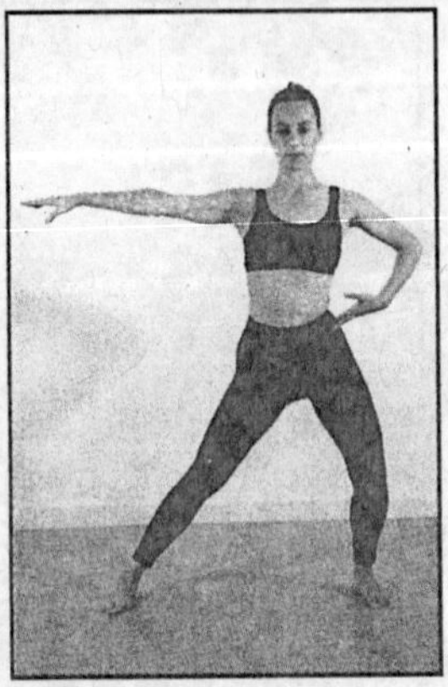
A-38

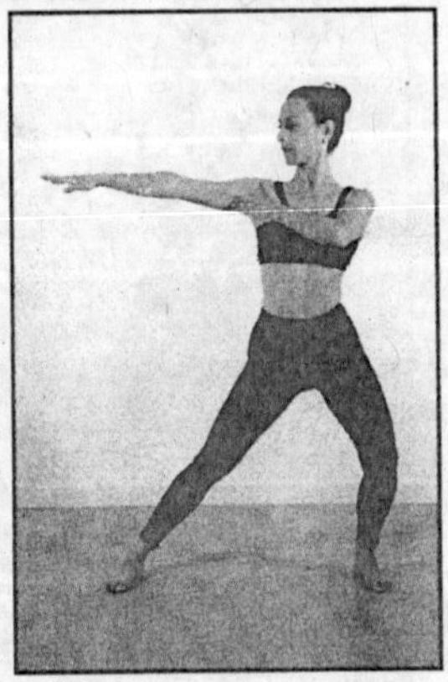
A-39

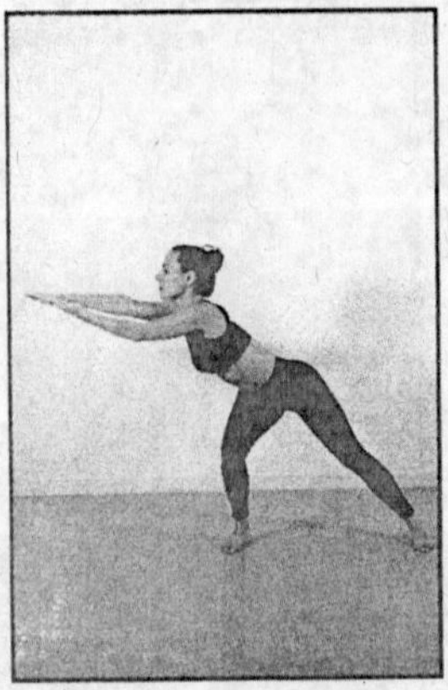
A-40

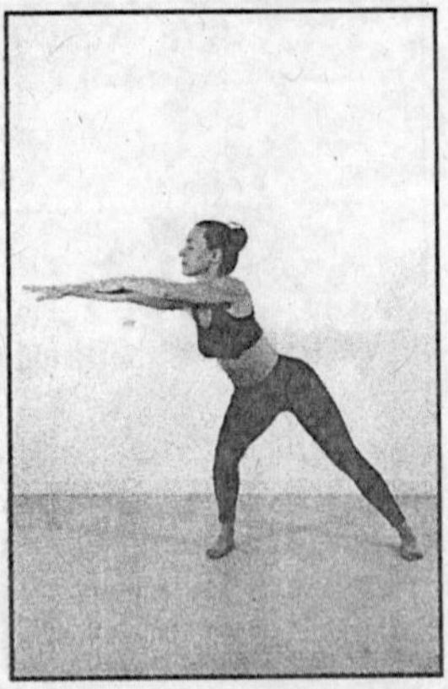
A-41

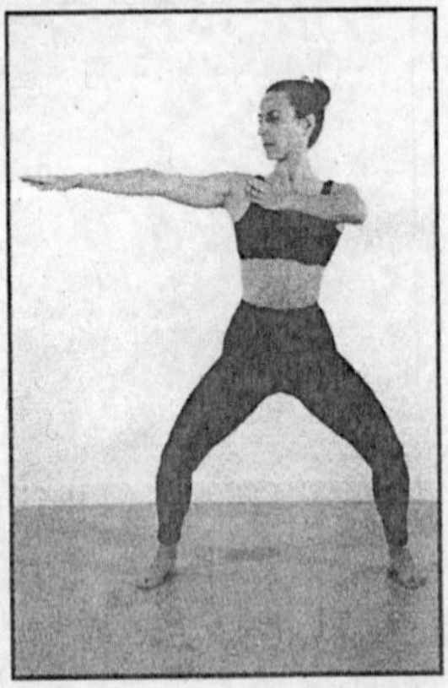
A-42

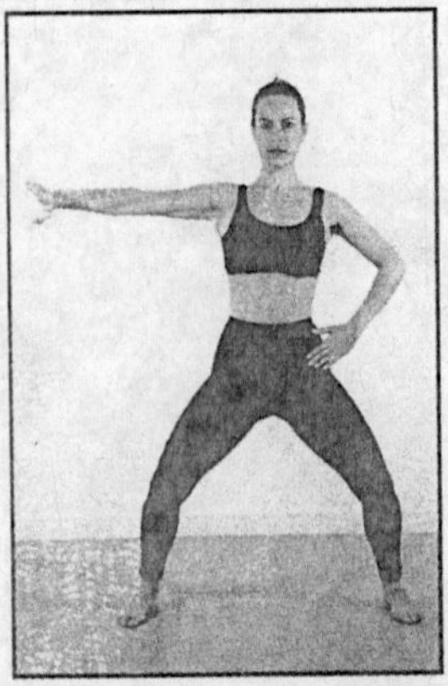
A-43

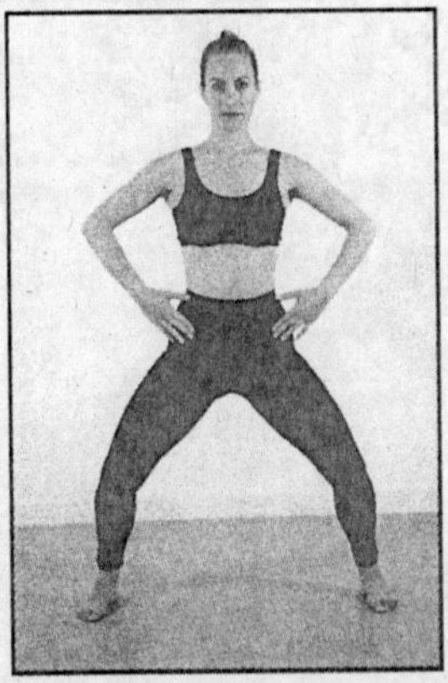
A-44

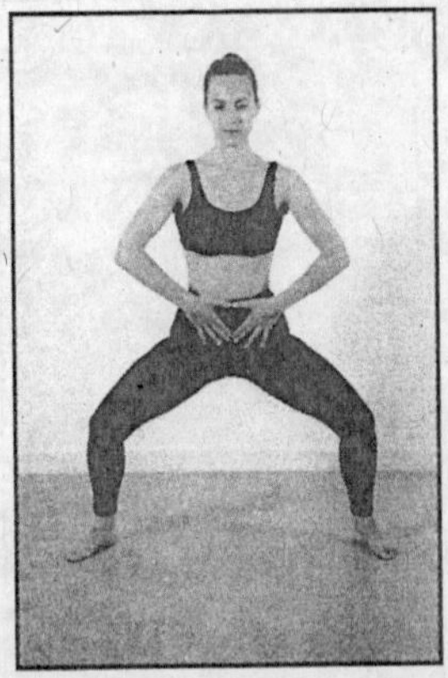
A-45

Repeat movements A-37 to A-45, projecting the opposite arm as demonstrated in A-38,39,40,41,42 and 43

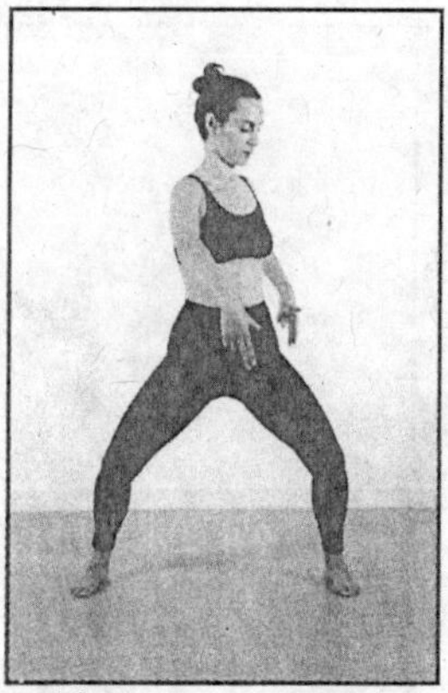
A-46

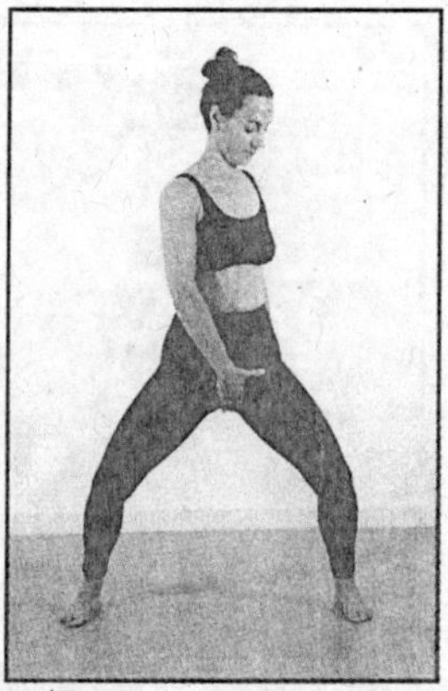
A-47

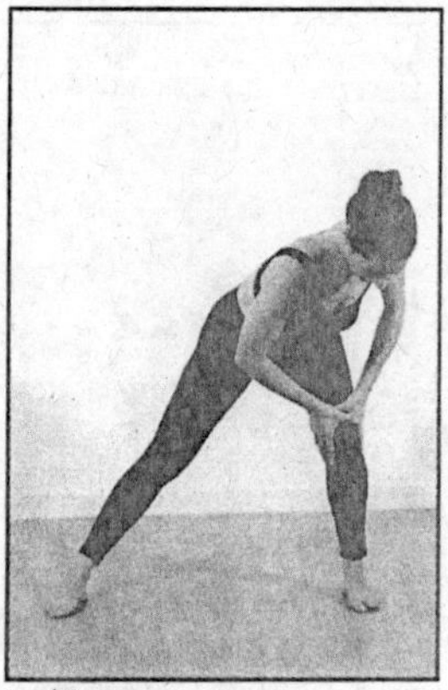
A-48

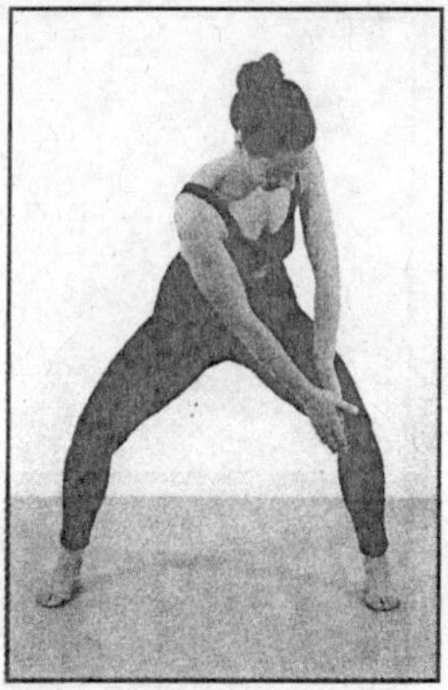
A-49

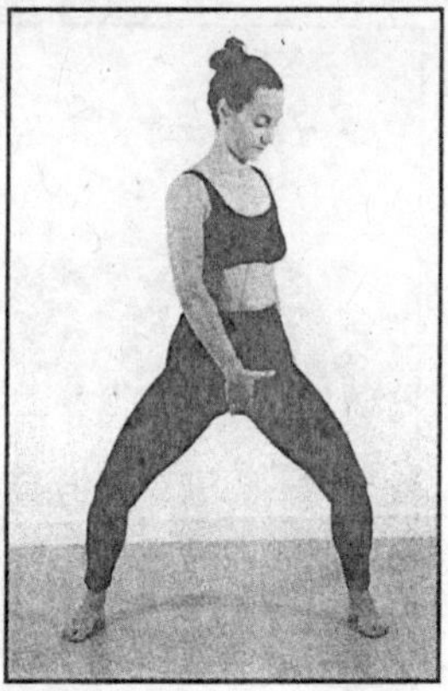
A-50

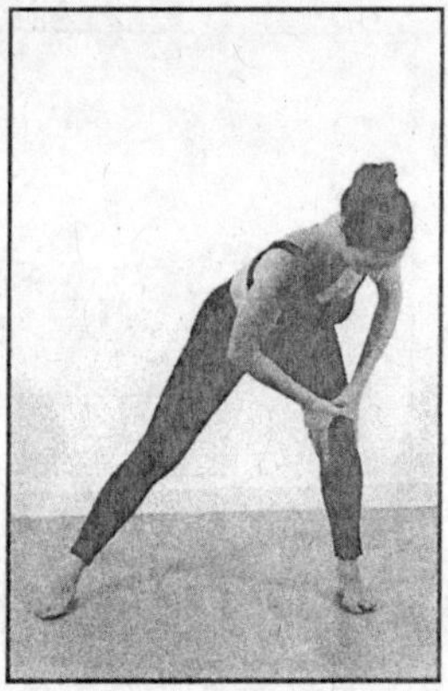
A-51

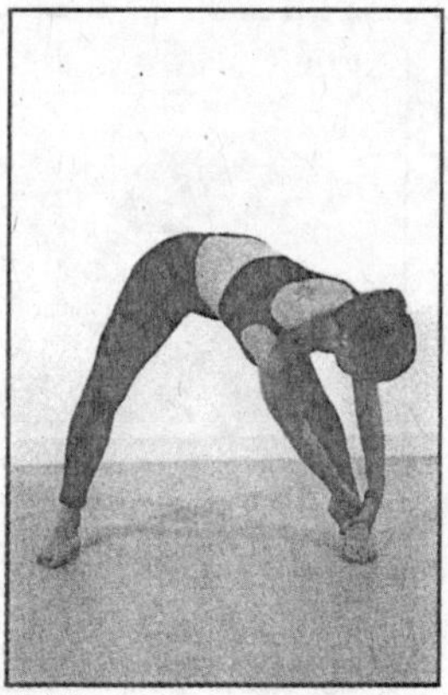
A-52

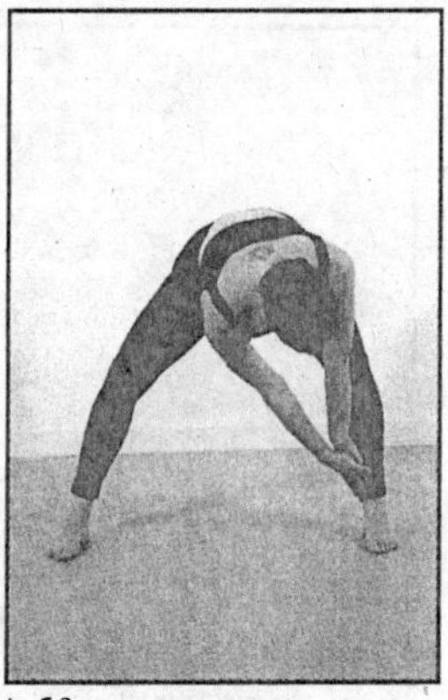
A-53

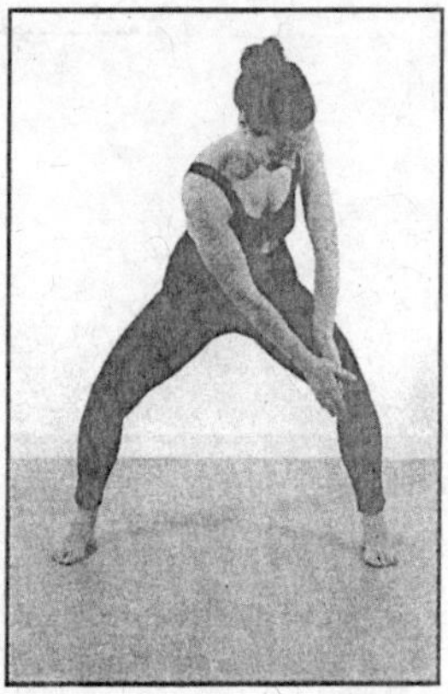
A-54

Repeat movements A-46 to A-63, this time performing the vyangas on the other leg.

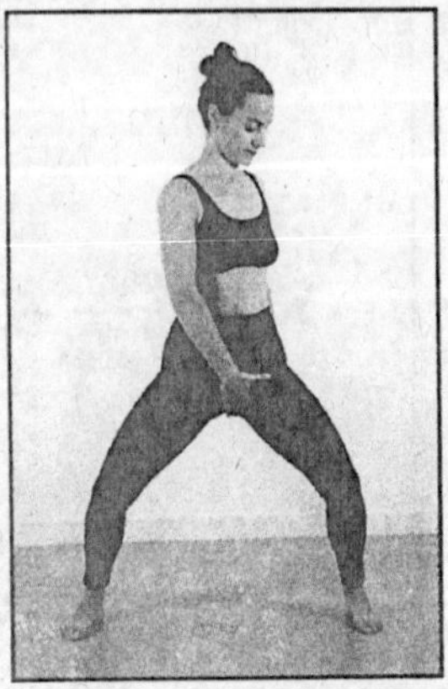
A-55

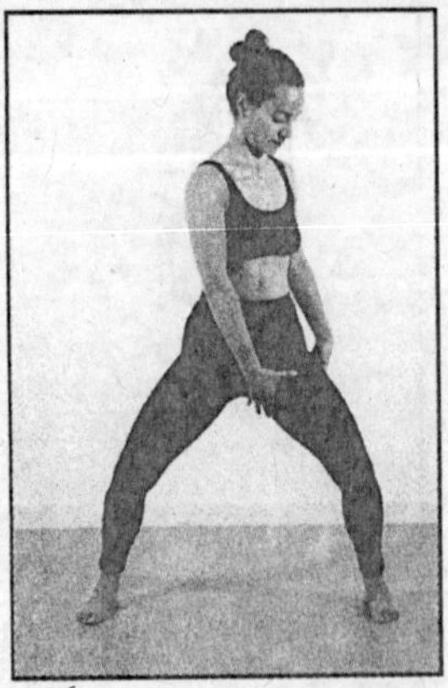
A-56

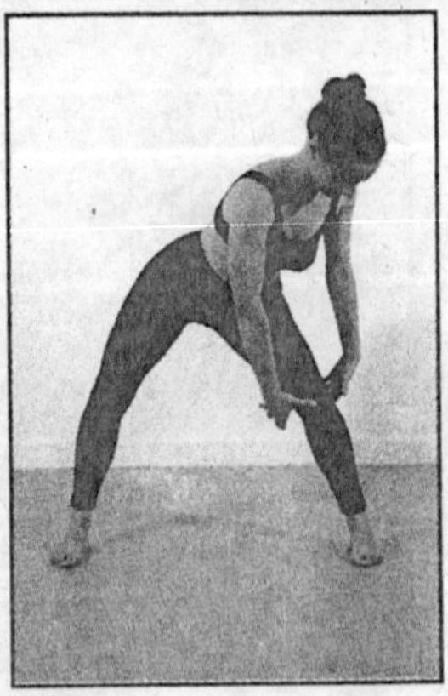
A-57

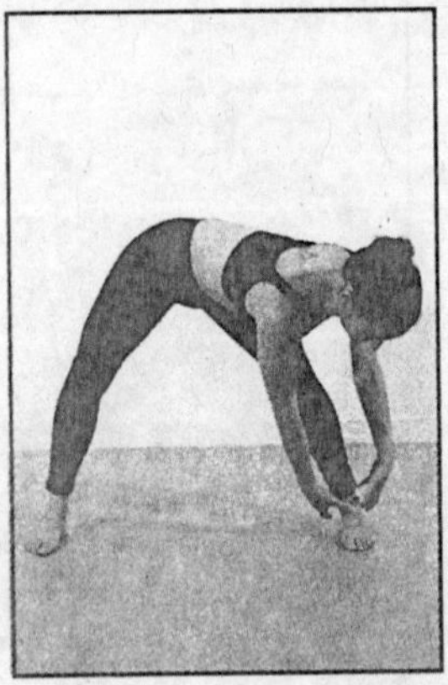
A-58

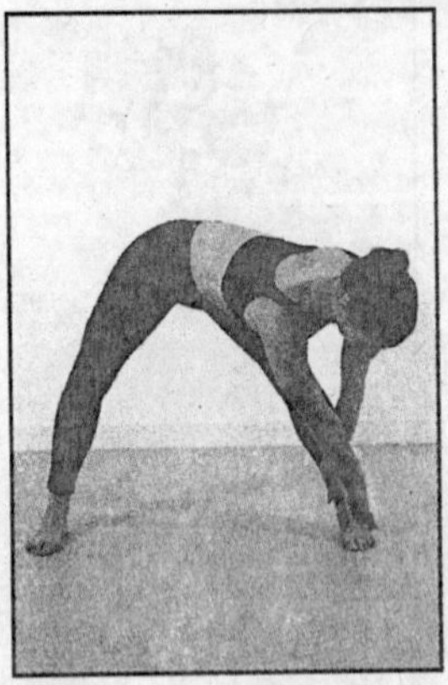
A-59

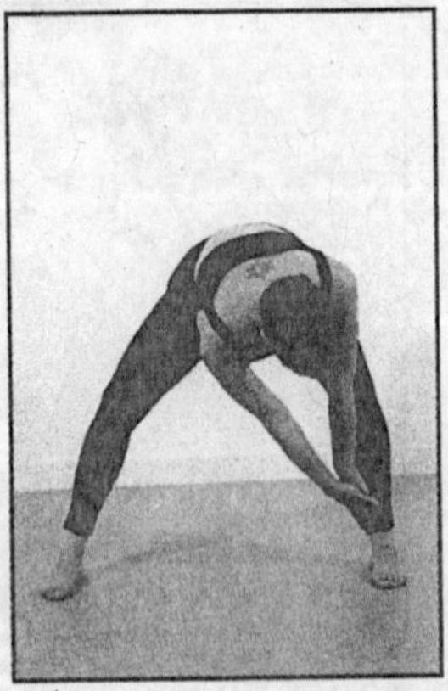
A-60

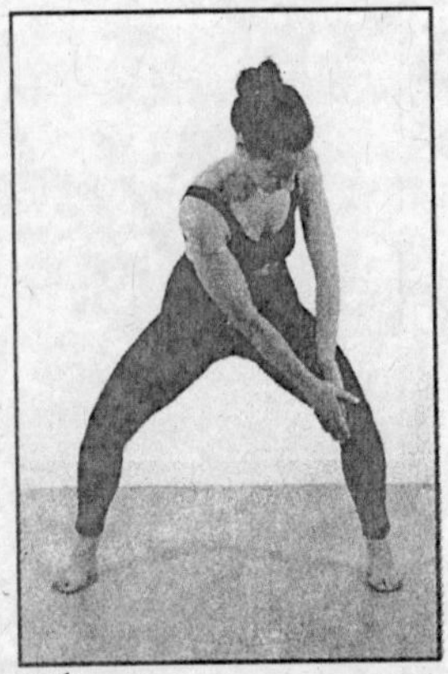
A-61

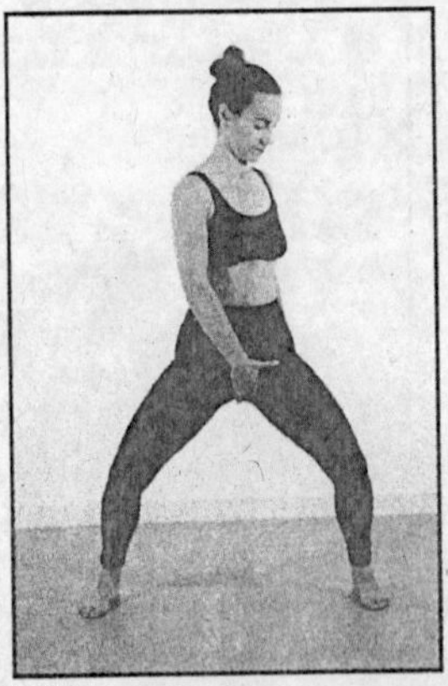
A-62

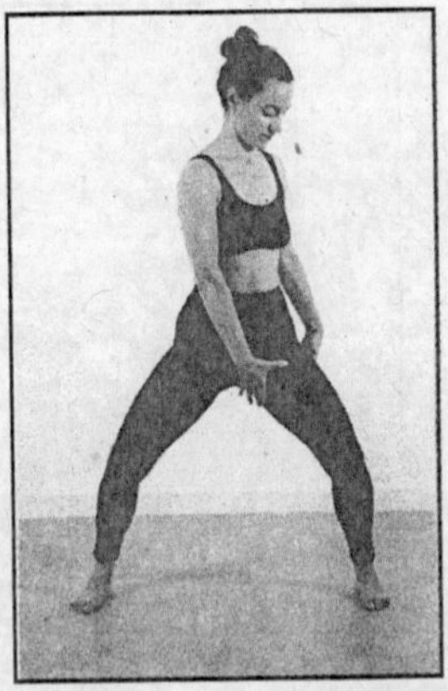
A-63

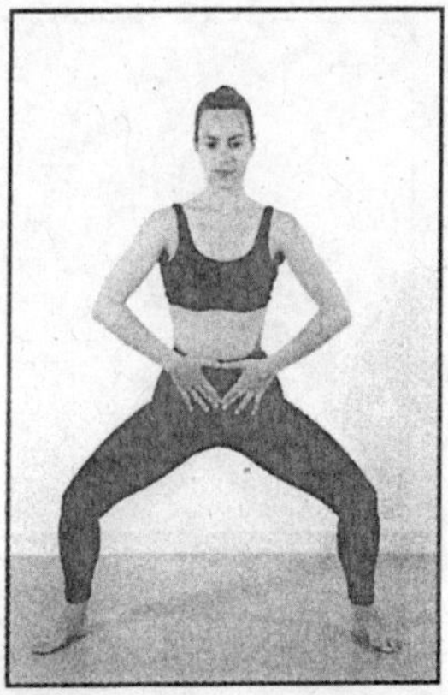
A-64

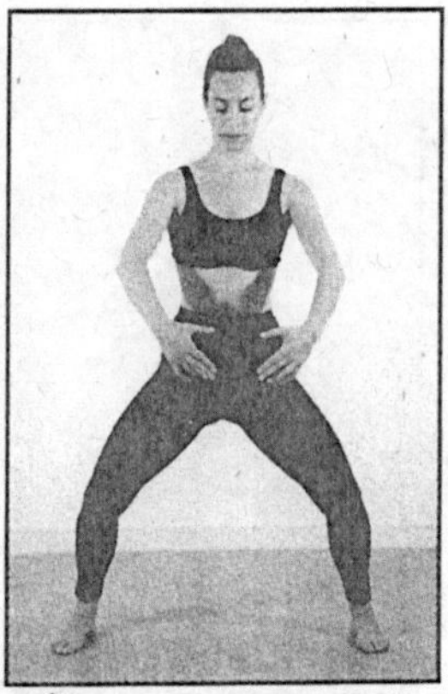
A-65

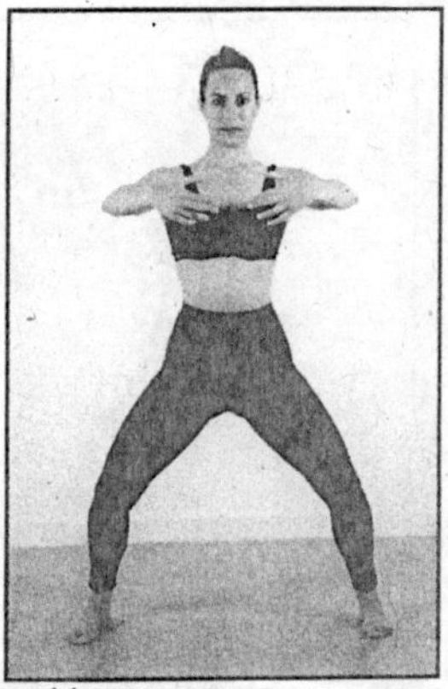
A-66

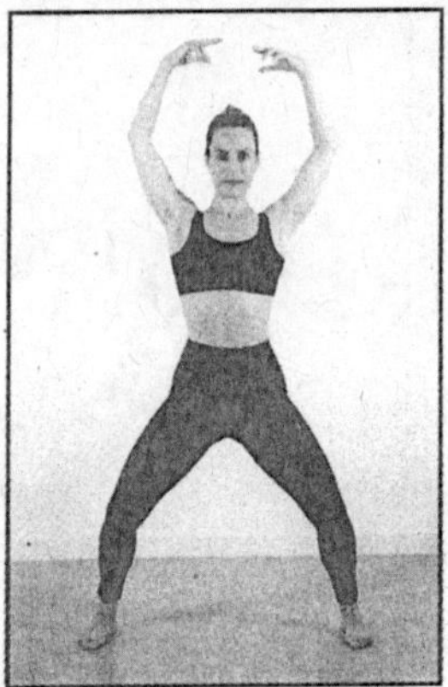
A-67

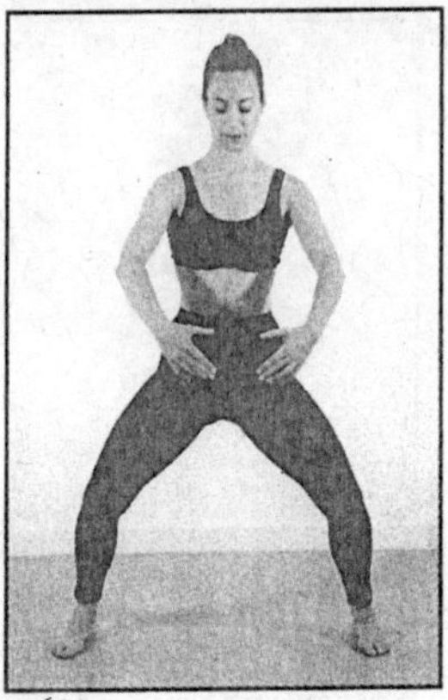
A-68

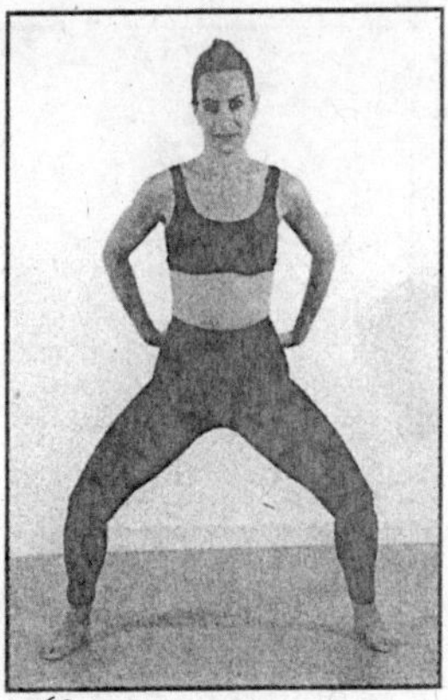
A-69

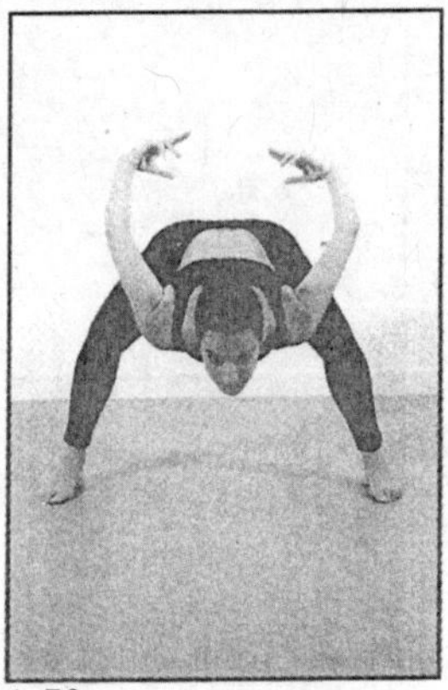
A-70

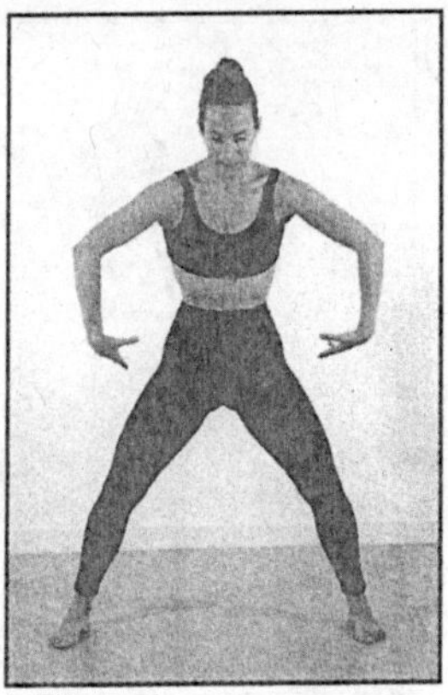
A-71

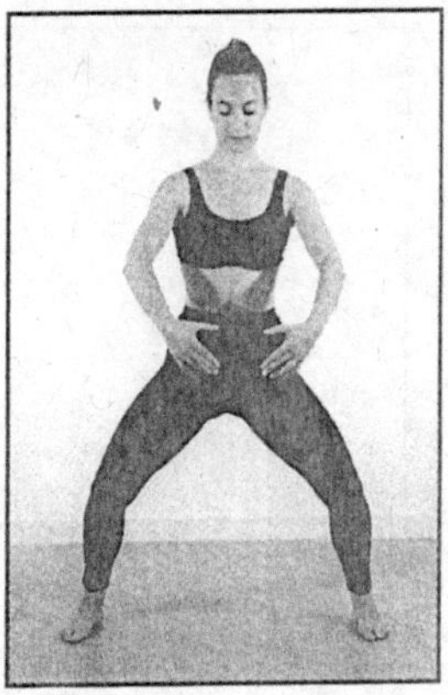
A-72

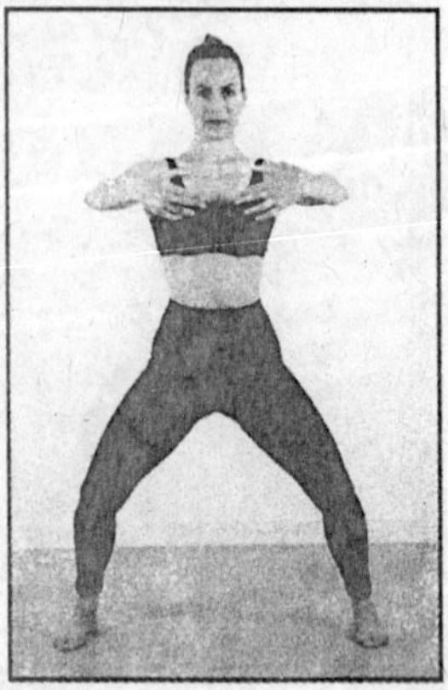
A-73

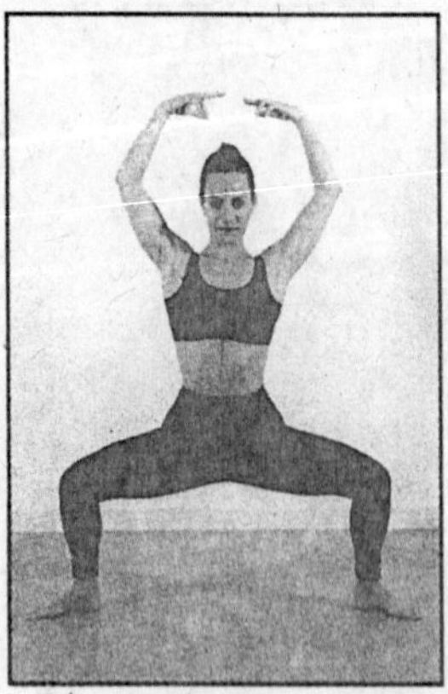
A-74

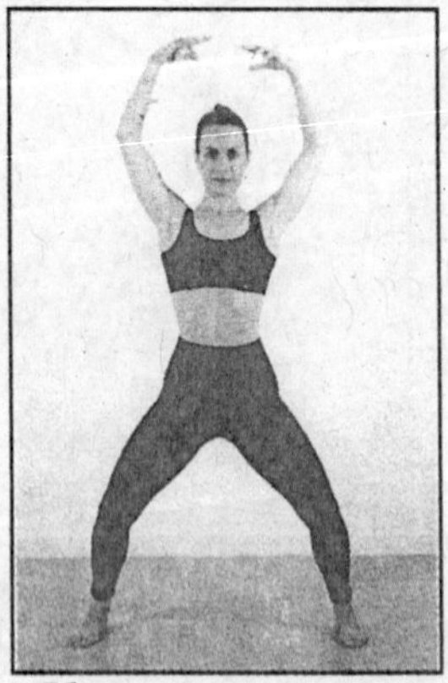
A-75

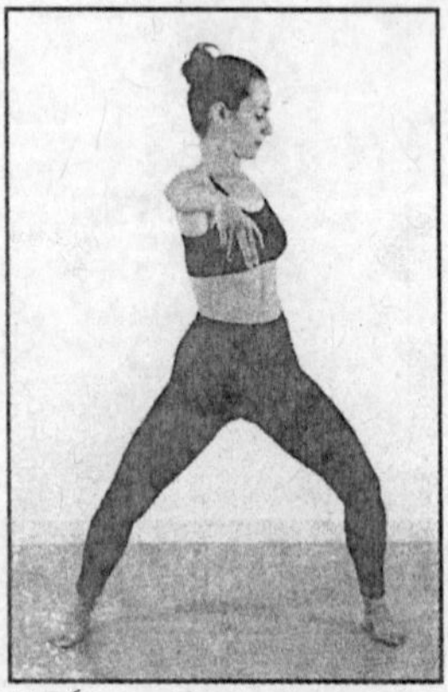
A-76

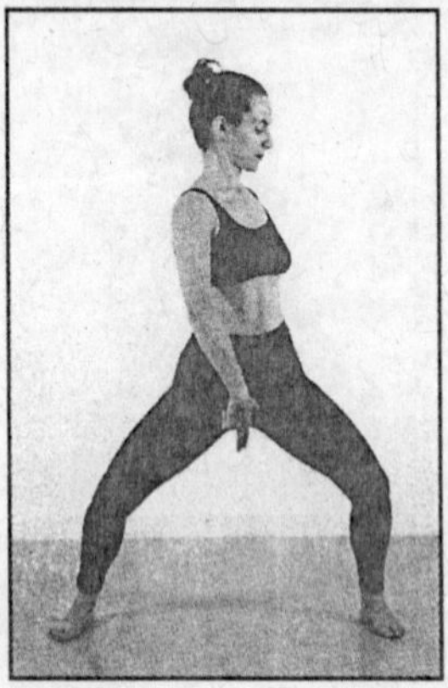
A-77

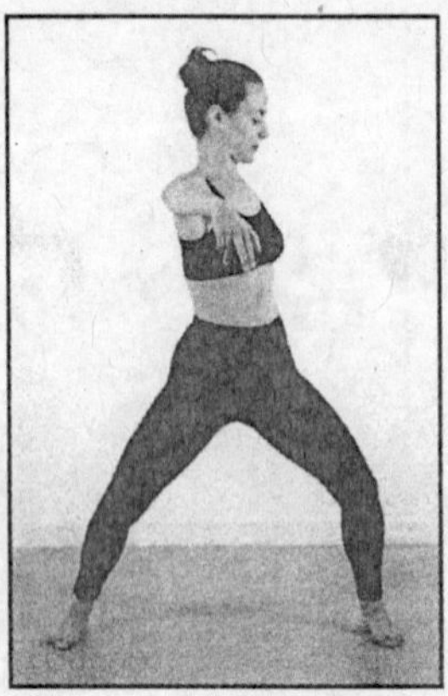
A-78

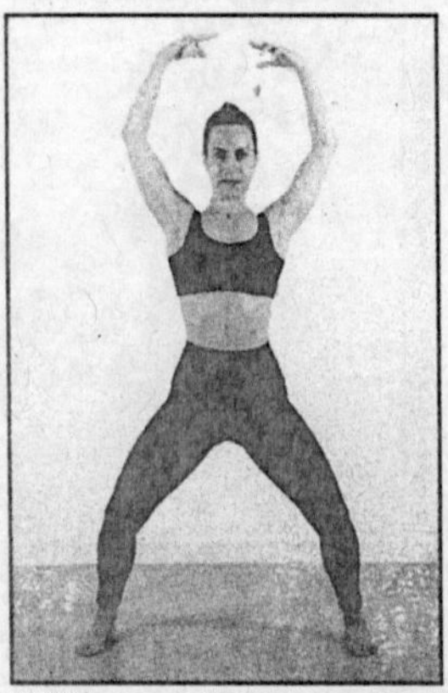
A-79

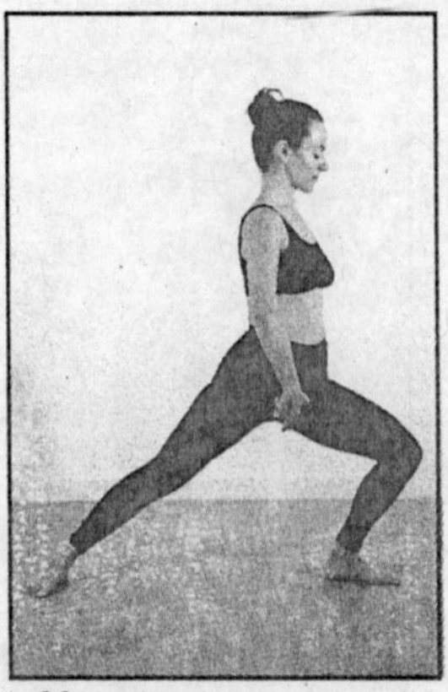
A-80

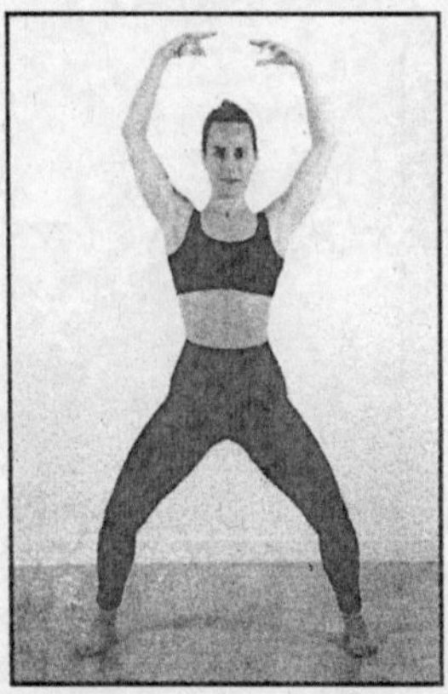
A-81

Repeat movements A-73 to A-81, this time performing the vyaṅgas on the opposite side.

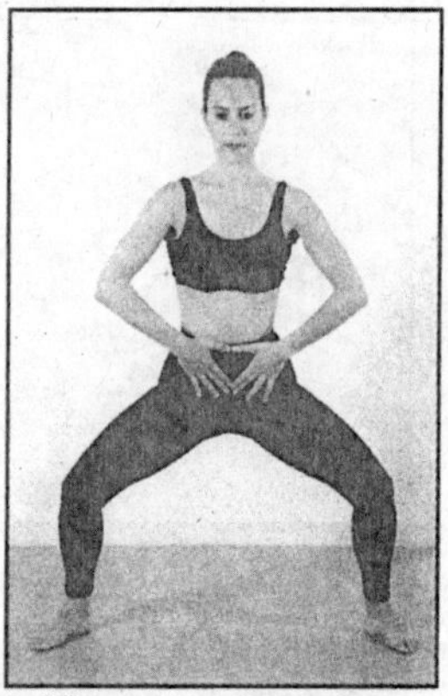
A-82

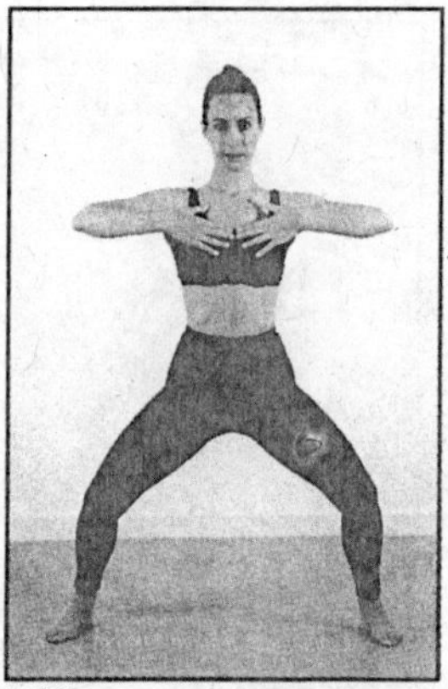
A-83

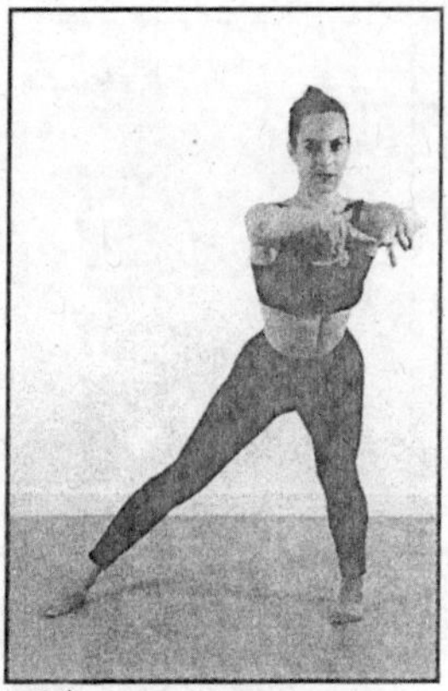
A-84

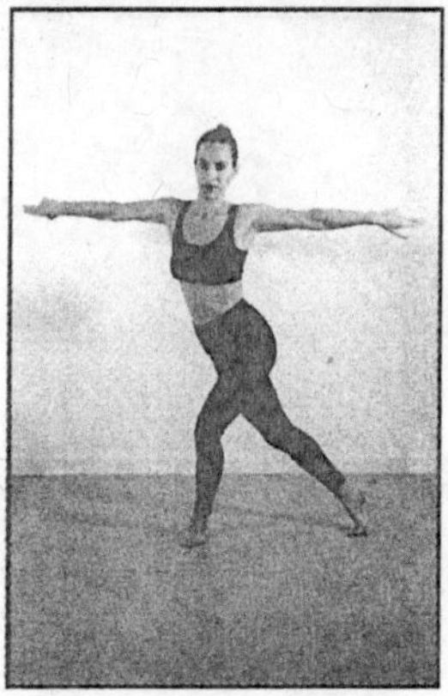
A-85

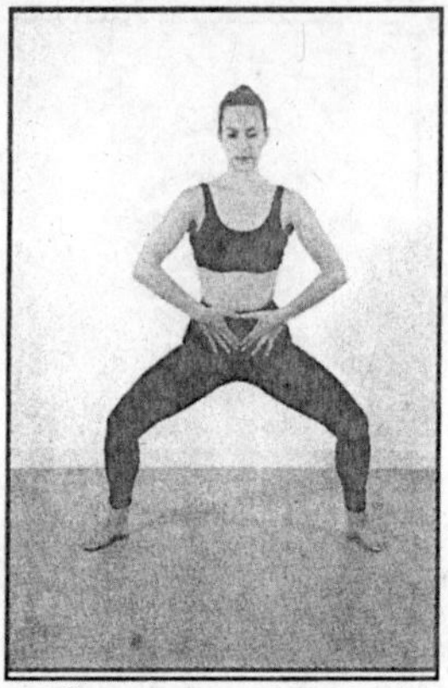
A-86

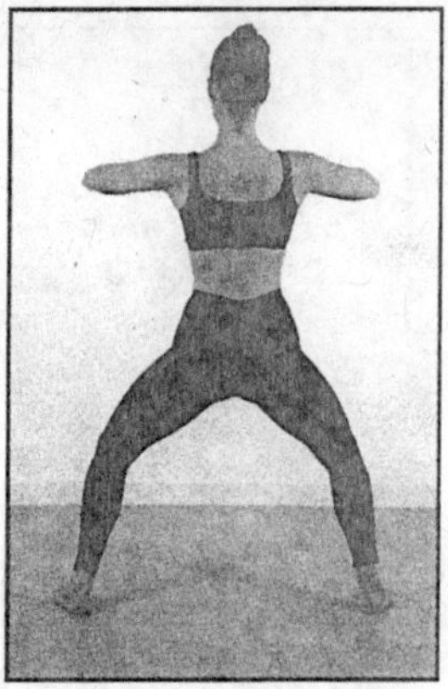
A-87

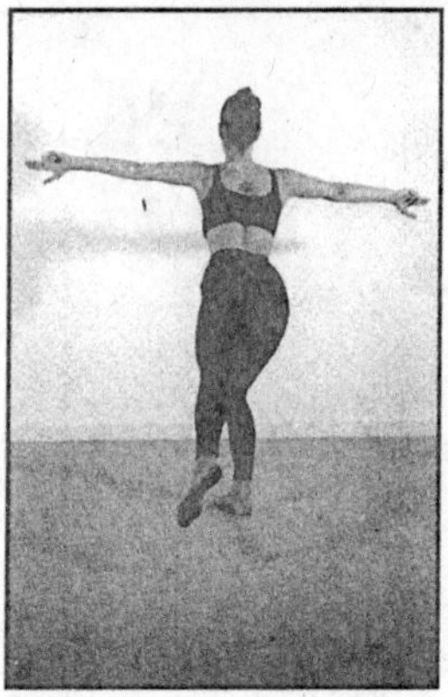
A-88

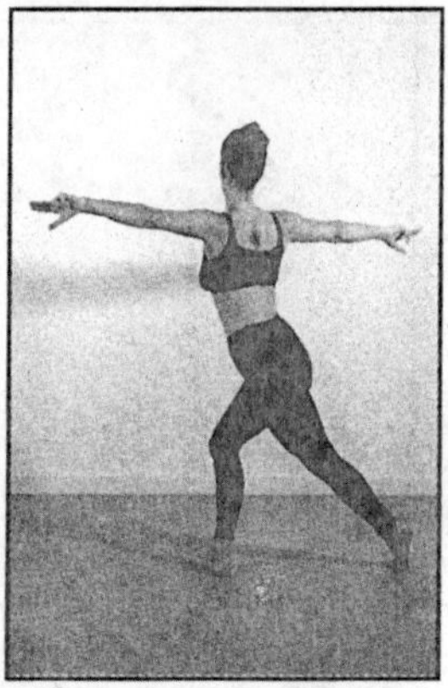
A-89

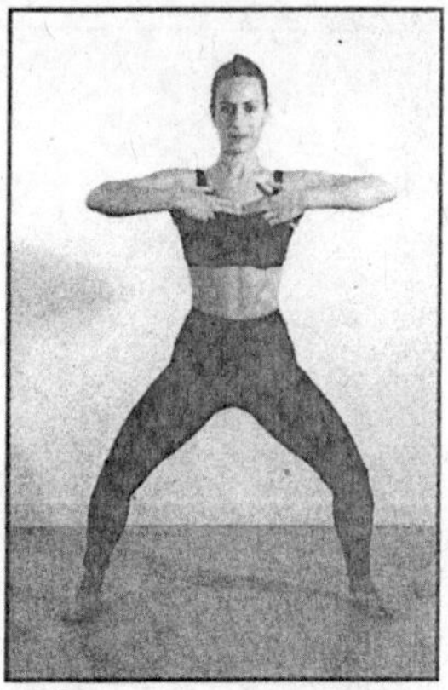
A-90

Repeat movements A-83 to A-91, turning the body in the other direction.

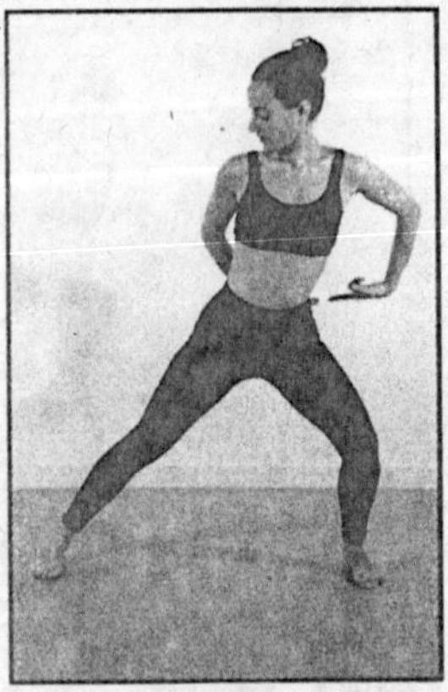
A-91

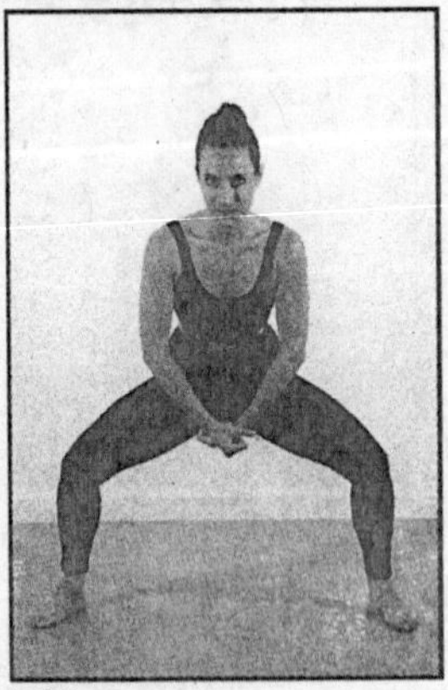
A-92

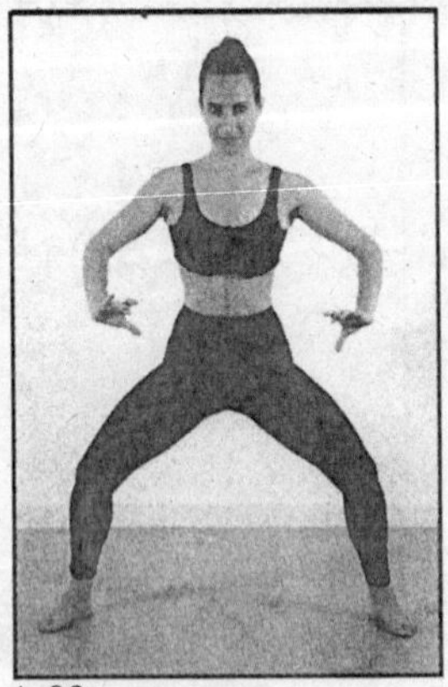
A-93

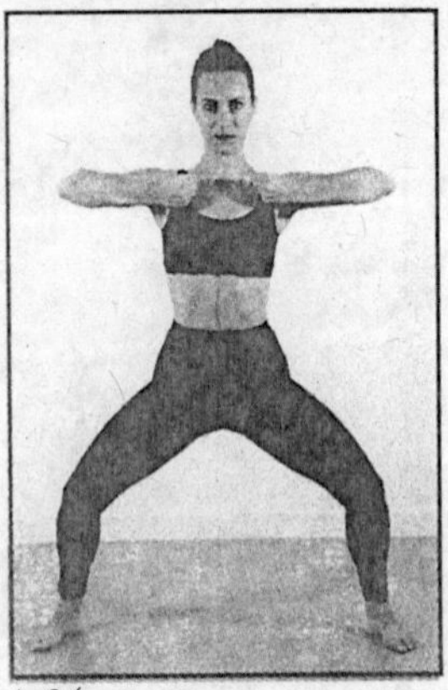
A-94

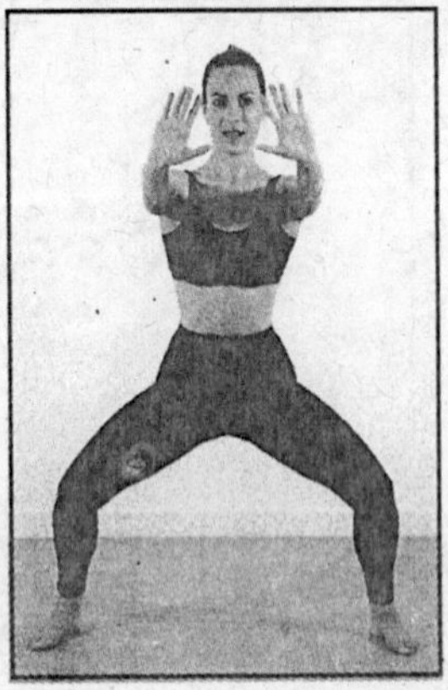
A-95

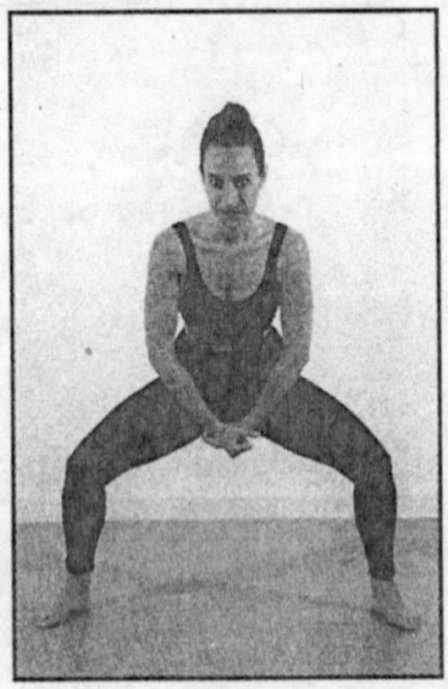
A-96

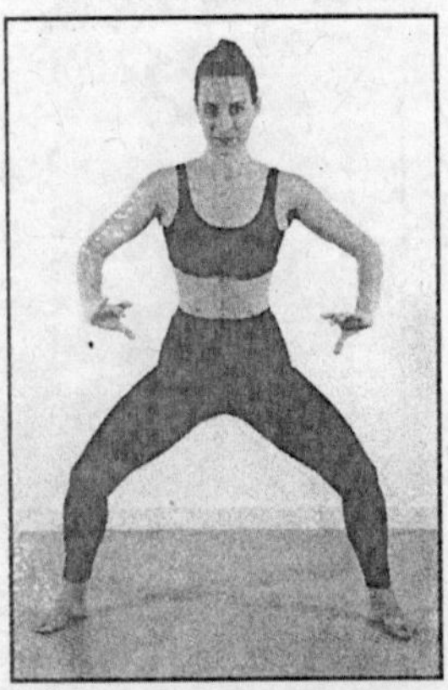
A-97

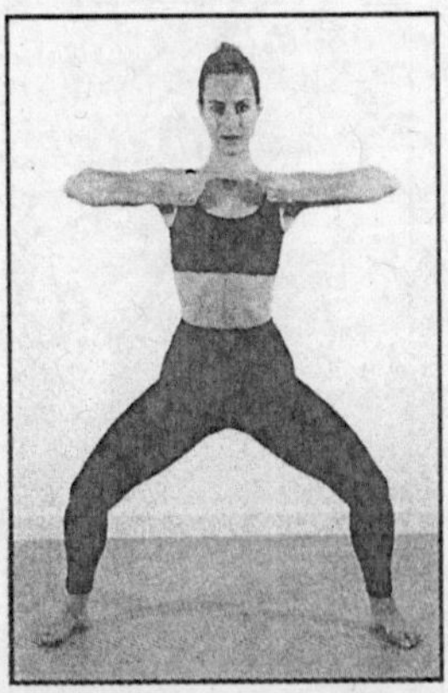
A-98

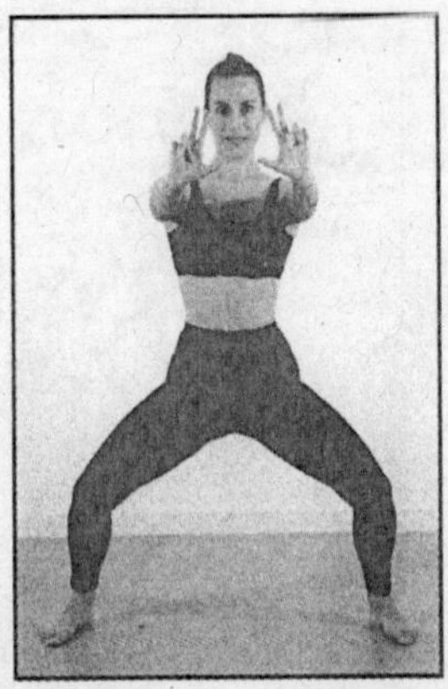
A-99

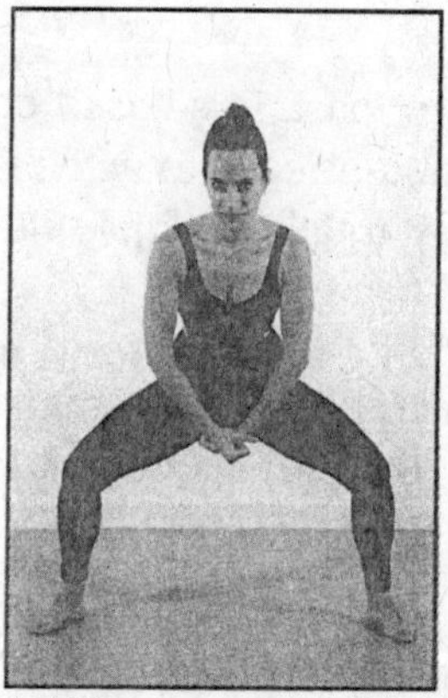
A-100

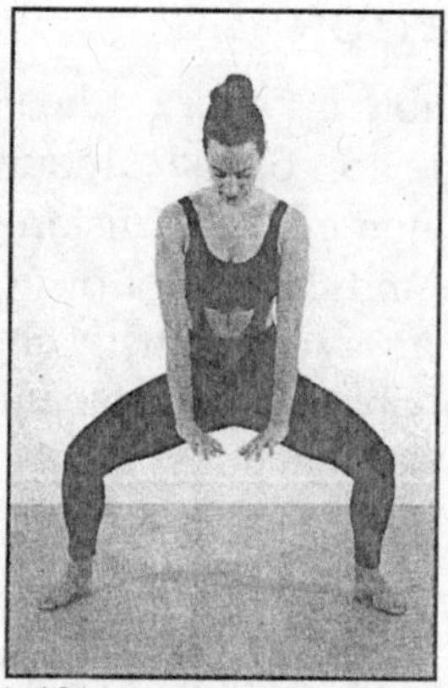
A-101

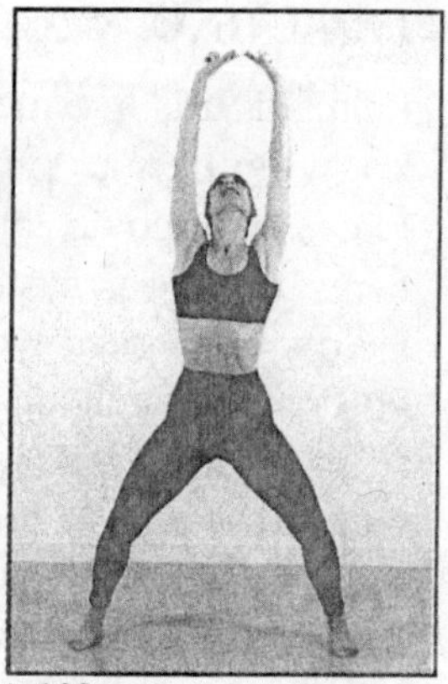
A-102

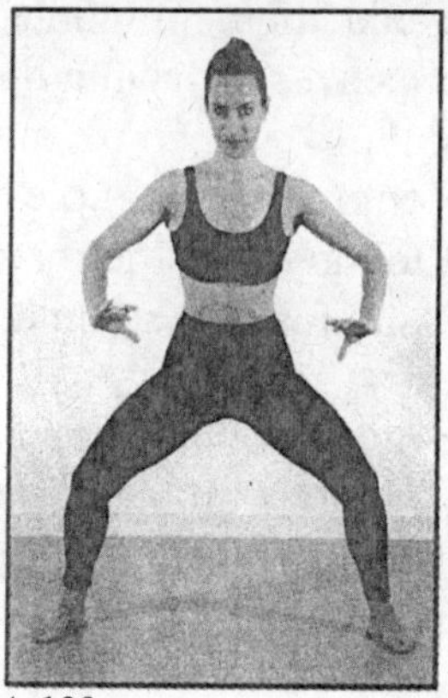
A-103

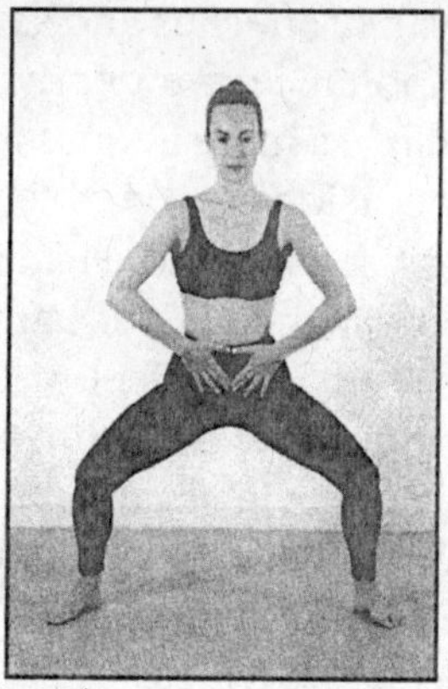
A-104

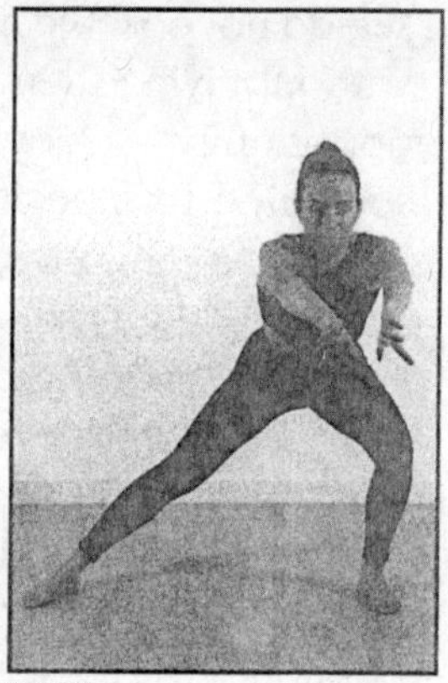
A-105

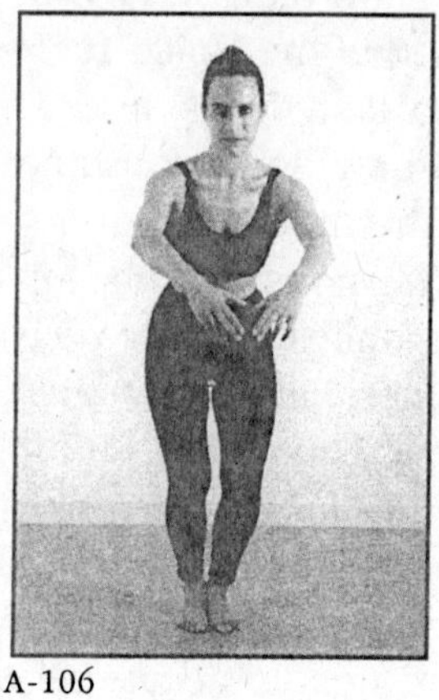
A-106

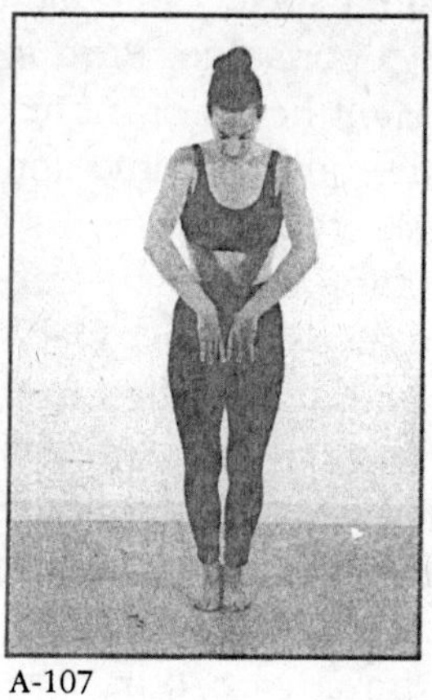
A-107

LEARNING RELAXATION

Relaxation is indispensable in order for health to exist. It is based on knowing how to put the appropriate amount of tension into activity. Excessive activity and unregulated tension may totally collapse our central nervous system and the rest of our organism.

In this respect, we can say that activity should be ruled by positive criteria that facilitate self-analysis. When the mind is obsessed, it cannot see the consequences of its actions, or notice the effort required to take action.

During the day we perform many activities that we assume to be mundane like breathing, eating, excreting, working or loving. We carry them out very mechanically, without adequate consciousness. We do not observe how they affect us and as we take them for granted without giving them importance, we deprive ourselves of having the opportunity to enjoy them in a more intense manner. We are constantly searching for special occasions to be able to enjoy, for example a holiday, a new love, a prize, a movie, etc. The tendency of the mind is to submerge itself in a dynamic of constant desire for new stimulus, each time more intense in order to feel pleasure.

It is true that everything that does not happen frequently has a special impact in our mind, having a stimulating and favourable effect, but we should not distort the value of our daily activities, as they occupy most of our lives and make up the basis that allows for the possibility of these special activities.

We live in a society in which we are harassed by an unmeasured eagerness to consume. Productivity is the voice resonating in our minds for eight hours or more on a daily basis, in order to generate wealth in the quickest time and to be able to consume according to the messages transmitted to us by the media.

This situation causes numerous tensions that end up generating a generalized state of stress, which is manifested in two ways: a sensation of euphoria and a feeling of emptiness. It directly affects our central nervous system and our hormonal system. Its physical and psychological consequences generate many types of disorders.

Stress treatment firstly requires a detailed analysis of the causes that motivate it. We should observe our approaches to life and the value we impart on our surroundings (objects, people, animals, activities). Once these factors are found, we need to re-educate our tastes and our tendencies, trying to avoid falling subject to the previous factors.

Relaxation has a preventive and therapeutic value and in both cases need to be accompanied by the following:

1. Adequate diet.
2. Adequate exercise.
3. Adequate breathing.
4. Positive thought.

Human beings develop their lives on three levels of existence: wakefulness, sleep and deep sleep, all of which require concentration of consciousness and vital balance.

When the activity we carry out in the wakefulness level is unmeasured and loaded with tension, it is possible for these tensions to be projected in our memory cells, keeping them from working in a correct way. It is also possible that the inertia in the mind prevents it from accessing the deep sleep state, causing sleep disorders.[3]

According to yoga and āyurvedic[4] medicine, there are three types of tensions: muscular, mental and emotional. All of them produce a general lack of energetic balance, which constitutes a serious disorder. They may be projected to a part of the body, but they also may move to another place and generate a number of illnesses.

There are more reasons to justify the need to practise, along with relaxation and the four previously highlighted points: adequate diet, adequate exercise, adequate breathing and positive thought. All of them will generate a dynamic that is capable of eliminating the potential for mental, muscular or emotional tension. We should point out that once a disease has already manifested itself due to stress or tension, it must be treated by adequate means. Relaxation and the other four practices are a fabulous complement for allowing a quick recovery and a barrier against possible relapses.

3. Man is a collection of realities and their underlying essence is what we call consciousness, which is projected through the mind and the body in three levels of existence: wakefulness, sleep, and deep sleep. In deep sleep, consciousness returns to its original state, but it is still linked to the mind as a consequence of action, karma. This link is what brings it back, projecting itself again to the sleep and wakefulness states. In deep sleep, the body is exclusively relegated to its vital functions, allowing it to obtain a profound rest. At an energetic level, consciousness becomes revitalized as it contacts its original source.

4. In Āyurveda, we can find a physical-psycho-energetic therapy that helps re-establish health. We can also find in Āyurveda the āyursiddha, a medicine based on tantra knowledge, also called magical, and āyurvidyā, a conventional medicine that employs drugs or surgical interventions when needed.
Āyursiddha puts emphasis on the strength of the therapist, siddha, or abhyāsin, someone who dominates the technique and practices it in a consistent way.
In āyurvedic medicine, the balance between mind and body is based on the stabilization of the essential elements or doṣas: vāta, dominated by air; pitta, dominated by fire, and kapha, dominated by earth.

In contrast to the sleep state in which the mind switches to another form of activity allowing the possibility of muscular spasm, breathing alteration and the mind acting in an incessant way, relaxation grants us a refreshing break and a harmonization of our organism. During relaxation, we consciously induce our organism into a state of rest. In the same way that unmeasured activity imprints a certain character into our cellular, mental and emotional memory, directed relaxation sessions do the same.

Relaxation sessions are a good start to promote a relaxed attitude that will allow us to transmit the adequate tension needed to our activities. By having the capability to induce our organism into a specific state, we gain the possibility of saying "stop" to activities whenever necessary.

Most people enter a depressive state when their moment of retirement arrives. This clearly shows a lack of profound spiritual values that permit the individual to detach their working activity from the meaning of their lives.

An adequate Vyāyāma Yoga practice can be a very helpful tool for these people to overcome such disorders. The smooth exercises accompanied by precise breathing will help to develop a contemplative attitude so that the mind can be unbound from external actions.

LEARNING POSITIVE THOUGHT

Meditation and positive thought are intertwined. We cannot have a positive mental attitude if we do not practise meditation. If we tried to do so under moral principles for a few days, we would surely fail and negativity would come back. Meditation is 'complete emptiness'. Positive thought is cultivated in silence. The emptiness of thought is created first and then positive thoughts emerge in the intellect.

Pañcha Tantra states: "In times of adversity, only the word "friend" is the balm that cures all wounds." To look after a friend is a necessity. This is the thought of the guru, the master thought. The virtuous transformation of positive thought is the transformation or virtue of the guru.

"Yoga is the firm control of the senses. Then, man is never again a victim of his worries. So Yoga is the beginning and the end" (Kaṭha Upanishad, II, 6, II).

The main characteristic of the mind is change, rajas; that is why it is known as mano raja. This means that the mind is constantly plunged in a constant activity that vibrates in three frequencies: serenity, sattva, excitation, rajas and inertia, tamas. Depending on the characteristics of the person, his mind will tend to vibrate more on one certain frequency than another.

When vibrating in the serenity frequency, sattva, a luminous state is produced, in which the knowledge of the world is based on the real knowledge that comes from profound analysis, vichara.[5] Due to this illuminated awareness, a state of serenity is produced, allowing us to develop our activity in an appropriate way.

When the mind is vibrating in the inertia frequency, tamas, a confused state is produced, dominated by a confusing energy, āvaraṇa, in which the senses and the intellect become bloated. Our knowledge is not based on the real form of the object. This kind of ignorance is intimately related to egoism, passion, aversion and attachment to life. Affective and ethic elements become involved and are manifested as unmeasured desires to enjoy the world, laziness and lack of commitment.

When the mind is vibrating in the excitation energy, rajas, a state of confusion is produced in which the main characteristic is lack of objectivity. The mind is impelled by a desire to act moved by a changing force, vikṣepa, a dispersed energy that impedes an evaluation of the consequences of its actions and its reflection lacks objectivity.

All the experiences we have are stored in our minds, leaving latent impressions, or saṁskāras. Memory intervenes in this process through the triple activity of fixation, retention and reproduction. When Saṁskāras are reproduced, they are able to generate tendencies or impulses that enslave our personality, should they be caused by the āvaraṇa or vikṣepa energies. Such slavery submits the individual to a constant attraction and repulsion on unfounded knowledge.

In order to control these states, the strength of positive thought is fundamental; so we must work our energy at the physical level with Vyāyāma and Haṭha yoga. At a psychological level, the essential practices of reflection are vicāraṇā, and meditation, dhyāna.

Vicāraṇā helps us to expel all the disturbing elements and thus examine them in their real form. Saṁyama provides us with the

5. Detailed analysis of the nature of something.

capacity to dissociate subject and object. In this way, knowledge will always be produced in an objective way.

The Vedic masters, whether āyurvedic or not, thought that earth and heaven had value for the individual, according to his or her way of thinking. We live our life according to our mental attitude and our way of thinking either elevates or degrades us. We look for alliances in similar ways of thought in order to justify our criterion. We have more or less perspective depending on how we live. Our thoughts may become sick, weakened, or on the contrary, strengthened. And according to our thoughts, we enjoy or we suffer.

The criterion for gaining knowledge might be influenced by our state of mind, which generally oscillates between two extremes, rāga and dveṣa, attraction and repulsion. When the criterion is not balanced between these two forces, thought becomes sick and phobias arise. We can understand phobias as things that are isolated from what is produced, by analysing the chain of thought and the criterion by which the subject is governed, in order to find its roots and possible solutions.

Be it as prevention or as a fundamental help in the treatment of possible disorders, it is necessary to exercise positive thinking and balanced thought that is able to discern diverse situations and relationships. It is fundamental to establish a vigorous vicāraṇā in order to detach ourselves from the problem, and from there, adopt effective solutions.

If we know that the energy that moves thought is the same energy that moves our physical functions, then moving the body is to mobilize and renovate energy, directly influencing our quality, our thought. In this way, breathing techniques and the practice of Vyāyāma are two great and powerful tools in the treatment of mental disorders.

Lastly, we should directly work with the fluctuations of the mind, with the imbalance between likes and dislikes, passions and aversions that affect criterion by disturbing them or even by destroying them in extreme cases. Yoga, by definition, is a suitable tool to help us. "*Yogaś cittavṛtti-nirodhaḥ*", a sentence from the Yogasūtra (I.2), means, "Yoga is the cessation of the fluctuations of the mind."

The force of positive thought transforms the life of an individual, bringing health and balance and is the fundamental tool in order to know how to develop activity in its diverse fields.

LEARNING CONTEMPLATION

A man who does not feel his affinity with the world, lives in a kind of prison whose walls seem hostile. When, on the contrary, he finds himself reflected in all things and is able to see easily that he is an eternal spirit, and discovers the most complete meaning of the world he lives in, he feels perfect, authentic and in harmony with everything. In this way the man becomes a witness.

—RABINDRANATH TAGORE

A balanced life is the consequence of a state of well-being that comes from the equilibrium between joy and transcendence.

Transcendental experiences provide us with the serenity and equanimity necessary when faced with the natural dynamic of the universe, full of joy and suffering.

Vital balance manifests itself in the body, mind and spirit of a person. We can conclude that in a balanced state, the body is healthy and the mind manifests a serene character through contact with the spirit or inner energy.

In this context, Vyāyāma Yoga is the process or mastery of pushing aside all that has to be moved so that order can be established in the body, mind and spirit. Thanks to breath control, the body becomes healthy, the mind calm and we are allowed to enter into the meditative state that leads us towards our inner self.

Through meditation, thought is absorbed in the desired goal through two means:

1. By attempting to adjust and adapt ourselves to that goal, without creating resistance, as if trying to float on water.
2. By transforming our nature, making it identical to what we are looking for.

This thought absorption in its two forms requires that haṭha, the force that is manifested through the senses that bind us to the world, is brought back to its original cause, prāṇa, by means of abstraction, or pratyāhāra.[6]

Pratyāhāra literally means, "to gobble up the senses." When we inhale, the senses are activated, expanded and when we exhale, they are gobbled up.[7] This is the process by which the senses are

---

6. Abstraction: pratyakṣa-āhāra. Āhāra: to eat, to gobble up. Pratyakṣa: the senses.
7. In order to achieve a good pratyāhāra when meditating, or if we just want to establish a stable posture, we can perform one of the following vāyukas:
   - A short, quick inhalation, and exhalation with a unblocking sound.
   - A short, quick inhalation, and a quick exhalation with a high pitched sound emptying the lungs. They both create emptiness and distract the senses.

disconnected from the world surrounding us when we close nine openings of the body: the anus, genitals, ears, nostrils, eyes and mouth. In order to do so, we must quieten the other organs, the hands and legs and control the breathing by slowing it down as much as possible to the point of being barely perceivable.

In this state of abstraction, introspection should be produced as a fundamental tension that drives the mind inside and makes it stay there without being affected by anything internal or external. In this way an effective meditative state is developed.

In order to achieve meditative absorption, we train ourselves in the art of contemplation, which consists of a differentiated observation between the subject and everything surrounding it, without any type of identification or analysis. The only relationship should be mere observation and nothing else.

The body can be still or move slowly. The mind, although projecting itself towards what it perceives, is not altered, it is only fixed on that which it perceives through the senses.

There should not be any type of thought or memory evocation.

Contemplative attitude introduces us into meditation and allows us to develop adequate activity of our essential vital needs. Its final effect is a constant state of serenity and balance.

The most basic technique in the practice of meditation and contemplation consists in our ability to become the witness of the mind and body. We should move our body in unison with the breath, and the mind is a witness that observes the movement of the breath and body.

When the movement between body and breath becomes one, it is like a centrifugal force that moves everything away, bringing our internal force to a unified state, and the mind is concentrated, absorbed.

The process of expanding the tan unifies balanced activity between mind, body and spirit. This process is known as tantrayoga and the process that teaches us to tame the breath in order to obtain the force necessary to expand the tan is called Vyāyāma.

LEARNING SAṀYAMA MEDITATION

Saṁyamas are guidelines for the acquisition of qualities that are present in someone or something by dominating the deep nature of the mind. It is a practice in which we are able to cultivate attributes we lack and to comprehend the nature of something or the personality of some one.

In a more profound sense, saṁyama is a practice used in order to understand phases of deep philosophical knowledge.

Rather than intellectually comprehending, the person who practises gains an understanding through living and experiencing.

In meditation, the objective is the concentration of the mind on a point to restrict all mental processes. Saṁyama is a meditation practice, with the goal of acquiring the nature of something. To do that, the mind fixes on something and tries to awaken its culture. It is not a process of acquiring intellectual knowledge, because only observation and mental attitude are involved.

The most elevated Saṁyama is to look for the essential nature of where we come from as individual beings. It encompasses concentration, meditation, and a perfect state of serenity, samādhi, in which the mind is not affected by anything.

Saṁyama process

1. Visualization of something we wish to cultivate. We should know everything possible about the object by using the five senses and by analyzing its properties. The senses and the mind are actively focused on the object.
2. Mind focus is a fundamental feature. In the next phase, the mind summarizes a collection of properties in a symbolic way. The mind passes from analysis and observation to syncretism.
3. Abstraction of the senses. The senses are withdrawn inside the mind, like a tortoise putting its limbs inside its shell and travelling inwards to its most profound layers
4. The mind rests on the essence or sense of the object. Impelled by the force of abstraction it remains focused, maintaining a state of alertness and receptivity.

The process of assimilation is similar to the one produced after having digested food. All the properties that food has are synthesized and transformed and become part of our organism.

To successfully achieve Saṁyama, the mind should allow for the transfer of essential qualities. The content of the meditation should be passed onto the meditator. However it is not a search in which the meditator is an active subject wanting to possess the contents of the object on which he meditates.This knowledge comes from the deep subconscious.

Saṁyama meditation is also applicable to Vyāyāma Yoga practice, in the different movements, vyaṅgas, keeping in mind that most of them are inspired in activities developed by man, animals or by the nature of plants and objects.

As Vyāyāma Yoga consists of the mobilization of the śakti by means of prāṇa in Saṁyama meditation, the objective is to acquire the śakti contained in the object of meditation. We can conclude that Saṁyama practice applied to Vyāyāma Yoga is a technique of śakti reinforced by śakti, which in turn provides excellent results.

The execution of Saṁyama is based on a fundamental relationship that adopts many dimensions:

1. By meditating on philosophical premises or important sentences of knowledge about the essence of existence
2. By observing the qualities of an object
3. By direct contact with the object

The importance of the hands in Saṁyama

The hands are concentrated on the tan, and the tan energy in the hands transforms the life of a person. In the text that talks about music and dance, Nāṭya Śāstra, says: "where the hands go, the eyes go; attention is where the eyes are; energy is where the attention is, and with it, the vibrating ecstasy". The hands are the part of the body that marks the directions of the movement. They are the cause of all the activity of transformation of the world around us.

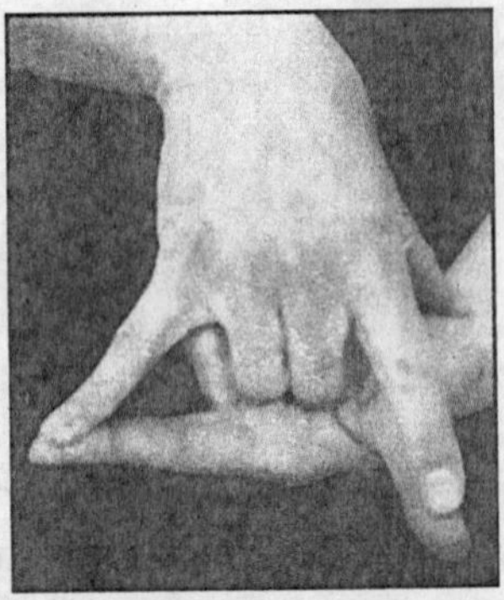

When the hands are sensitive, strong and full of energy, they are capable of transmitting many types of feelings and are also capable of perceiving them. Subtle ducts of energy, nāḍīs, flow through the hands and channel the vital breath; prāṇa, decompressed in its main functions. Through touch, the śakti of objects can be perceived and it can also be transmitted, functioning as energy acquisition and transmission bridges.

Different ways of acquiring energy through Saṁyama

Through contact:

By touching, hugging, kissing, breath, saliva and semen transfer.

Through sight:

The eyelids are semi-closed as if in deep concentration or meditation. It is not necesary to look directly.

Through thought:

Thinking of a person, focusing the attention on a part of his/her body, in order to strip away their energy, or to give or balance their energy.

The practice of Saṁyama is different from meditation practice in that the breath, vāyu, gradually fades out, may be even coming to a point of total retention, kumbhaka. In Saṁyama, the breath, Vāyu, is essential and is the director of the śakti. Vāyudeva is the God that blesses the practice of Saṁyama, and besides being one of the five essential elements, vāyu is the God of Imagination. Vāyu is located in the physical body at the same level as the third cervical vertebra and is known as the place of the wind, vāyu kanda, influencing emotional balance due to its relationship with the heart. According to knowledge found in the energy distribution centres of the body, ādi tala,[8] where they come together is known as the point of life and death. Physiologically, the heart receives sympathetic fibres, which originate at the neck and whose nucleus is placed near the third cervical vertebra. That is why it is recommended to perform breathing and neck exercises in order to strengthen the heart.

There is a breathing technique called vāyuprāṇāyāma saṁyama that improves sleep, relaxation, breathing and creativity. By adopting a relaxed posture and the gesture of knowledge, jñāna mudrā,[9] the following directions must be observed: the inhalation is made through the nose and the exhalation through the mouth with a low sound. The breathing is deep diaphragmatic. The inhaled air is sent to the tan as a discharged breath and then the breath is dragged simulating a light sound produced by the partially closed glottis, during both the exhalation and inhalation. This should produce the sensation of the breath being dragged through the throat. By putting the lips in a 'OU' form, a deep sound is made while exhaling. Inhalation is thoracic-clavicular and the exhalation is in the form of bhrāmarī, as indicated.

8. The different physical points in which the *talas* are projected.
9. A gesture made with the hands by joining the thumb and index finger tips together.

LEARNING AWARENESS OF THE THREE BODIES

There is certain knowledge about energetic anatomy we must be aware of in order to sensitize ourselves to be able to practise Vyāyāma Yoga in a profound way.

According to Tantra, man is made up of three bodies that contain five forms. These three bodies are: the dense body, sthūla śarīra, the energetic body, sūkṣma śarīra and the causal body, kāraṇa śarīra. Each one of the three types of Vyāyāma corresponds to these bodies and acts upon them. Dense Vyāyāma, sthūla Vyāyāma, works mainly on the physical body; energetic Vyāyāma, sūkṣma Vyāyāma, works mainly on the subtle body and magical Vyāyāma, kāraṇa Vyāyāma, works mainly on the causal body.

The existence of man depends on a correct and harmonious relationship between the bodies he is made of.

In the wakeful state, all three bodies are active, in the sleep state, subtle and causal body are active and in the deep sleep state, the causal body is principally active.

Beyond these three states of consciousness, there is a fourth state, known as the one that breaks the perception of the other three, turīya avasthā. In this state the perception of the senses is interrupted and consciousness directly perceived without using the body, the senses or the mind. This state is accessed through deep meditation.

The first of the bodies, the physical body, sthūla śarīra is dense and visible, formed by multi-cellular groups of organs and a number of diverse systems. Its only form, the substantial, annamaya kośa, is formed by the energies extracted from food. It is built of the five elements, predominantly solids, liquids and gases. In it, the five main action organs are placed: hands, feet, mouth, anus, genitals and the nine doors. It functions by interacting with the universe around us.

The second body, the subtle body, sūkṣma śarīra is the most complex. Three forms develop their activity in it: the vital, prāṇamaya kośa, the intellectual, vijñānamaya kośa and the mental form, manomaya kośa.

The vital form, prāṇamaya kośa, better known as the astral body, is a replica of the form of the physical body and is formed by the five vital breaths, pañcaprāṇas: Prāṇa allows for the functioning of the lungs, apāna for the excreting organs, samāna for the digestive system, udāna for the swallowing organs and vyāna, for blood circulation, other bodily fluids and nerve currents.

Each one of these vital breathes or prāṇas have, in turn, diverse sub-breathes that vitalize other parts of the physical body. We can locate their activity in the following areas of the body: prāṇa: head and heart, apāna: anus and genitals, samāna: from the genitals to the heart, udāna: from the throat to the heart and vyāna: the whole body, mainly in the extremities.

The substantial form, annamaya kośa and the vital form, prāṇamaya kośa, are connected, making life possible as we perceive it with our senses. When this connection is broken, death occurs. On some occasions, the vital form can separate from the substantial form, but still remain linked by a thin cord of energy known as the silver cord. This form (prāṇamaya) expresses itself through the five organs of action and is the uniting nexus between the substantial form and the rest of the forms contained within the subtle and causal body.

The mental form, manomaya kośa, is the second form contained in the subtle body. In it, we can find the functions of the inner organ, antaḥkaraṇa,[10] which are known as: conscious mind, manas and subconscious mind, citta.

Manas receives information from the outer world through the senses, from the subconscious and also in a direct way, what we know as intuition. Manas is constantly vibrating in three states: sattva, rajas and tamas, which are: luminosity, passion and inertia. The perception of information is conditioned by the vibration state. When the mind is vibrating in tamas, it lacks the strength necessary to correctly perceive the information received through the senses. It is as if the lenses of our glasses were dirty or misted over, keeping us from seeing with clarity.

Citta is the subconscious mind where all information is stored, either processed by the intellect or directly received through the conscious mind. In the subconscious we can find not only the experiences of this life, but also thousands of experiences of past lives. These are accumulated in the form of seeds, or saṁskāras and tendencies, vāsanās, formed by groups of saṁskāras of the same nature.

10. Antaḥkaraṇa is the organ of investigation available to the Being, ātman, which is manifested in a body, in order to get in touch with the external world around him. This organ of investigation expresses itself through four main functions: the transmitting and receiving capacity along with the thinking function, manas; the ability to store all the impressions received in this and other lives: chitta; the identity associated with a physical body, ahaṁkāra; and the ability to discern, buddhi.

The third form of the subtle body is the intellectual form, vijñāmaya kośa. It contains the other two functions of the mind or antaḥkaraṇa: intellect, buddhi, and ego, ahaṁkāra.

Buddhi is the intellectual function that processes all the data received through the mind, classifying them according to the trends and tastes that characterize its personality. An illuminated intellect represents the possibility of being able to deeply discern reality in our lives. This allows us access to a large number of tools that provide us with harmony and serenity.

Ahaṁkāra is the unifying force function that provides an identity to the collection of bodies. Its function is similar to that of the government of a nation, organizing and regulating the different functions of the various individuals that form the social group, giving them an identity.

The third body, kāraṇa śarīra, is the causal and the origin of the two previous bodies. This is the body through which the ātman, the very Being, is projected. It only has one form like the first body and a triple constitution: priya, moda and pramoda.

Priya is happiness experienced in the presence of that which is desired. Moda is the happiness experienced when possessing the object of desire. Pramoda is the happiness obtained while enjoying what is desired. This triple quality is produced due to the blessed nature of the Being, ātman. When it loses its self-perception and projects itself as the false ego, it is constantly looking to attain the blessed state through the causal body form.

Due to the material nature the false ego can experience, the attributes of the causal body form are subject to their opposite pairs. Apriya is the suffering caused by the possibility of losing what one desires; amoda, is the suffering produced when the enjoyment of what one desires is consumed; and apramoda is the suffering from having lost what was desired.

These three bodies with their distinctive forms are closely related among themselves. Any negative or positive affectation in any one of them has an impact on the rest. By practising Vyāyāma Yoga we influence the three bodies, in a direct or indirect way, gaining great amounts of strength and balance and the opportunity to obtain a state of awareness in which recognition of the true nature of the ātman[11] is easier.

The three bodies of the living entity Jīvātman		
The physical or dense body **Sthūla śarīra**	**Subtle body** **Sūkṣma śarīra**	**Causal body** **Kāraṇa śarīra**
State of consciousness Wakefulness **Svapna avasthā** Substantial form, Annamaya Kośa. Formed by food substances.	State of consciousness Wakefulness, sleep **Svapna avasthā** Vital form, Prāṇamaya Kośa. Formed by the five vital breathes, Pañca prāṇas: prāṇa, allows the functioning of the lungs; Apāna, excreting organs; Samāna, digestive system; Udāna: swallowing organs; Vyāna: the flow of all body currents. Intellectual form, Vijñānamaya Kośa. Formed by: Intellect, Buddhi and Ego, Ahaṁkara. Mental form, Manomaya Kośa. Formed by: conscious mind, Manas, and subconscious mind, Citta.	State of consciousness Wakefulness, sleep and deep sleep **Suṣupti avasthā** The form of eternal bliss, Ānandamaya Kośa. Formed by three attributes: Priya, happiness experienced by perceiving the desire. Moda, happiness experienced by possessing the desire. Pramoda, happiness experienced by enjoying what is desired

(11) ***ātman***: my self, that which determines my existence. It is the primary consciousness where existence and eternal bliss reside. The *ātman* is self-luminous, it doesn't need reflection in order to know itself, however, due to the illusory power it contains, it stops perceiving itself as it is, to start identifying with something different and not whole. In this process of false perception where the false ego emerges, it constantly looks to experience the properties of the *ātman*: happiness, consciousness, and existence, because it has risen from such attributes. In this way, the false me is submerged in a reflective process, developing itself in a universe of forms that is constantly acting as a mirror, in order to perpetuate its attainment. Soul is often identified with ātman, which is inexact, because the soul is associated with the properties of understanding, wanting and feeling. The soul can be modified in its nature depending on the relationship with the world around it. If we agree that the soul is the essence of man and so should therefore be protected, the need for a series of moral principles that keep the soul from falling from its state of purity and supreme beatitude is implied.

Desire leads the soul to project itself on the world and it is affected by the many experiences produced by such projection.

Here we can find a big difference between Christian and Vedic morality. While Christianity prescribes a salvationist morality in which the soul must avoid becoming contaminated with the bad of the world, in order to reach heaven. Vedic morality is based on the regulation of the life of man in such a way that a balanced process of self knowledge could be followed and the last aspiration of which, is that the ātman recognizes itself. Two basic principles underlie Vedic morality:

1. Ahimsā: the principle of non-violence that should lead us to limit the evolution of all living beings that are related to our subsistence.
2. The need to carry out and satisfy the basic needs of our life in terms of our economy, relationship with the universe in which we live in, senses and self-knowledge.

Vedic morality is applicable to all aspects and needs of the life of man, providing a path of harmony and balance.

LEARNING THE IGNITION OF THE SIX POWERS

The energetic centre, Tan

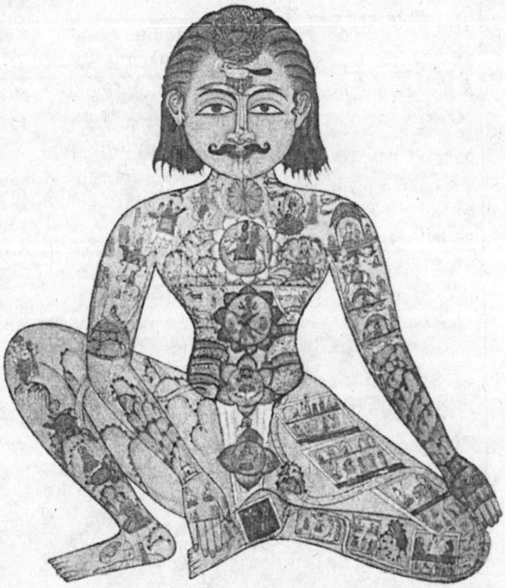

It is the internal and singular manifestation of the Mahā Śakti, the energy from which everything originates. It is the energetic heart of every individual being and regulates energy movement throughout the whole body. It provides the personality and characteristics of each person, making the benefits of Vyāyāma practice different for every person who practises.

In its projection, Mahā Śakti manifests itself as a force that propagates igniting and generating heat. It glows, emitting radiance and the capacity to transmit energy. Self-improvement beyond our capabilities, personal limitations and karmic conditioning is produced due to the force of the tan when it expands. In it, we can find the secret of what we are, beyond mind and senses and its balanced state means health for our body, mind and spirit.

The projection and concentration of the tan in the physical body is located four fingers below the navel and from there it projects towards the back area.

Because the majority of work done in Vyāyāma is concentrated in the tan, large amounts of heat are generated, large doses of sweat and toxin elimination occurs, while will power, resistance and perseverance are increased.

The originating power of all that exists, Mahā Śakti

The term śakti comes from the Sanskrit root 'śak', which means "power, doing". It indicates activity and capacity. Śakti is power in general and in any particular form of power.

It is the essential energy from which the whole universe and all that exists originates, visible or invisible, either manifested or non-manifested. This śakti energy is submerged in constant activity by means of its triple capacity: icchā śakti, the capacity or power of determination, where the possibility of time, space and action comes; kriyā śakti, the power of the action that manifests in everything, projecting itself in time and space and jñāna śakti, the capacity of recognition which allows for the individuality of all that is manifested. It is present everywhere and in everything, in the same way as water is present in a drop as much as in the entire ocean. This makes it possible for everything to be, to move, to be generated and reproduced, being the origin of all the forces.

The individualized generating power, Kuṇḍalinī

This is also known as the power of the serpent. Symbolically, it is said that kuṇḍalinī adopts the form of a sleeping serpent that is coiled up three and a half times, dwelling in a spot that is located at the base of the spine, called the kaṇḍa.

This symbol has various meanings, one of them explaining that śakti penetrates the three modifications of essential nature, prakṛti which are: knowledge, sattva; passion, rajas and inertia, tamas. The remaining half of the serpent, its head, represents that although immersed in these natures, its power completely transcends them and it is ready to be awakened.

Kuṇḍalinī is the latent power of Mahā Śakti, which is condensed and manifested in all beings. Its power is expanded through the tan.

Prāṇa, vital energy

Its basic manifestation in the body produces the functioning of the lungs, swallowing, digestion and excretion and allows for better body current flow. It is the manifestation of Mahā Śakti that makes it possible for individualized life to exist. In its decomposition it is manifested as the haṭha force.

The polarized force, haṭha

Ha, is the force that regulates the anabolic processes in the organism. It is identified with the energy of the Sun, heat and all that is positive.

Ṭha, is the force that regulates the catabolic processes in the organism. It is identified with the energy of the Moon, the cold and all that is negative.

The force requires a constant and balanced ha-ṭha exchange.

Cakras: generation and regeneration energy centres

There are six fundamental energy centres not perceived by the eyes, which generate and regenerate prāṇa and its different manifestations. As well as regulating body energy, they also regulate all the psychic and spiritual processes. In their physical projection they are located one on top of the other along the spinal column, coinciding with the location of certain vital centres or glands.

Svādhiṣṭhāna cakra is called 'the seat of vital force', situated in the sacrum plexus, at the root of the genital organs.

Maṇipūra cakra is known as the 'bejewelled city', located in the solar plexus, forming the important union between the right and left sympathetic chains, Iḍā and Piṅgalā with the spinal-brain axis.

Anāhata cakra is located in the cardiac plexus.

Viśudha cakra, all that is 'pure', situated in the laryngeal plexus.

Ājñā cakra, the 'government' is placed in the cavernous plexus, in the space between the eyebrows.

And above all the other cakras, there is the Sahasrāra cakra, the 'thousand petals' cakra.

These cakras are represented as lotus flowers with 4, 6, 10, 12, 16, 2 and 1000 petals respectively, each corresponding to a converging nāḍī. The sum of the first six is 50, corresponding to the sounds of the Sanskrit alphabet.

The amount of petals in each cakra is determined by the amount of nāḍīs that converge in them, and the location of each letter in the petals corresponds to the vibration produced. For example, in the Viśuddha cakra, the vibration produced in the nāḍīs corresponds to the vibration of the 16 vowels contained in the Sanskrit alphabet.

Nāḍīs, the subtle channels of prāṇa energy

The term nāḍī comes from the root word 'naḍ' meaning movement. There are also other meanings like river, flow or current.

Prāṇa flows through the subtle channels, nāḍīs, in its many manifestations. There is a large number of nāḍīs and if they could be seen by the naked eye, they would appear as a very complex flow graph.

According to the Bhūta Śuddhi Tantra there are 72,000 nāḍīs. Other texts, like the Śiva Saṁhitā, indicate the existence of 350,000, but the most important ones are Iḍā, Piṅgalā, and Suṣumṇā. Prāṇa flows as Ṭha energy through Iḍā nāḍī, and as Ha energy through Piṅgalā nāḍī. Both nāḍīs interweave in each of the first five cakras along the spine, and end by joining with the Suṣumṇā, which covers the whole spine in a straight line. From here, Suṣumṇā ascends alone to the Sahasrāra cakra.

Inside Suṣumṇā the Vajriṇī nāḍī is found, and inside this, the Citriṇī nāḍī is located. The Brahmā nāḍī is inside Citriṇi nāḍī. At the end of the citriṇī, there is a door known as Brahmādvāra, which opens the way to Kuṇḍalinī in its ascension toward the Sahasrāra cakra.

Talas, energy distribution centres

Talas are energy distribution centres that come from the cakras. They are points at which energy converges, is managed and directed to other areas. We have a great number of talas, which coincide with āyurvedic medicine acupuncture. The nāḍīs arrive in the talas forming blocks. Some of them are fundamental and have to be aligned so that in its physical projection they provide stability to the body, whether in movement or stillness. Unless the nāḍīs and the talas are aligned in order to take and project energy, the movement will not be effective, as the force will not flow sufficiently.

In Vyāyāma Yoga, the talas that are placed in:

1. The soles of the feet, regulating the vitality of the organism.
2. The tip of the big toes.
3. The knees, giving strength to the legs.
4. The hips.
5. Below the ribs.
6. At the entries to the armpits.
7. In the centre of the chest.
8. At the base of the throat, from where the breath departs and oxygen is polarized as ha and ṭha.
9. The chin.
10. Over the shoulder blades. The strength of the inner breastplate comes from here.
11. The shoulders.
12. The elbows.
13. The wrists.
14. The palms of the hands, known as mahā talas or great talas.

15. The five fingers. The main ones are the index, middle and thumb fingers.
16. The space between the knees, which emerges from the tan.
17. Four fingers above the head, coinciding with the previous one in its inflection point. These last two are ethereal talas, which allow the maintenance of perfect equilibrium.
18. Four fingers below the navel, known as tan tala, mahā tala or tan hara, and its projection toward the back, tan śakti.

Energy connection cores, marmas

Marmas are connection centres in which the subtle energy flows in the astral body and are projected to the physical body, allowing motor impulses to function. According to the Suśruta Saṁhitā, the 108 marmas are very vulnerable areas where muscles, veins, ligaments, bones and joints meet.

Disorder in these areas causes an increase in the vāta humour, nāḍī blockage, pain, limb or blood loss, choked breathing, collapse and even death.

Tantra teaches the knowledge of energy in its sublime, pure and divine form. It even tells us that God is energy, that consciousness is energy. It teaches us that this energy is present in the body, in the mind, in the Being itself, ātman, and in God. It teaches us that liberation or self-realization means experiencing this knowledge and in order to do so, we need a method, yoga, knowledge, jñāna, experience and assimilation of one thing by another and an intense desire for liberation, mumukṣutva.

Tantra provides us with enough energy so that we are able to carry out all of the above. In the Durlabhasāra Tantra we find the following explanatory sentence: "*Tanyate vistrīyate jñānamanena iti tantram*", which means: "That by which knowledge and its powers are achieved, prolonged and perfected, is Tantra." The mind is both the tool of knowledge and the field of knowledge. The universe is perceived by the mind in the same mind, but the core of the mind is its own divinity, and that is why the body is the temple of the divine[12]. In the Rudrayāmala Tantra we can find the following quote, which clearly states Tantra's attitude to life and its way to attain wisdom: "*Bhukti-mukti-vidhāyakam*", which means: "Wisdom is the right combination

12. It is here we find the reason why Tantra doesn't disintegrate a person; in fact it does just the opposite. It looks to reintegrate them with their own reality, formed by the body, mind, and ātman.

of pleasure and transcendence." To reject the body or the mind in favour of the spirit would be to deprive oneself of knowing the divinity within them.

The fruit of tantra practice is to obtain a life that is perfectly regulated by the four puruṣārthas, which are the values of the life of man, the puruśa. Dharma, the value of balanced relationships; artha, the value of economic satisfaction; kāma the value of the balanced satisfaction of the senses and mokṣa, the value of liberation. Its foundation rests on two pillars: balance, kauśalya and harmony, samattva, as set by the tradition: "*Mahājano yena gataḥ sa panthāh*", "You shall journey by this great path behind the steps of those who preceded you."

In the first stages of awakening the inner power, Kuṇḍalinī, work is principally done on the Mūlādhāra and Svādhiṣṭhāna cakras. This work is known as Kuṇḍalinī yoga and it consists in awakening the sleeping dragon,[13] Kuṇḍalinī, the essential energy. Kanda means base or support and linī means 'coiled up'. Kuṇḍalinī has the power that lies coiled up three and a half times. Each one of these times corresponds to one of the three bamsic energies that derive from it.

Icchā śakti, the energy that arises from will power.
Kriyā śakti, where the power of action arises.
Jñāna śakti, where the power of knowledge originates.

These three energies generate the three bodies with their forms, including the five breathes, the five senses, the five organs of action, and the faculties of knowledge: The faculty of knowing through the organs of the senses, the faculty of knowing by inference from previous knowledge, the revelation and the inner experience.

The remaining half coil of the serpent is inside the tan and from here it expands, allowing the 'I' to transcend the state of purity, sattva, excitation, rajas and inertia, tamas. The awakening of the Kuṇḍalinī adopts two aspects: the Bhairava producing a ferocious state and Rudra, which produces a state of happiness.

To awaken it, we have to activate the six cakras, where the six fundamental powers of this energy are gathered.

In Vyāyāma Yoga there is a practice called, "The ignition of the six powers", in which we work on the root, ascendant and determining cakras. This is done by performing mobilizations, vyaṅgas, certain

13. The dragon is a mythical being that has the head of a lion and the body of a snake. It slithers along and can make itself invisible. It has its eyes and mouth open and is symbolic of Kuṇḍalinī energy.

types of meditation combined with hand gestures, mudrās, the repetition of powerful words, bīja mantras, strong body postures, haṭhāsanas, in which a number of body postures, āsanas, gestures, mudrās, and breaths, svaras, are combined.

The determinant cakra mainly regulates all the common psychic and physical functions. This is the cakra with which the main work is done and where all the energy for the practice comes from. Its use becomes an important dynamo that provides great doses of energy to develop the qualities it regulates.

The key cakra establishes the rules of behaviour. This cakra is needed to channel the energy obtained in the other practices to everyday activities.

The exercised cakras are chosen according to the characteristics set at the date of birth. Their description follows:

In Mūlādhāra, the root sounds or bījas that dominate are: hram mu, ni, sa. Its gesture or mudrā is the trident, triśūla and its shape or yantra is a square inside a circle with an inverted triangle in its centre. The surface on which it is formed is blood red, the same as the inner area, and the lines of the shapes are of a smoky white colour.

In Svādhiṣṭhāna, the root sounds or bījas that dominate are: hrim, sva, da. Its gesture or mudrā is water, jala and its shape or yantra is a circle over which a quarter crescent moon rests. The surface on which it is formed is white, the circle is orange and the moon is pearl-white.

In Maṇipūra, the root sounds or bījas that dominate are: hrum, ma, pa. Its gesture or mudrā is the heart, hṛdaya and its shape or yantra is a circle with an inverted triangle in its centre, with its angles touching the circle. The surface on which it is formed is blood red, the colour of the inner area is an intense sun-like yellow and the lines of the shapes are white.

In Anāhata, the root sounds or bījas that dominate are: hraim, an, na. Its gesture or mudrā is knowledge, jñāna mudrā and its shape or yantra is a circle with a pair of opposing triangles embedded in it. The surface on which it is formed, the inside area and the lines of the shapes, are all sea-green.

In Viśuddha, the root sounds or bījas that dominate are: hraum, vi, ga. Its gesture or mudrā is the void, śūnya and its shape or yantra is a circle with an inverted triangle in its centre, with its angles touching the circle. In the centre there is a small circle that expands. The surface on which it is formed is light blue. The inside area and the lines of the shapes are mother-of-pearl white.

In Ājñā, the root sounds or bījas that dominate are: hrah, ag, sa, re. Its gestures or mudrās are chin and the earth, bhūmi and its shape or yantra is a circle with an inverted triangle in its centre, with its angles touching the circle. In the centre there is a small circle. The surface on which it is formed and the inside area are white. The lines of the shapes and the small circle are indigo-blue.

Ignition of the Six Powers Set of Exercises

Ṣaṭ Cakra Agnipatha Krama Vyāyāma

This series consists of six movements, each of them directed to a specific cakra. Although its main benefits are energetic, its psychological and physical benefits are of equal importance. We should not forget the great influence produced by each cakra over many secretion and hormone production glands, the hormones being the substances that regulate a large number of physical and biochemical processes and a number of disorders can occur if these are not secreted in the correct way. The glands are the physical and dense equivalent to the cakras. Their activity and relation to each cakra will be described in each particular movement of the Ignition of the Six Powers Series.

This Vyāyāma Yoga may be performed in a sitting position, standing still without moving, by opening and moving the feet and with projections in order to improve the coordination of the physical and psycho-physical body movements.

Working on these cakras helps with the improvement of disorders, diseases and psycho-physio-energetic disturbances caused by their possible dysfunctions or energy blockages.

Movement on the *Ājña Cakra.*

Vyaṅga pictures: B-1-2-3-4-5-6. This movement opens the following subtle channels, nāḍīs: the central nāḍī of conception (as the hands raise from the tan to the centre of the forehead). It also opens the pericardium and heart (placed in the frontal and external, lateral side of the arm). It strengthens the muscles of the shoulders, arms and higher dorsal area and enhances lung capacity.

The execution of the gesture, mudrā, on this cakra, positively activates it in the development of intuition and spirituality. It improves the capacity of observation and motivates self-absorption. It helps to heal disorders and diseases associated with this cakra, like headaches, lack of memory, colds, sinusitis, haemorrhoids, ear inflammation, deafness, cervical and vertebral pain and personal attitudes like indifference, lack of creativity, fantasy, depravity, mental rigidity and anguish.

By stimulating this cakra, the person tends to reduce his sleep hours. He might be even able to achieve and enjoy the conscious sleep of yogis.

Its development stimulates the functions of the cerebellum or lower brain and of the central nervous system.

Ājñā cakra is related to the pituitary gland, which produces various and important hormones that regulate the functions of the body. Therefore, the conditions of these hormones and of this cakra associated with the pituitary gland can be treated by the practice of this movement or vyaṅga.

Movement on the *Viśuddha* Cakra

Vyaṅga pictures: B-7-8-9-10-11-12-13-14-15-16-17-18-19-20-21. This movement provides strength to arms and shoulders and releases muscle tension in the dorsal area. It opens the subtle channels, nāḍīs, which are located on the external side of the arm and corresponds to the small intestine, the three humours, tridoṣa and the large intestine. This opening allows better circulation of energy and is an excellent treatment for diseases related to these organs. When this movement is done with expansion, almost all of the muscles of the back are also engaged and worked.

It helps to overcome diseases originating from the malfunction of this *cakra*, such as repeated throat and ear infections, hayfever, colds, lack of defences, cervical pain, angina, pharyngitis, bronchial disorders and unhealthy tendencies like melancholy, depression, excessive worry, creative and comprehension difficulties, pride, individualism, fanaticism, and lack of self-respect.

It also stimulates the following personal behaviour: awakening the consciousness, understanding personal problems, Nature and the Universe and how to examine personal attitudes like arrogance. It revitalizes the lungs, throat, vocal chords, tonsils, salivary glands and the thyroid gland and allows for better creativity expressed through the written or spoken word.

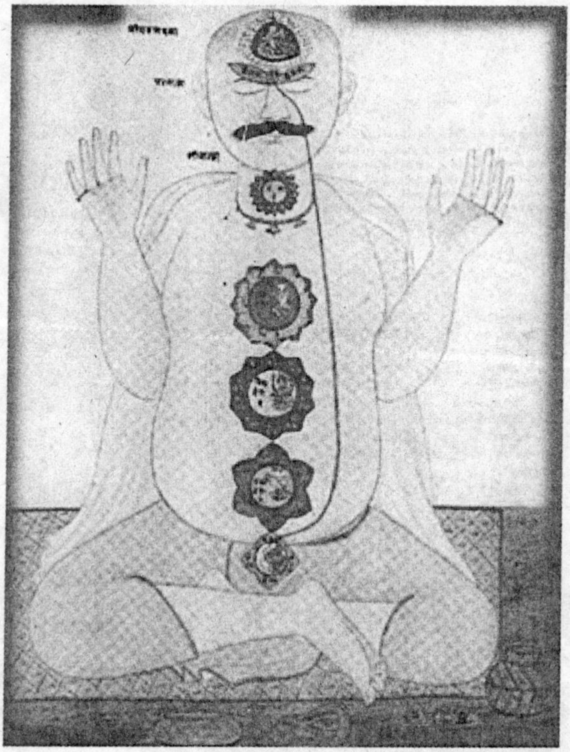

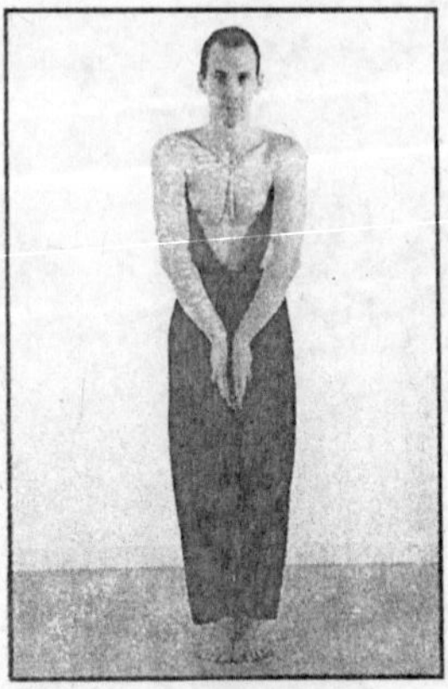
B-1

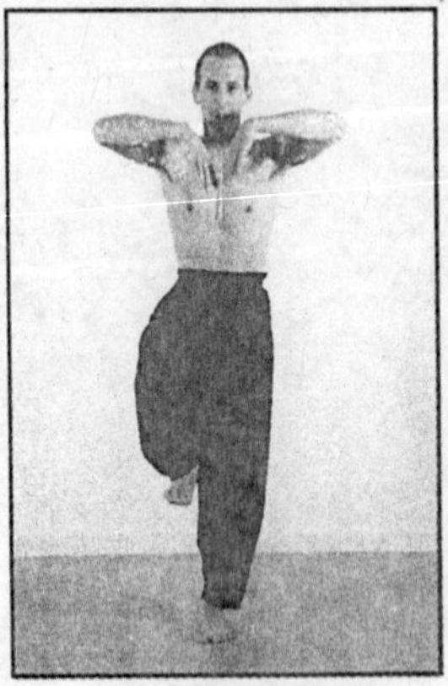
B-2

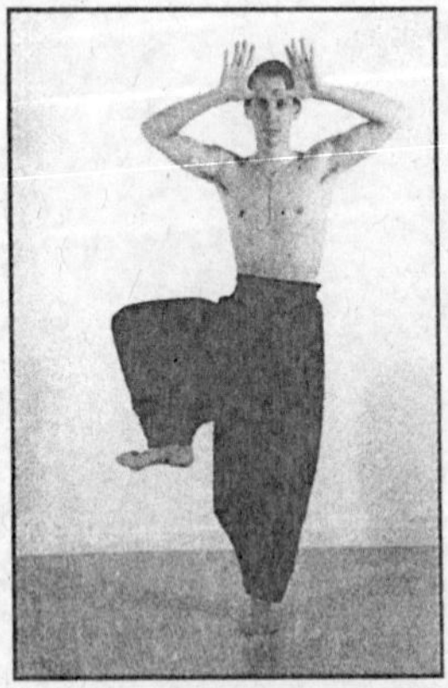
B-3

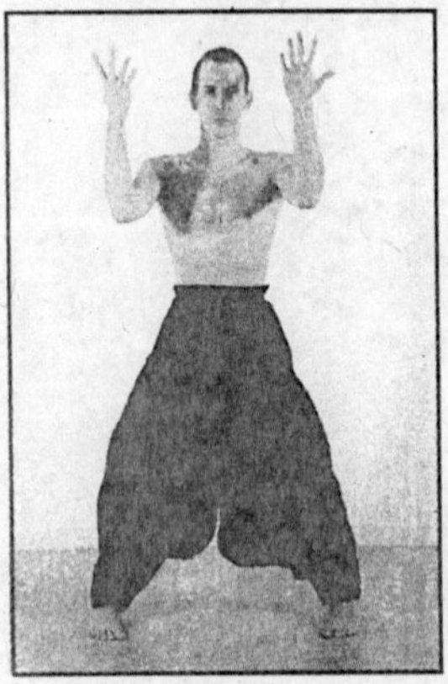
B-4

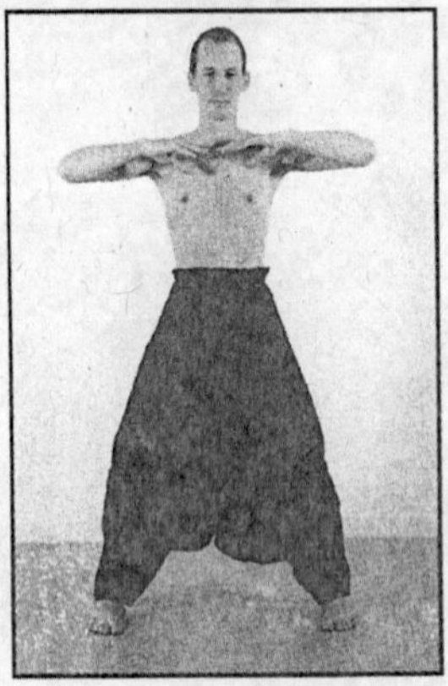
B-5

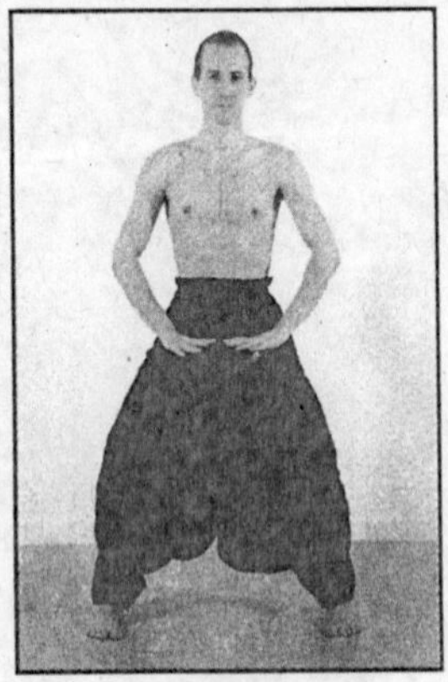
B-6

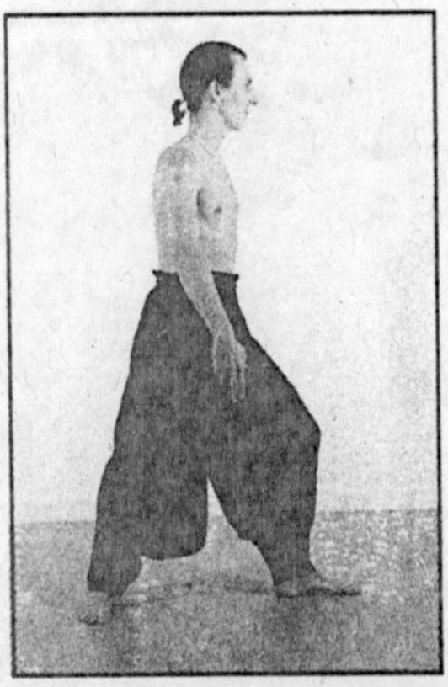
B-7

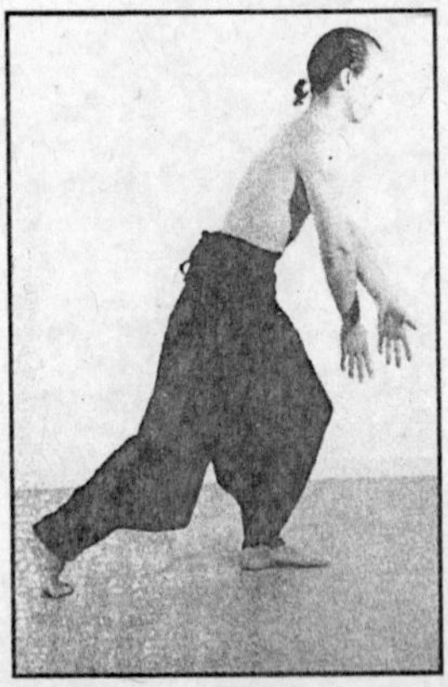
B-8

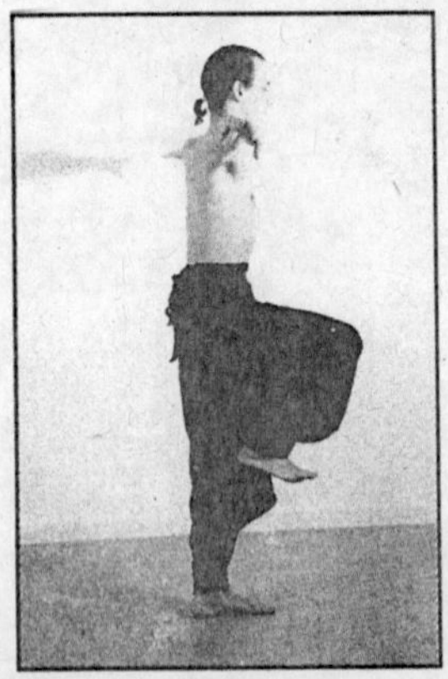
B-9

The movements from B-7 to B-21 are repeated on the other side.

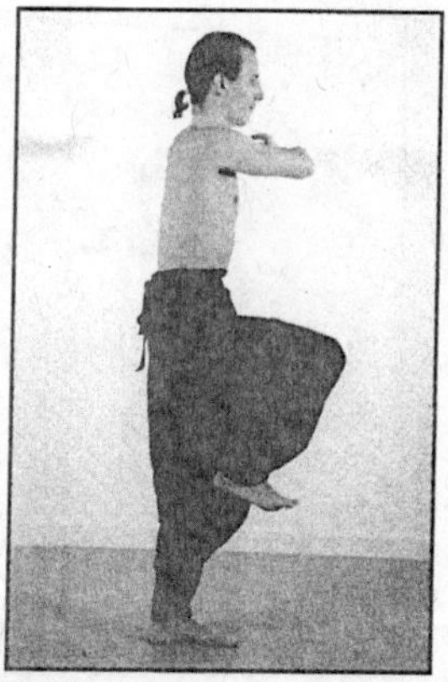

B-10a

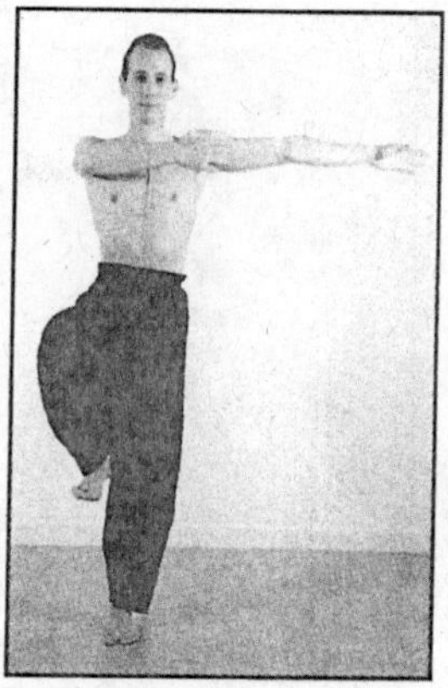

B-10b. Frontal view of the previous movement.

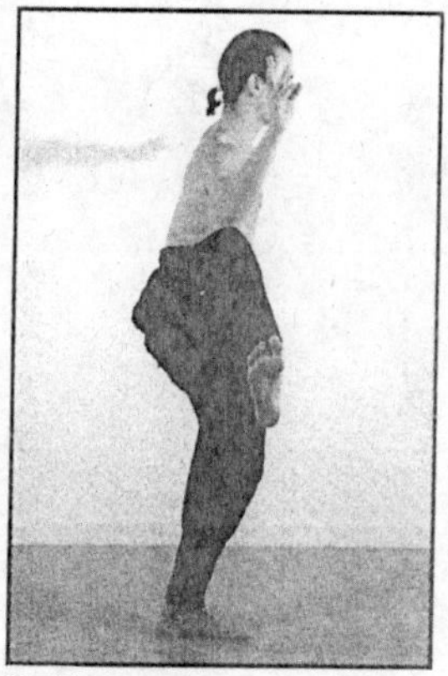

B-11a

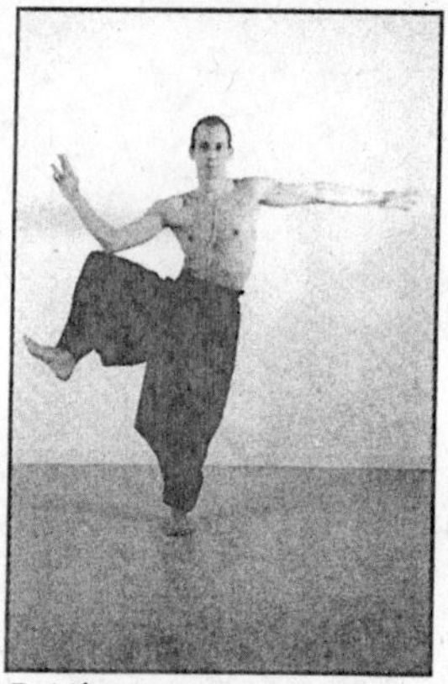

B-11b. Frontal view of the previous movement.

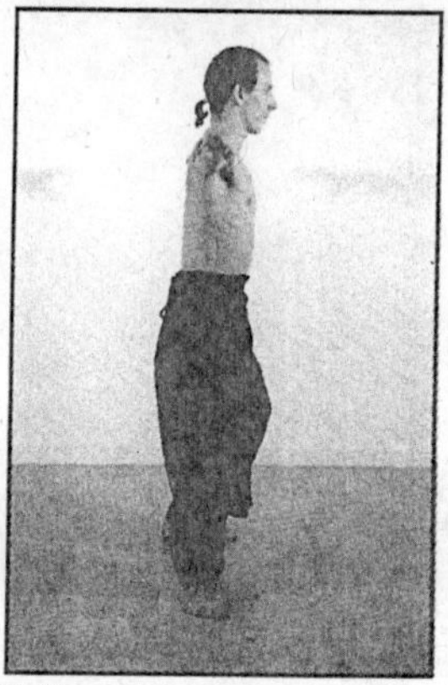

B-12a

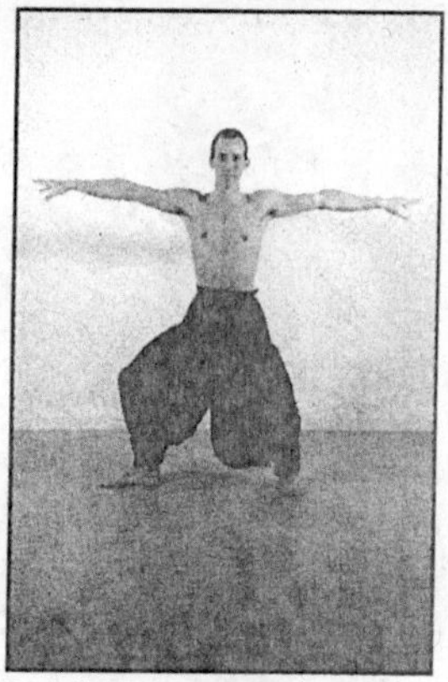

B-12b Frontal view of the previous movement.

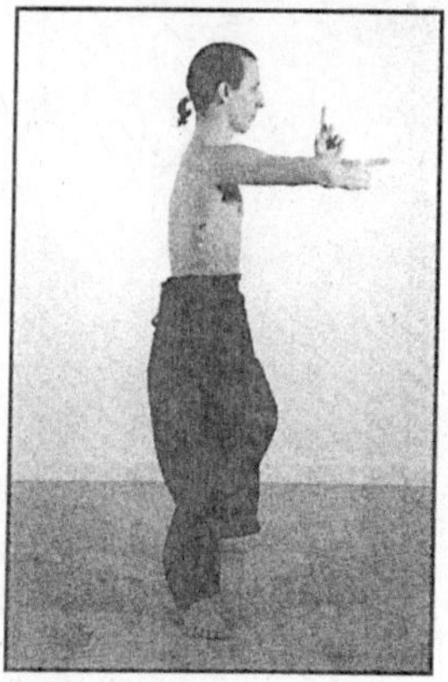

B-13a

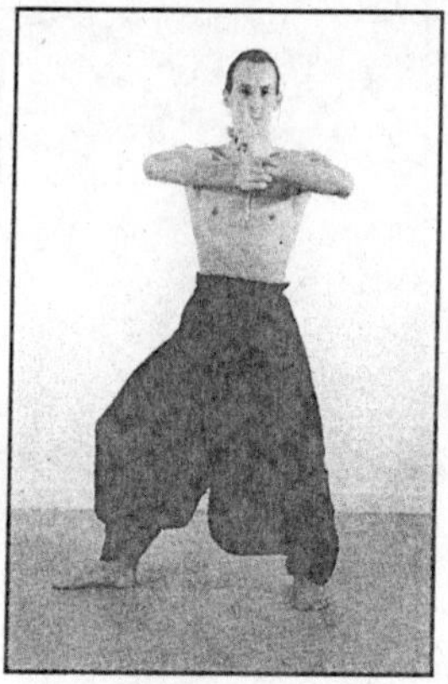

B-13b. Frontal view of the previous movement.

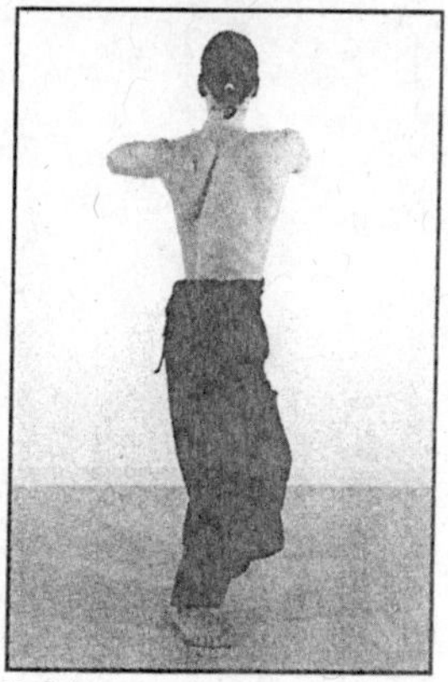

B-14

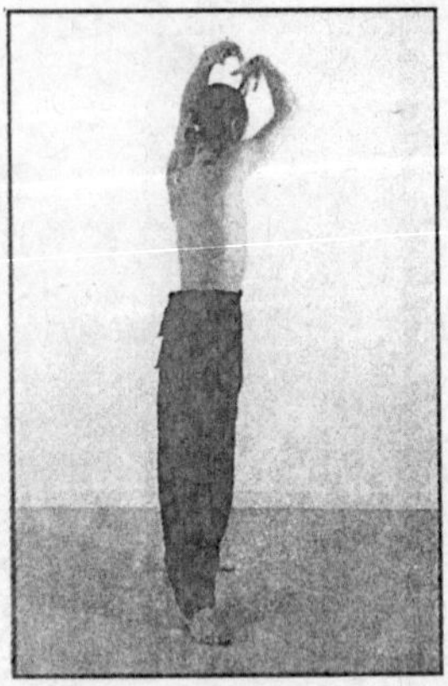
B-15

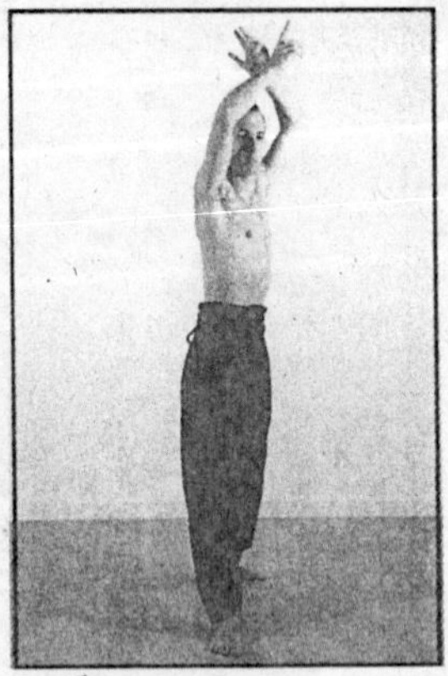
B-16

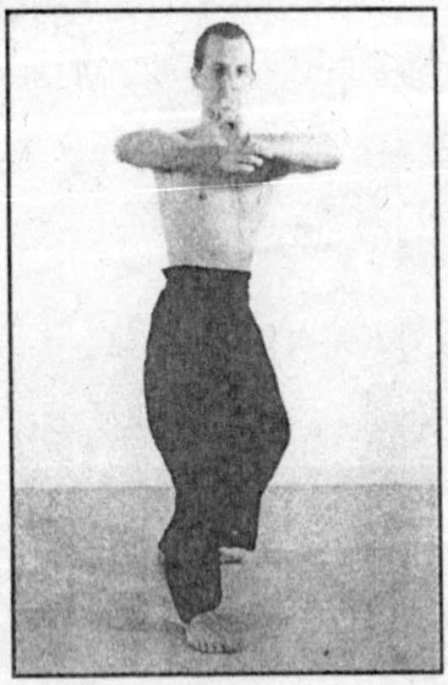
B-17

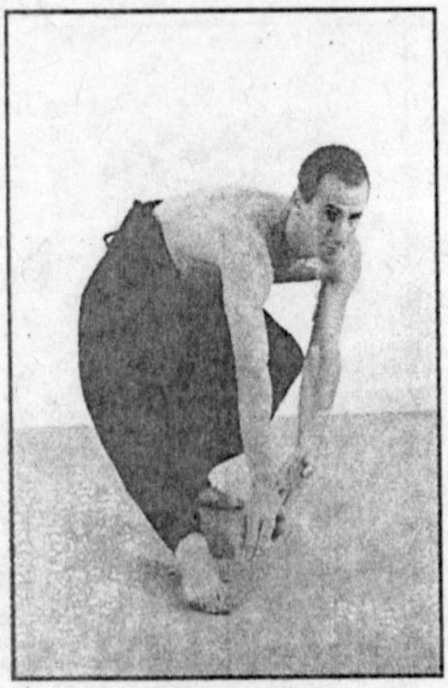
B-18

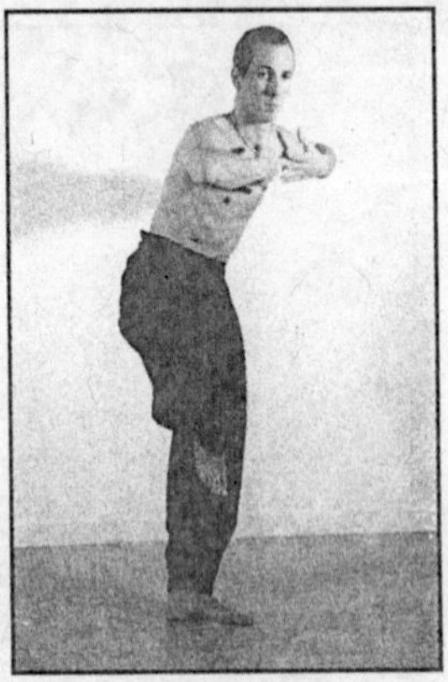
B-19

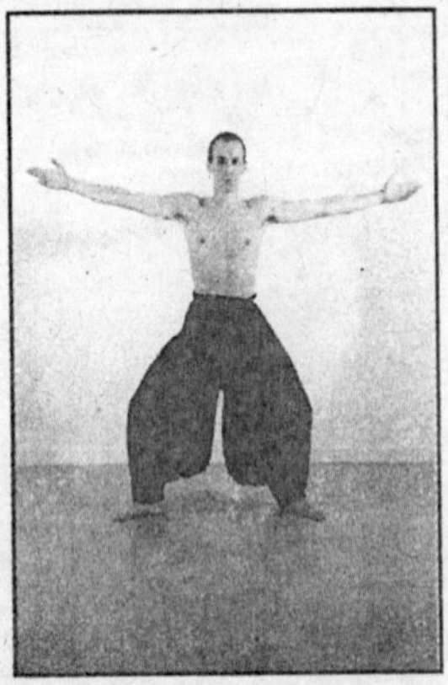
B-20

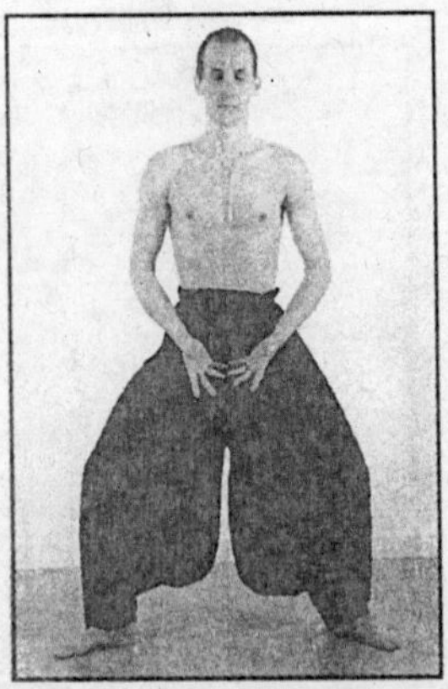
B-21

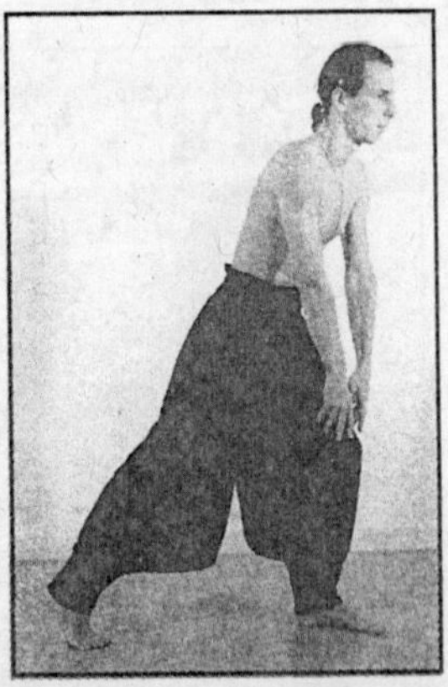
B-22

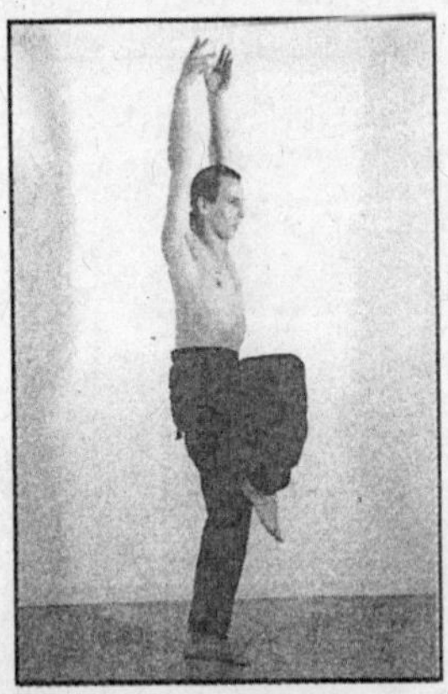
B-23

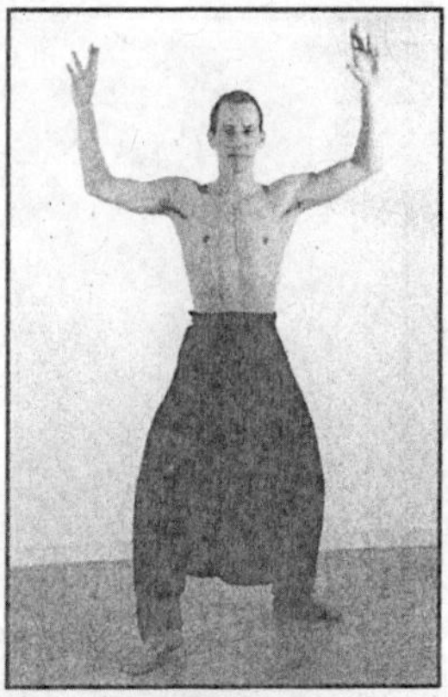
B-24

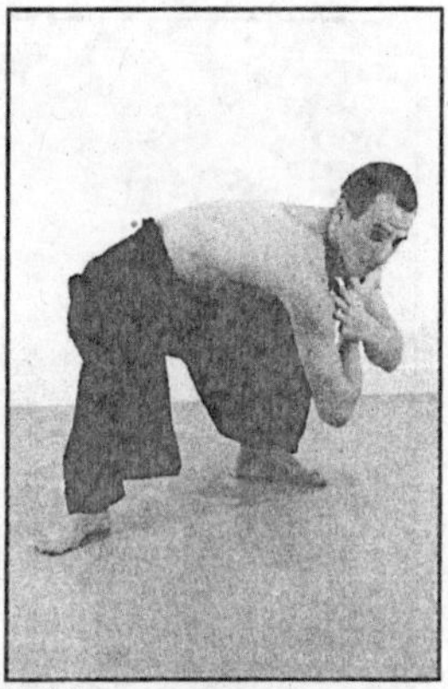
B-25

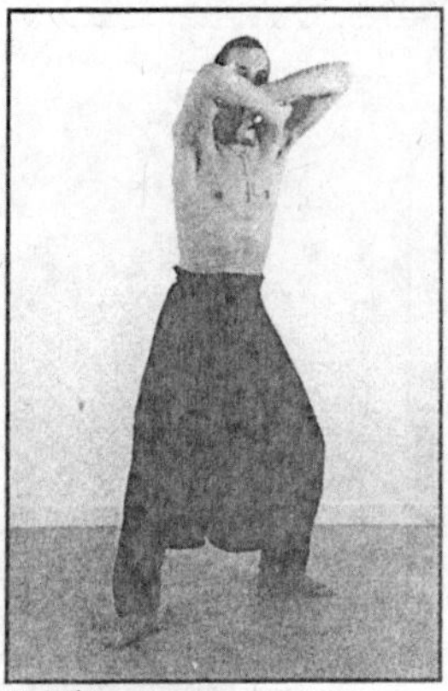
B-26

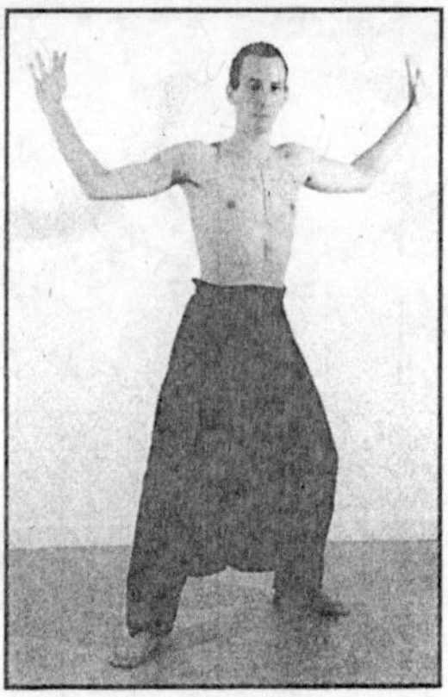
B-27

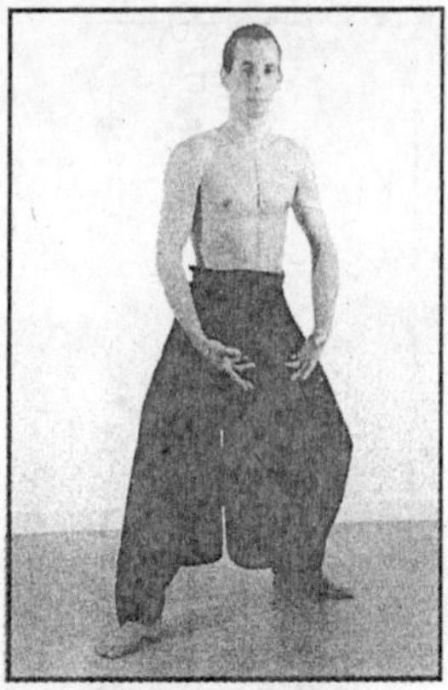
B-28

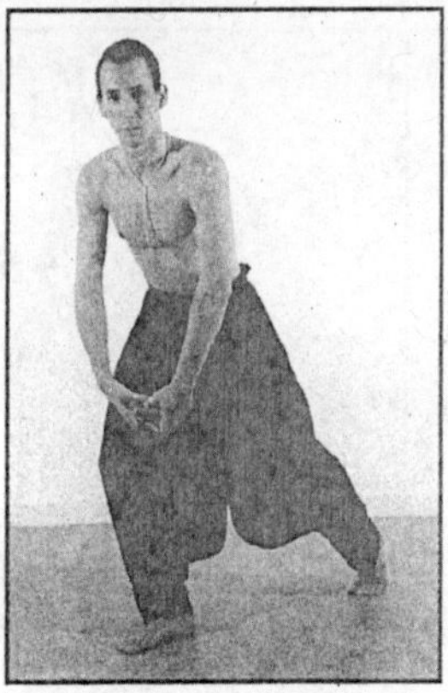
B-29

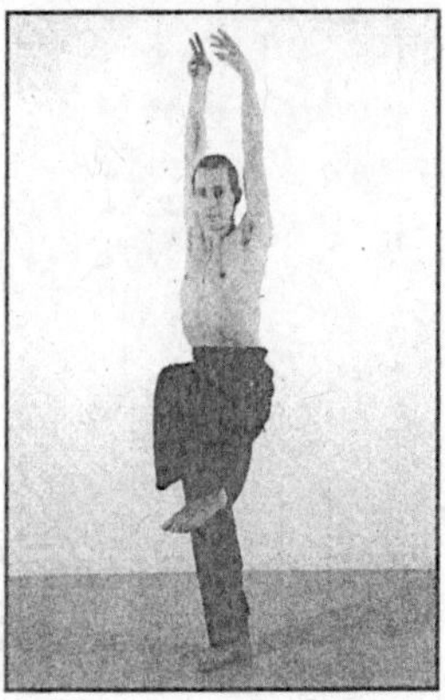
B-30

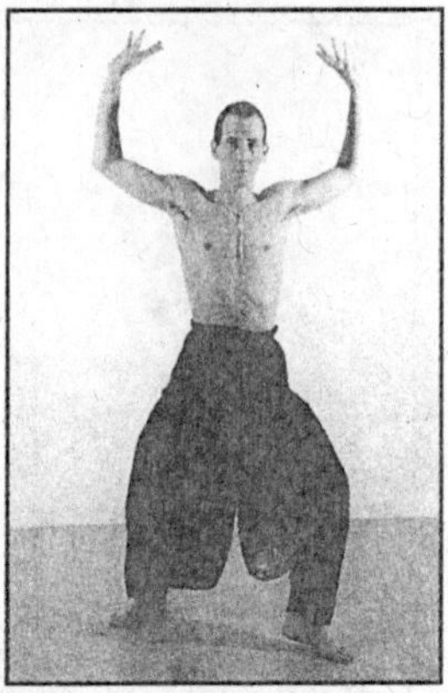
B-31

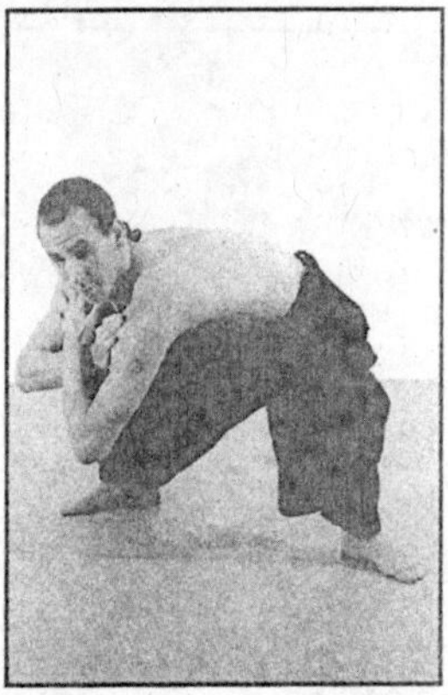
B-32

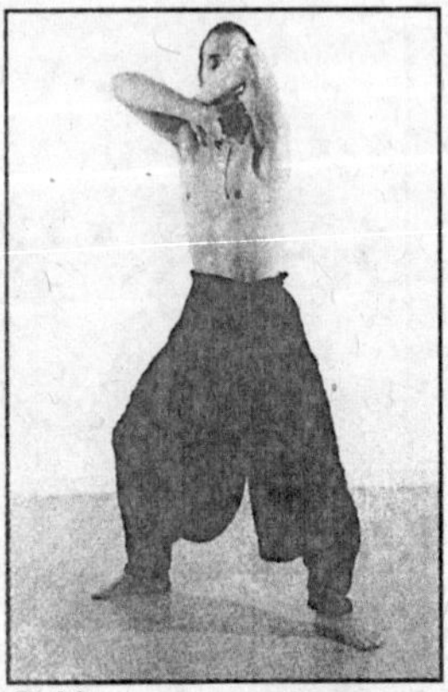
B-33

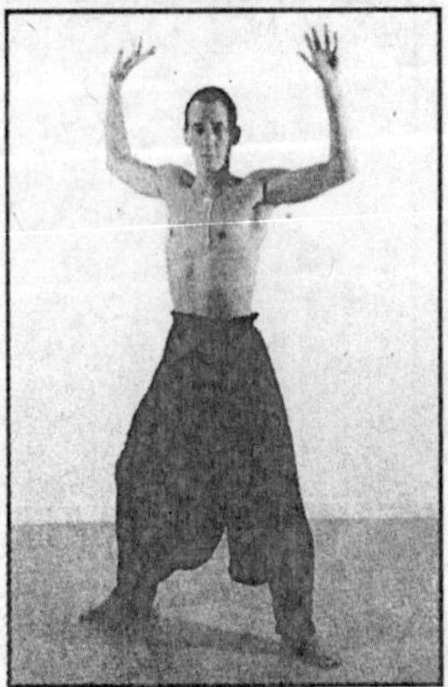
B-34

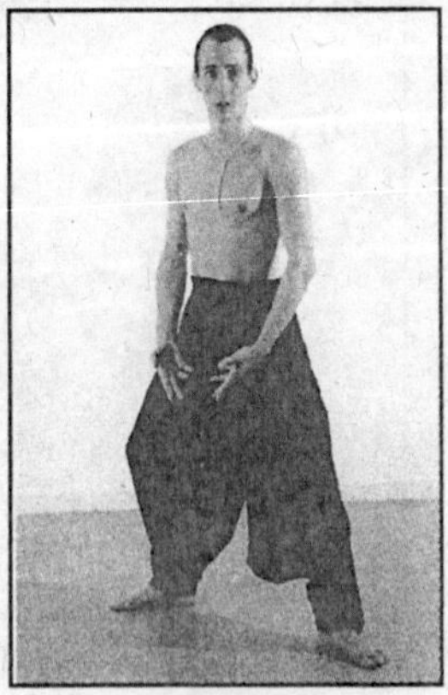
B-35

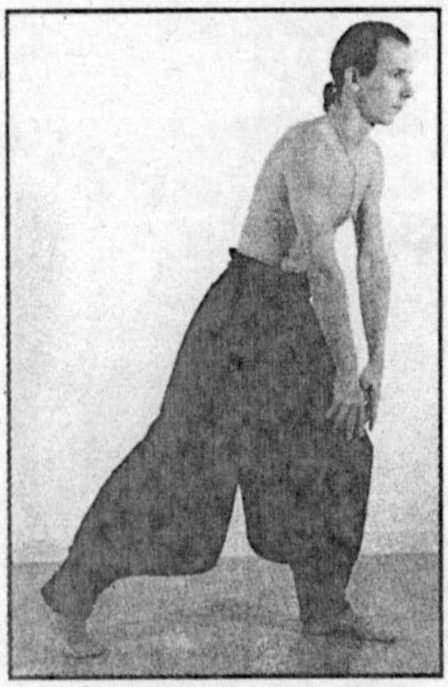
B-36

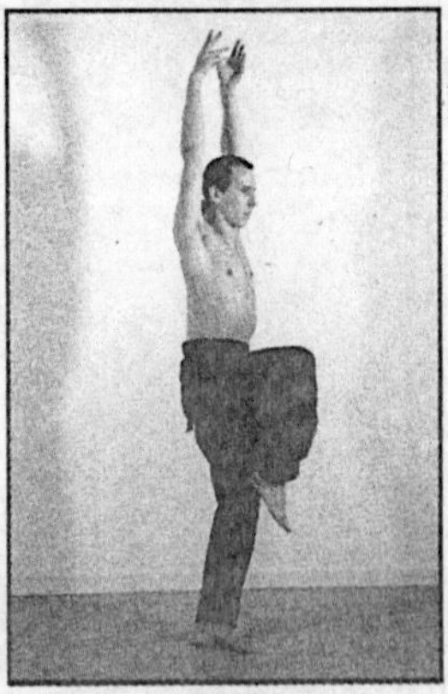
B-37

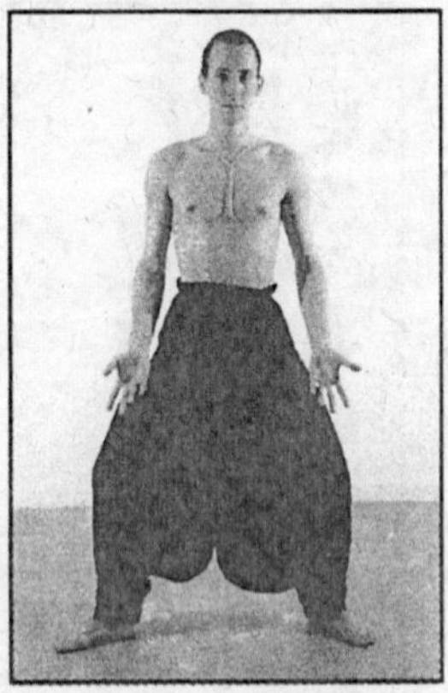
B-38

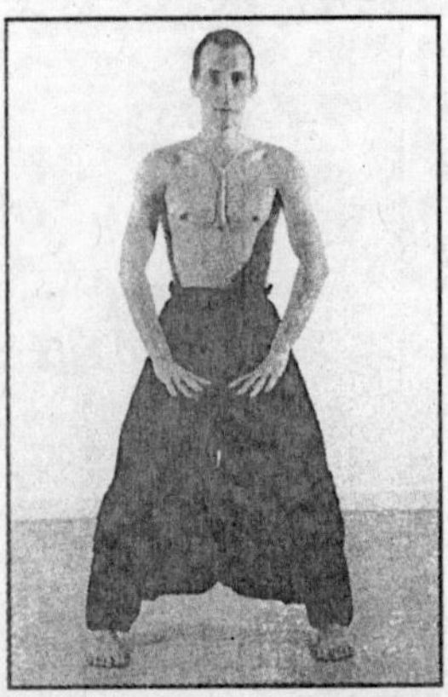
B-39

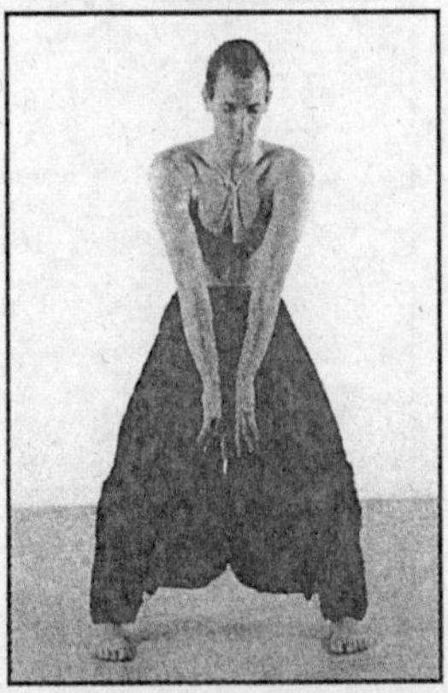
B-40

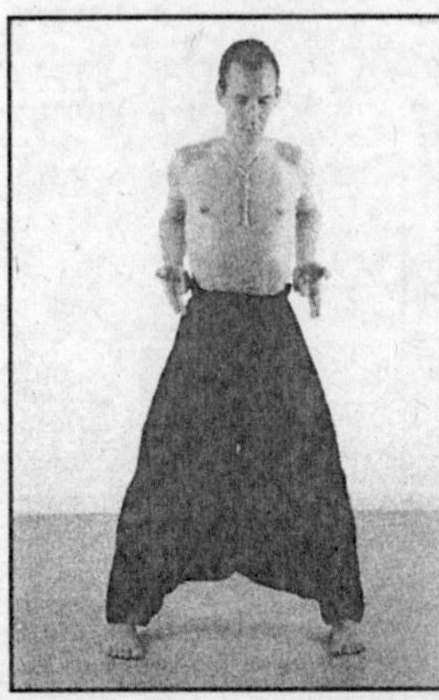
B-41

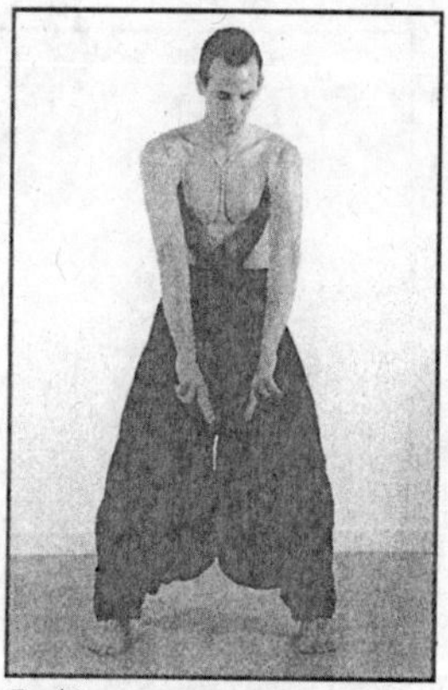
B-42

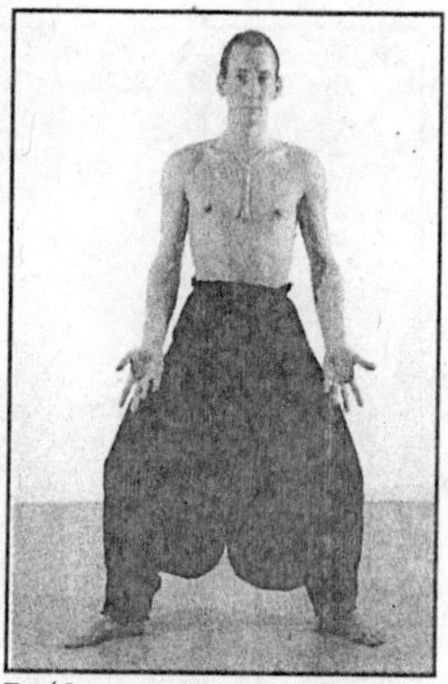
B-43

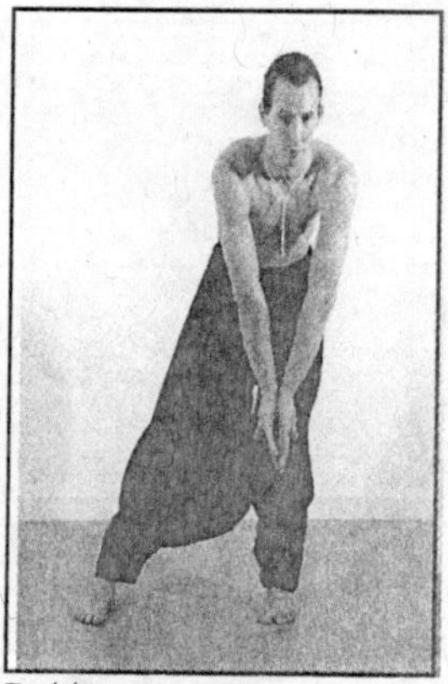
B-44

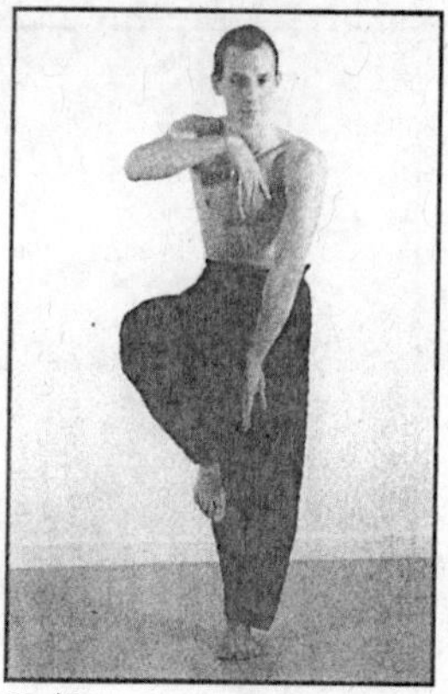
B-45

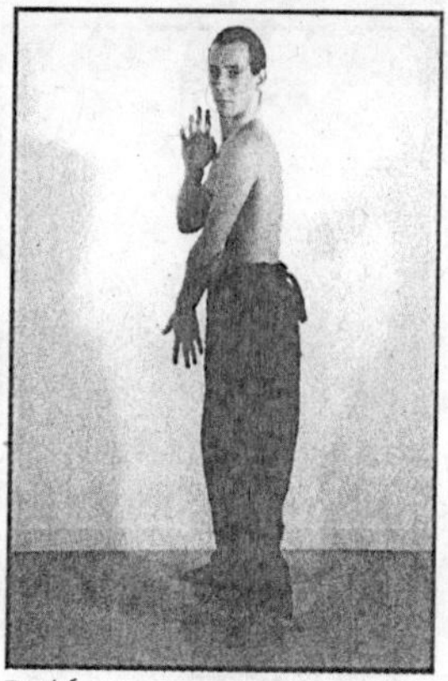
B-46

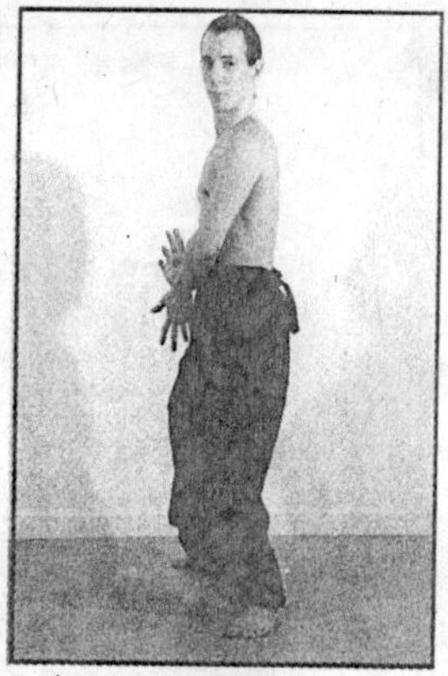
B-47a

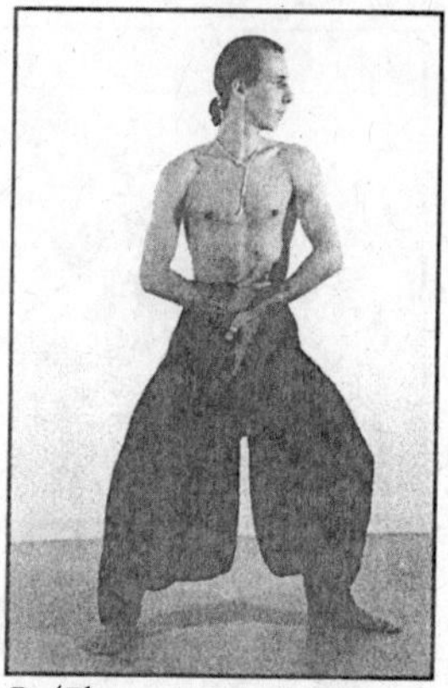
B-47b

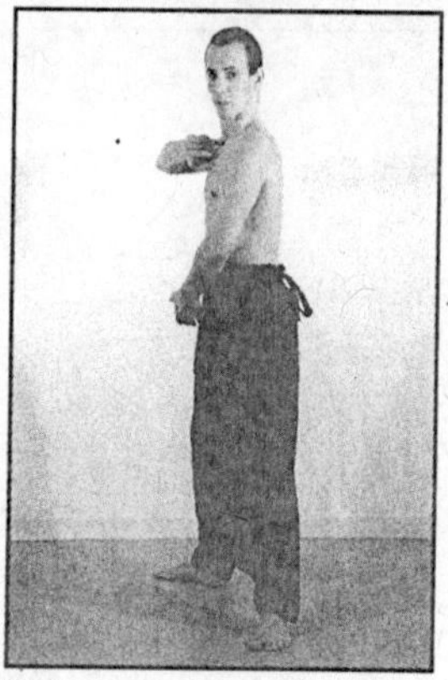
B-48

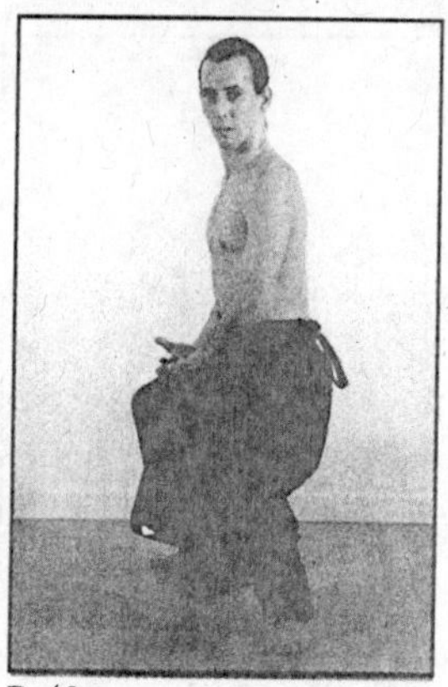
B-49

The movements from B-44 to B-51 are repeated on the opposite side.

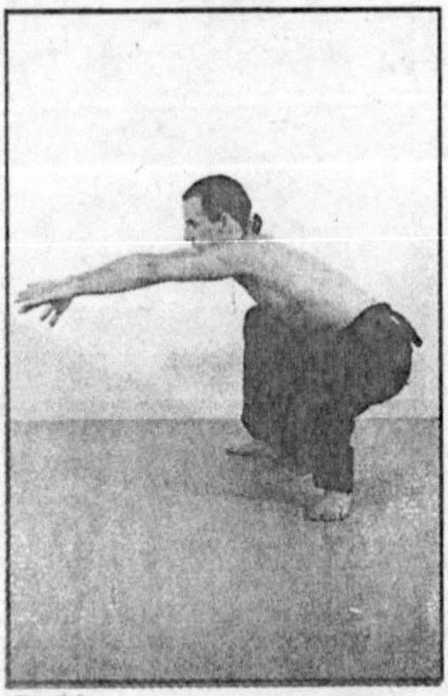
B-50

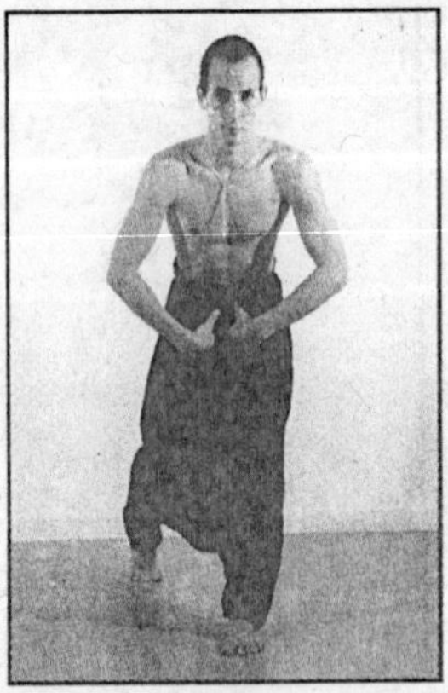
B-51

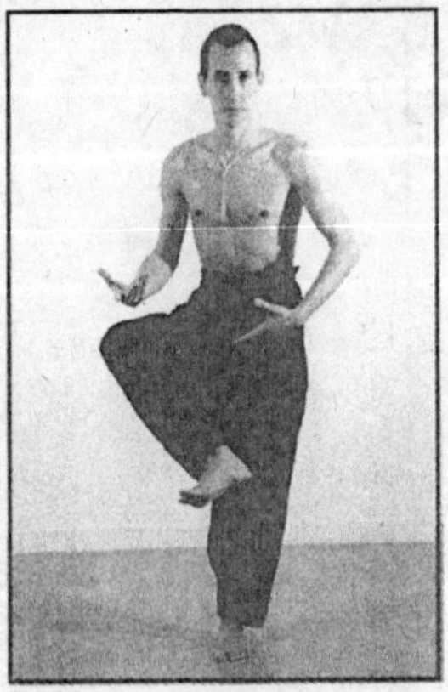
B-52

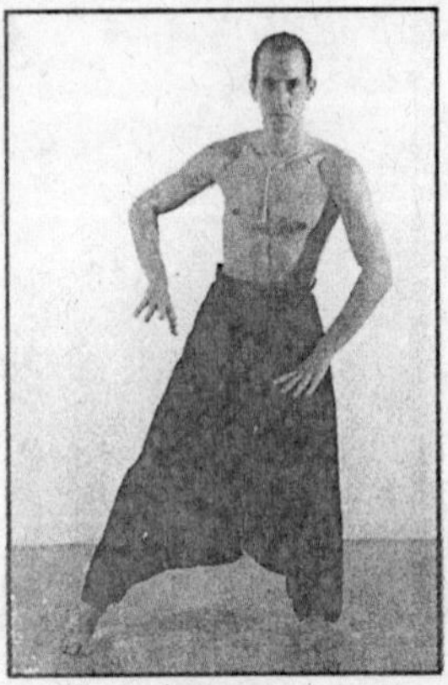
B-53

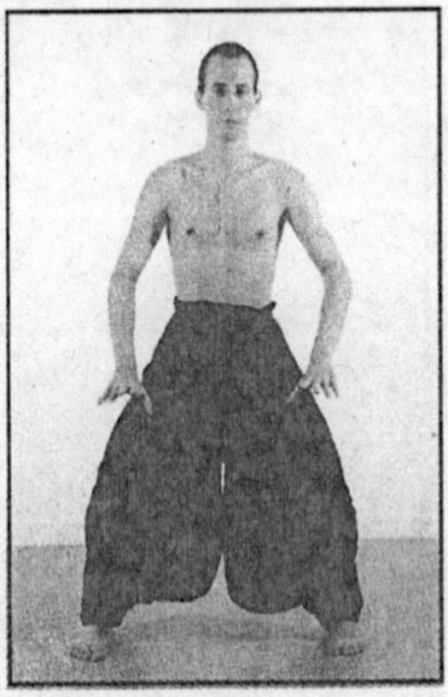
B-54

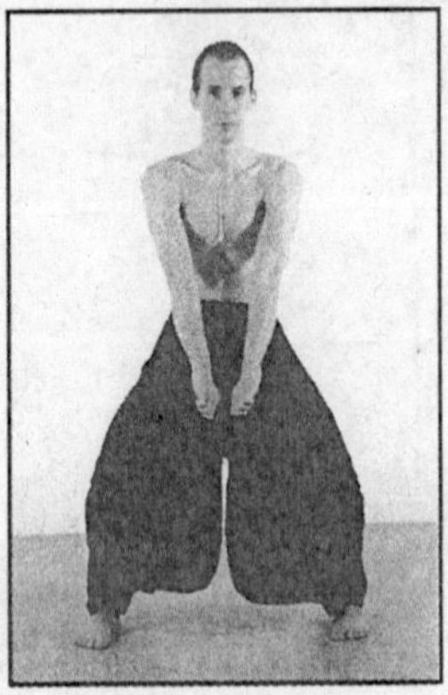
B-55

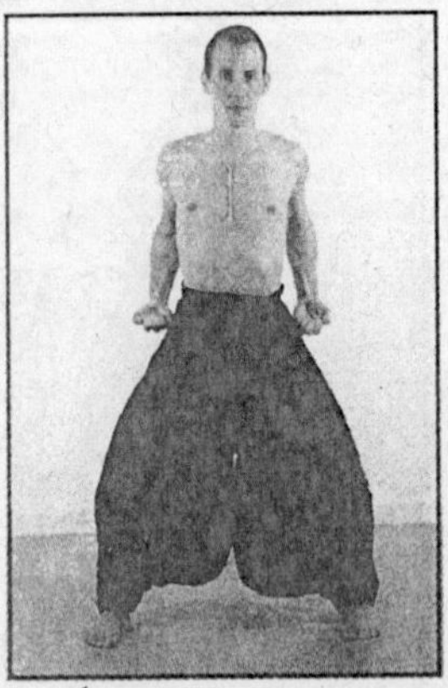
B-56

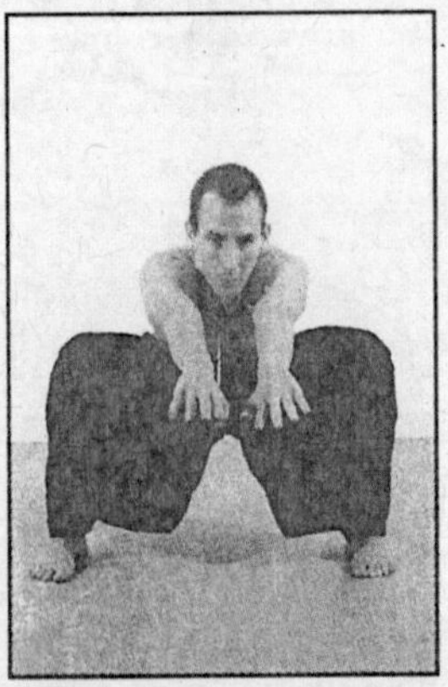
B-57

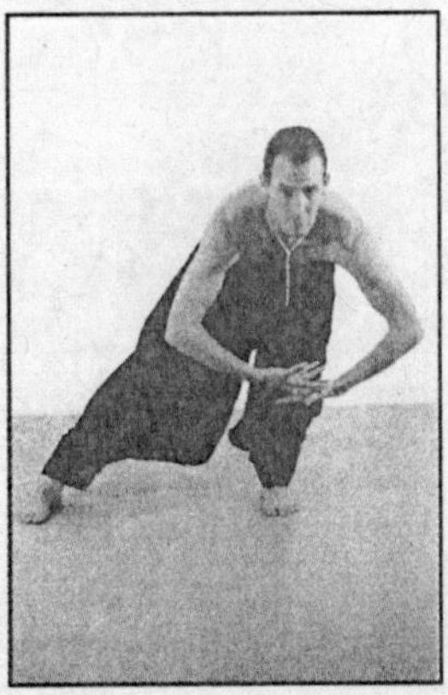
B-58

The movements from B-55 to B-70 are repeated on the opposite side.

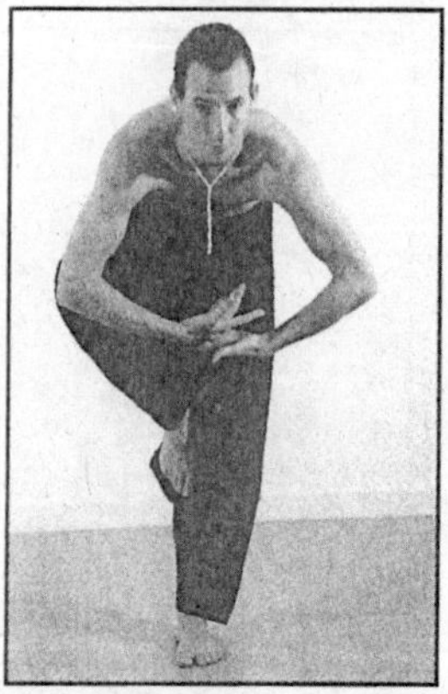

B-59

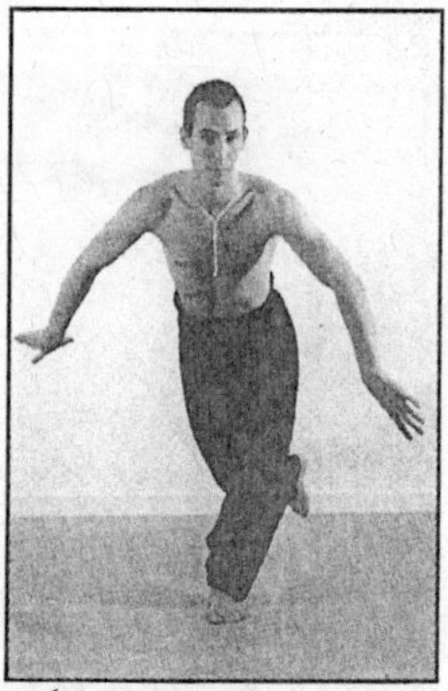

B-60

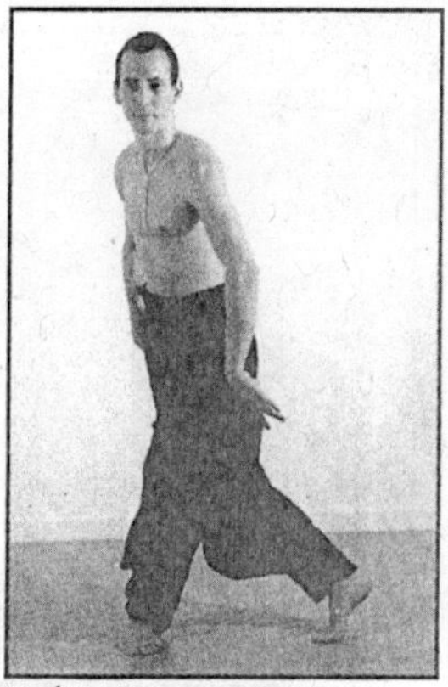

B-61

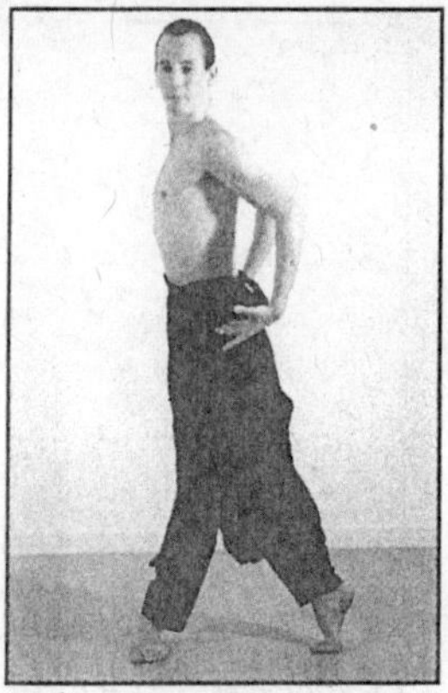

B-62

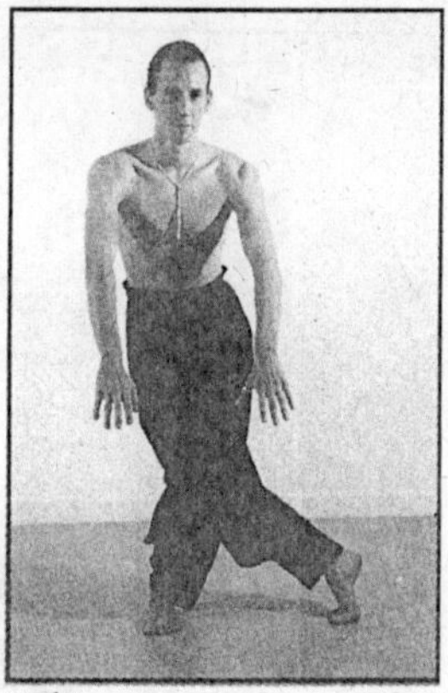

B-63

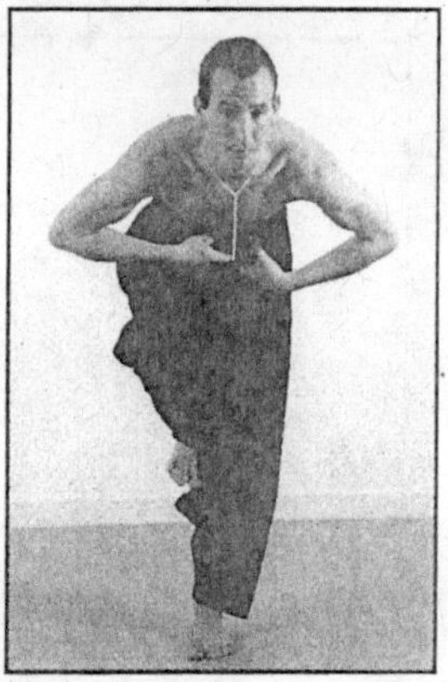

B-64

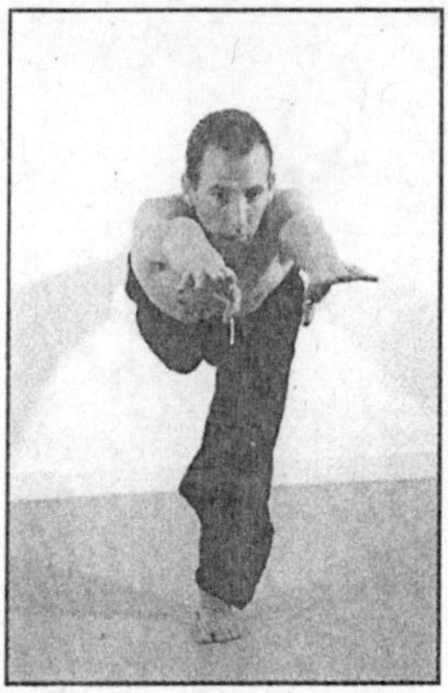

B-65a

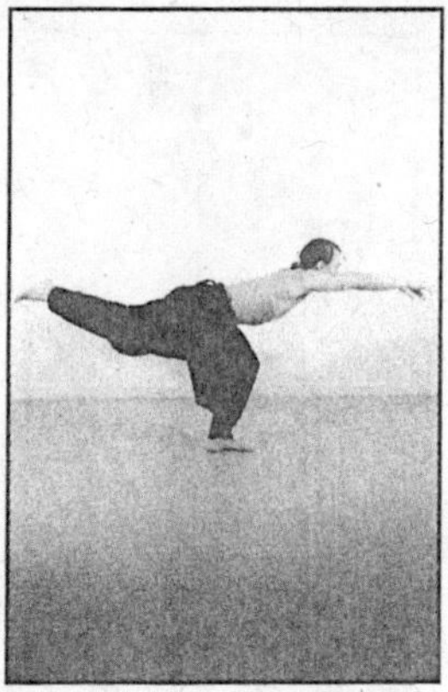

B-65b

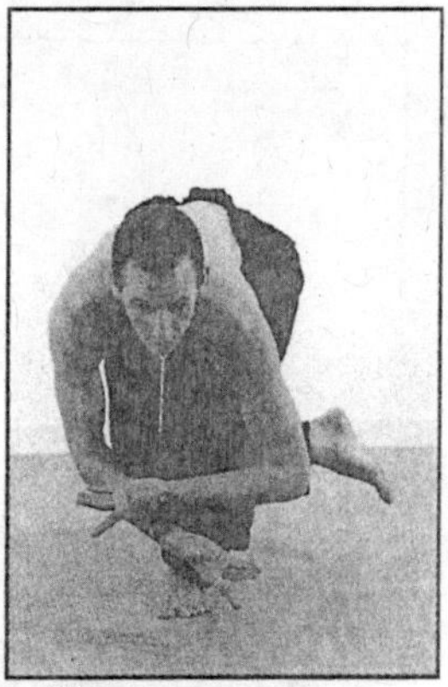

B-66

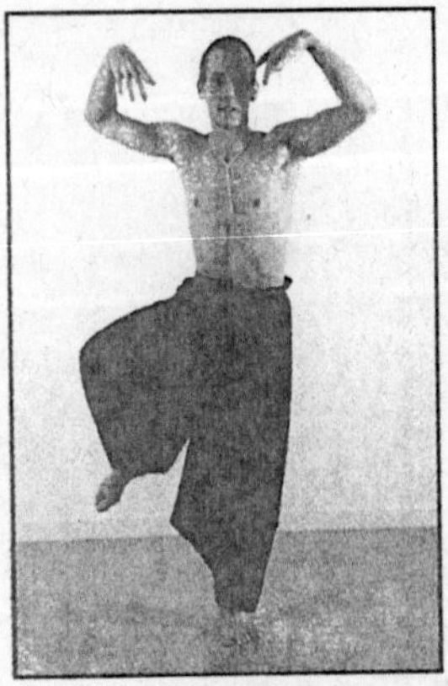

B-67

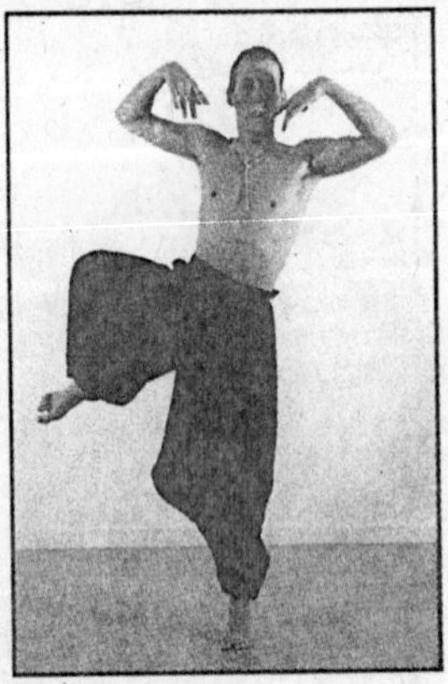

B-68

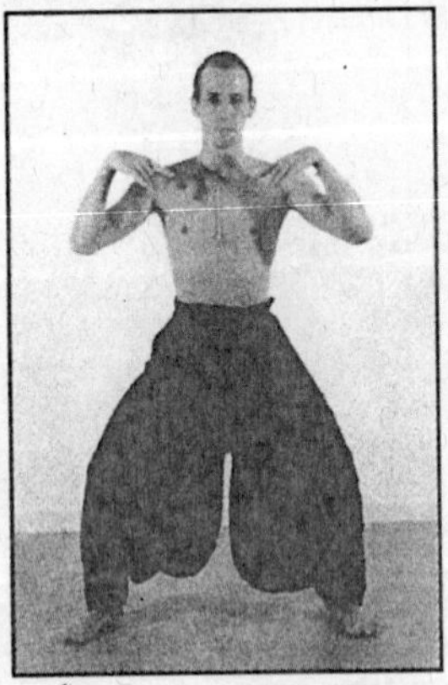

B-69

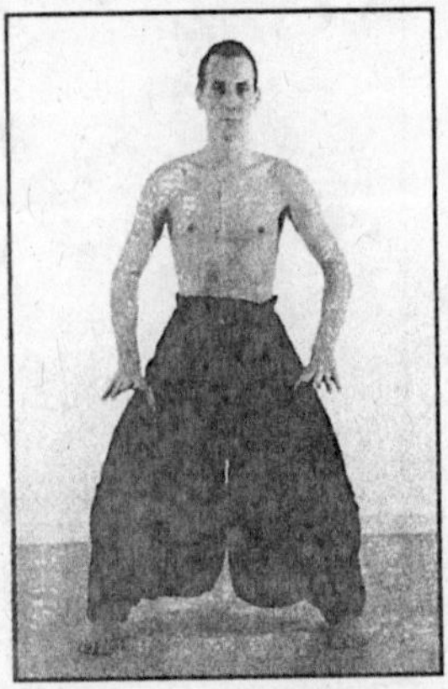

B-70

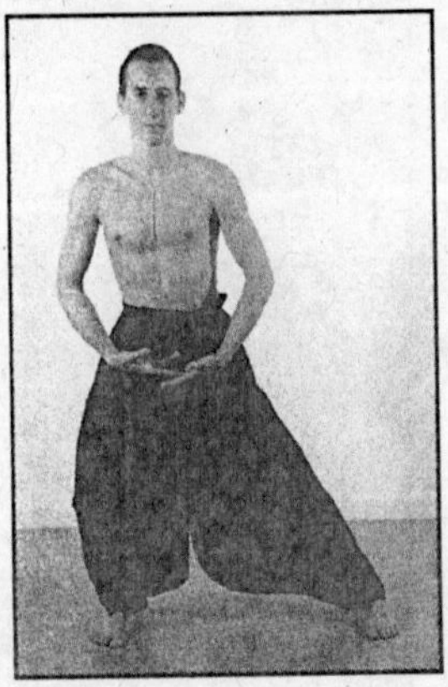

B-71

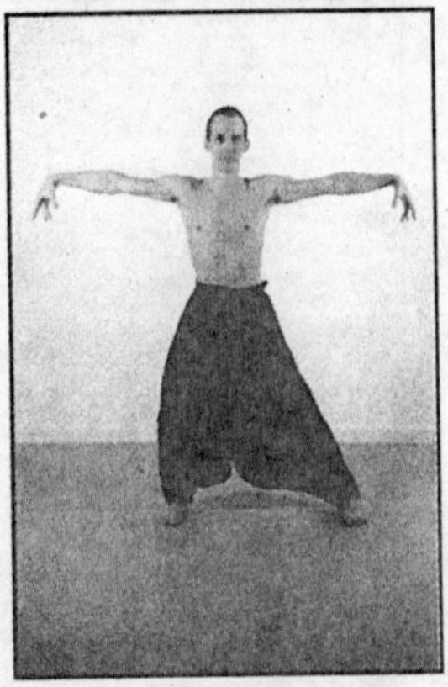

B-72

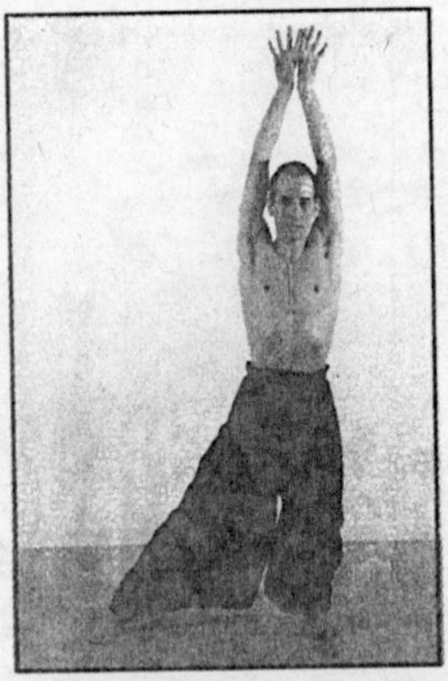

B-73

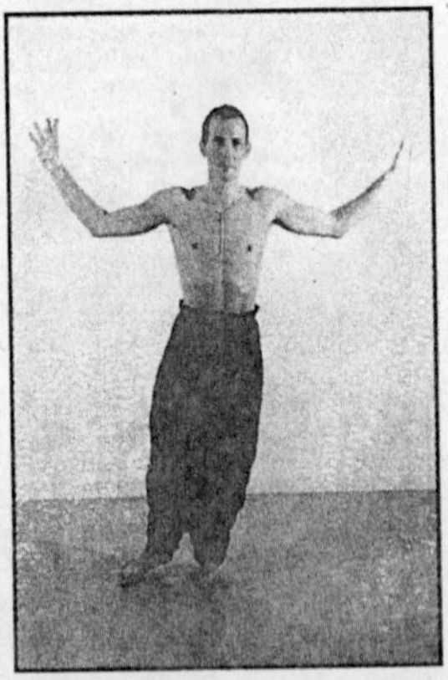

B-74

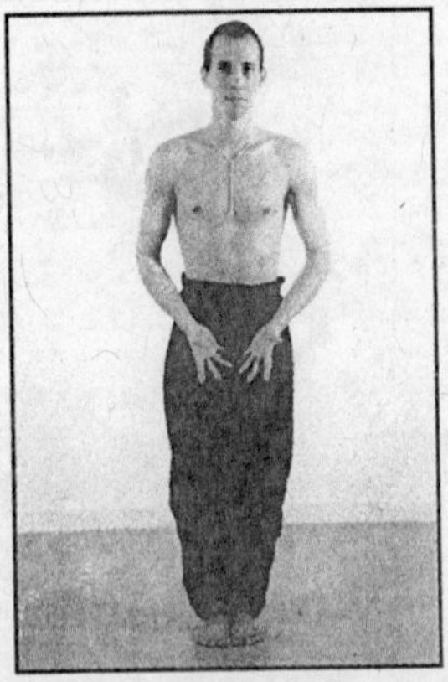

B-75

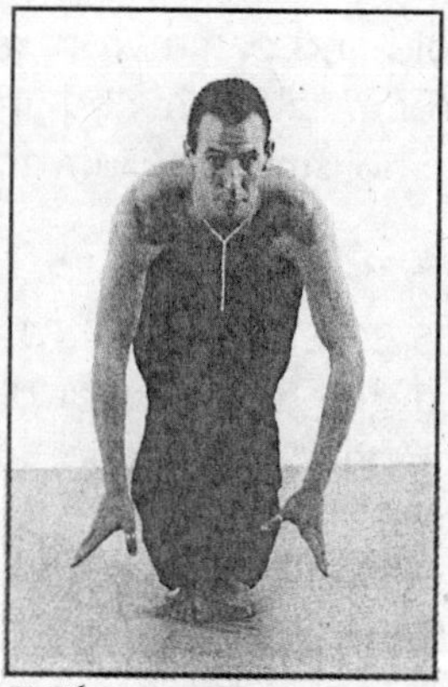

B-76

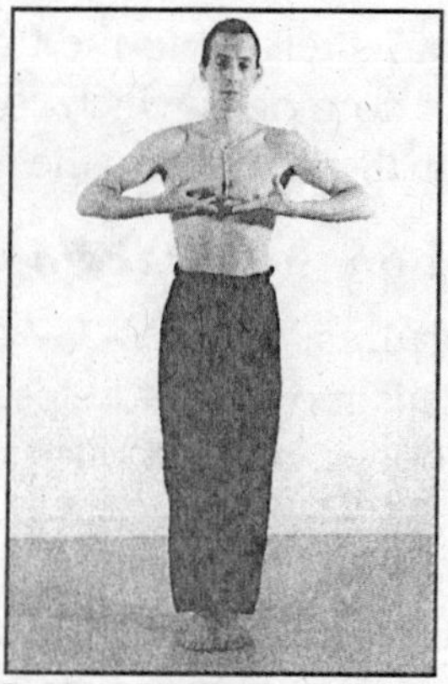

B-77

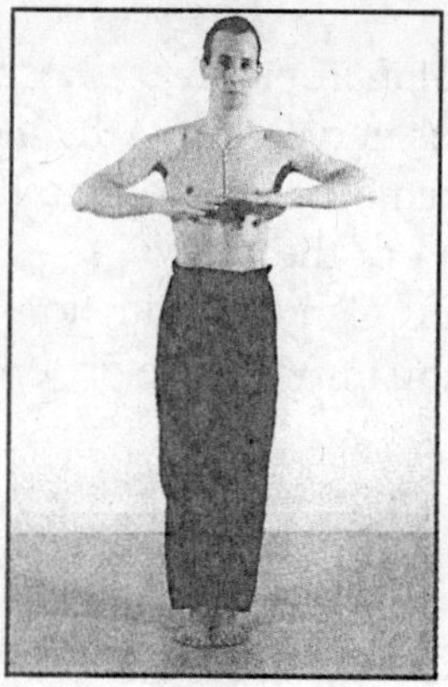

B-78

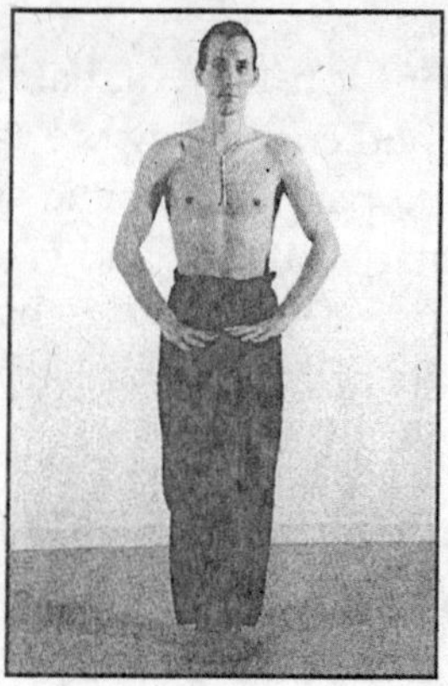

B-79

This cakra is related to the thyroid and parathyroid glands, which produce the hormones which control metabolism and growth and the hormones that contribute to the metabolism of calcium and potassium.

Movement on the *Añahata Cakra*

Vyaṅga pictures: B-21-22-23-24-25-26-27-28-29-30-31-32-33-34-35-36-37-38. This movement helps with the disorders or diseases of the cardiac, blood, nerve, emotional or pulmonary types and especially asthma. It contributes to the correction of inappropriate behaviour such as ingratitude, instability, distraction and drug addiction. On the other hand, with the practice of hand gestures, mudrās, behaviour related to understanding, forgiving and tolerance of others are reinforced.

Work done on the Anāhata cakra revitalizes the organism, by stimulating and controlling the vagus nerve, one of the most important nerves of the parasjimpathetic system. It regulates the functioning of the involuntary muscles and viscera of the body.

This cakra is related to the thymus gland. Its function is not known exactly, except that it has a great importance in emotional and immunological processes.

Movement on the *Maṇipūra* Cakra

Vyaṅga pictures: B-39-40-41-42-43. The effect of this movement is to open and regulate the functions of the cakra, which are related to spleen, liver, pancreas, stomach and adrenal gland diseases, as well as digestive and intestinal disorders, constipation, colitis, ulcers, abdominal swelling, cirrhosis, hepatitis and diabetes. It invigorates and stimulates the sympathetic nervous system. It helps to improve personal behaviour related to vanity, pride, eating and drinking in excess, intolerance and anger. It also stimulates self-affirmation behaviour, desire to control life situations, ambition and the desire for respect.

The glands related to this cakra are the pancreas and liver and the hormone secreted by certain cells of the pancreas, insulin, contribute to the accumulation of glucose in the liver, drops the level of sugar in the blood, influences the hydro-electric body balance, and is the primary factor in the regulation of the transfer of glucose to the cells, which is essential to its life. It also produces a hormone which contributes to stimulating the emission and the outflow of glucose from the liver. Working on this cakra helps to regulate all these functions.

Movement on the Svādhiṣṭhāna Cakra

Vyaṅga pictures: B-44-45-46-47-48-49-50-51-52-53. This movement helps in the recovey from diseases of the kidney, lymphatic glands, hormonal secretions and sex organs, like venereal diseases, sterility, menstrual disorders, impotence, frigidity, urinary infections, oedema and chronic fatigue. It works on personal behaviour like jealousy, desire, anger, sexual perversion and lying.

It also regulates the following personal behaviours: search for pleasure through food and drink, sexuality and exaggerated sensations.

This cakra is related to the sexual glands. Their hormonal secretions intervene in the preparation of the uterus so that the ovule remains fertile. They stimulate and maintain the secondary masculine and feminine characteristics and prevent abortion.

Movement on the Mūlādhāra Cakra

Vyaṅga pictures: B-52-53-54-55-56-57-58-59-60-61-62-63-64-65-66-67-68-69-70. This movement influences and intervenes by helping to get over bone, muscle and fat related diseases such as obesity, thinness, decalcification, vertebral problems, jaundice and anxiety with no apparent cause. It also improves behaviour related to the excessive influence of tamas in our body, which causes heftiness, fat, congestion, laziness, carelessness and cowardice. It stimulates and sets problems related to self-confidence and other needs such as food, drink, and accommodation.

Mūlādhāra is considered to be related to the adrenal glands, which are responsible for the control of glucose, protein control and general metabolism. They also control mineral balance, mainly sodium and potassium and excite the nerve and circulatory systems, increasing metabolic speed and they also intervene in the contraction of the blood vessels. Working on this cakra provides benefits to all these processes.

LEARNING OF THE HEALING ENERGY

"All disorders are caused by the phobia of human thought" ***Caraka Saṁhitā*** [14].

Health is everything. It allows for everyday social, emotional, work and religious life. When frequent disorders arise disease arises. It is very common to become accustomed to many disorders from a young age, not giving them the importance they deserve. Afterwards, they manifest themselves as a much more complex problem, which could have been prevented if at the time they were treated appropriately. Looking to be healthy should be a constant aim in our lives, paying attention to possible disorders and their possible solutions, because health integrates the person with his or her self.

Healthy energy and good health are based on diet, breathing, exercise, relaxation and positive thought.

Diet

According to the principles of yoga on which Vyāyāma practice is based, the diet should be moderate, which means balanced. It must include processed and raw food, and abundant liquids.

We should find a balance between the combination of protein, carbohydrates, vitamins, minerals and trace elements. An excess or deficiency in any three will produce a disorder. Fresh and raw vegetables provide, among other elements, the necessary fibre for our digestive processes to be carried out normally.

Inappropriate diet is the cause, in most cases, of constipation, which is a very common disease nowadays and this carries a high possibility of contracting infectious diseases.

Looking for balance in the diet is fundamental, starting with the choice of food, taking care of its preparation, its final presentation and lastly, its ingestion and assimilation, including allowing enough time for digestion to be completed. We should observe and analyze which types of food and ways of eating make us feel good and which do not. This will lead to a natural habit of choosing the proper food and ways of eating that are better for us.

There is another type of food, which is subtler, that we ingest through our senses. When we relate through some of them, or through all of

14. Classic āyurvedic medicine text, attributed to the wise man Caraka.

them, with something or someone, an energy exchange exists, in which we give or receive in some occasions, this exchange is revitalizing, in others, it debilitates us, according to our mental and energetic state. In the same way, we should pay attention and learn which types of relationships we should establish.

Breathing

Breathing is one of the most important sources of nourishment, providing essential oxygen to our entire organism. In the initial chapters we saw how breathing not only facilitates life, but how our health and vitality also depend on the quality of our breathing. For example, poor breathing has a direct influence on problematic digestion because it prevents our organism from eliminating all the unnecessary waste and this accumulation will contribute to the appearance of infections and other illnesses. Oxygen-rich breathing regulates the good functioning of our organism and prevents possible diseases.

By practicing Vyāyāma Yoga we learn how to enrich our breathing and use it in different ways according to our needs. We can establish the basis of breathing learning about the four basic types.

1. High breathing is done with the upper part of the lungs by lifting the shoulders and collar bones. It is the poorest type of breath and can for some people lead to a tendency to breathe through the mouth bringing a higher risk of contracting infectious diseases. When the air enters through the nostrils, it is dampened, heated and filtered, retaining dust particles and possible germs it may contain. If the air enters through the mouth, filtering is not done. This type of breathing is unconsciously done by many people, mainly women and is the cause of great anxiety. It produces the feeling of breathlessness. In Vyāyāma Yoga, we use it when we want to fix the mind on an external point.
2. Middle breathing is produced at the side of the ribs. The diaphragm elevates, the abdomen is contracted, and the ribs expand to the sides. It is more complete than the high breathing, but still insufficient. In Vyāyāma Yoga, it is used when we want to calm down and relax.
3. Lower or diaphragmatic breathing is produced with the inferior part of the lungs, where the most capacity lies. The diaphragm

muscle moves downward inflating the abdomen, the lungs feel free and air enters their lower area.

In Vyāyāma Yoga we use this type of breathing when we want self-control, to control the body and expand the tan. It is the best breathing of all three, although the most perfect is the complete breath, because it uses all three of the previously indicated parts. In it we work all the muscles, so it creates a greater expansion of the thoracic cavity. In order to practise it, it is not necessary to completely fill the lungs in each inhalation, but to take the air equally to the three parts.

This produces more oxygenation, prevents colds and exhaustion, enlarges the capacity of the thorax, enhances the immune system and invigorates the nervous system.

Exercise

When exercise is practised with breath control it provides great physical benefits to our organism and prevents possible diseases. The many muscles, ligaments, tendons and joints receive rich oxygenation and are able to eliminate waste more easily. Regularly practiced, it increases elasticity and invigorates the muscles. It also helps the internal organs to receive more oxygen and reduces the amount of fat, a possible cause of cardiovascular illness. The heart benefits the most of all the internal organs when we exercise.

By practising diverse Vyāyāma Yoga exercises, the muscles, tendons, ligaments and joints are exercised with micro tension, which permits a greater blood influx. In Vyāyāma Yoga, we should try to observe many points that will help us obtain maximum benefits: be constant in the practise, try to practise in a well ventilated area, avoid practising outdoors in excessive heat; if possible, try to perform Vyāyāma Yoga at sunrise or sunset, use comfortable natural fibre-made clothes like cotton and maintain good hygiene, before and after exercising.

Relaxation

Any tension produced during exercise should end with a period of relaxation, so that the organism can acquire appropriate muscular tone.

Relaxation, unlike sleep, does not imply any type of activity, except for the vital signs that maintain the body. It consists in consciously taking the body to this state of relaxation and saving a great amount of energy. During relaxation, the whole body is in harmony and is recharged with vitality. After a relaxation session we feel a state of well-being. Relaxation directly cases the stress-provoked tensions and acts upon the whole nervous system by draining it.

Positive thought

Thought has a direct bearing on the nervous system, which regulates the activity of our organism.

A balanced and calm thought allows our nervous system to be in a state of harmony, which directly influences the rest of the bodily functions.

A depressive thought produces a progressive devitalization, leading to self-destruction. Euphoric thought drives us to a quick consumption of our vitality, unmeasured worry and agitation. A balanced and profound thought knows the consequences of our actions and their impact on our lives and we find the necessary means to develop ourselves with the greatest possible satisfaction.

Positive thought, through the practice of magical Vyāyāma Yoga, karaṇa Vyāyāma, teaches us to directly enter in contact with the fundamental structures of our mind and to transform them.

Healing energy has its base in the strength of the mind. A strong mind is able to help balance one's own disorders and those of others. The strength of the mind resides in electro-magnetic energy, which is explained in yoga as the vibration of all that exists. In Sanskrit it is described as the three ways of manifestation of the Śakti through vital energy. They are:

1. Rajo guṇa, the vibration of the mind and its faculties
2. Sattva guṇa, the vibration of the 'I', free from any type of movement
3. Tamo guṇa, the vibration that makes up the body

Rajo guṇa moves on top of tamo guṇa, and in the upper part sattva guṇa is found.

Electromagnetic energy manifests itself in everything, specifically in the central nervous system through vital breaths, prāṇas. It generates impulses and affinities that alter our body and mind.

The therapist or person who wishes to help another become balanced, must always keep in mind that this electromagnetic energy is the basis of his work and that he should transmit his own energy, the quality of his thought and the reflection of the energy to the other person. This will allow the patient to feel self-esteem without becoming dependent on the therapist.

Give and take are fundamental exchanges in the practice of healing energy. If this is not produced then communication and interaction is impossible. These are the basic principles of prāṇotherapy.

One of the methods that healing energy uses is massage. In āyurvedic medicine, which is related to Vyāyāma Yoga practice, it is called śāntala, that which provides peace and balances the energy of the talas. Its benefits are multiple and we can highlight them in the following list: general balance of the organism, improved blood circulation to the stomach, better digestion, better rest and deep sleep, an increase in appetite, life extension, delays in the ageing process by hydration of the organism, the elimination of muscle oxidation and fatigue, elimination of excess air, improved vision and the perception of the senses in general, strengthening of the skin, resistance to disease, calms illnesses caused by air and mucus, improves the colour, texture and pigmentation of the skin.

LEARNING THE INVOCATION OF THE POWER OF THE THREE GODS AND THE THREE GODDESSES

Tantra is a complete, complex and very advanced method of obtaining spiritual powers, siddhis, material powers, ṛddhis, and liberation from karma,[15] mokṣa.It is fundamental in the elevation and transformation of the polarity, ha and ṭha, consciousness and energy, Śiva and Śakti, and the expansion of the inner power.

This tantra is taught from master to disciple. It is a method of knowledge whose expression depends on the particularities of the master who teaches it and on the student who learns it. That is why tantra is not a closed knowledge system as it is constantly renovating itself.[16] It honours the female energy in conjunction with the male energy. Keeping in mind this veneration as a fundamental principle, the student seeks that the union of the two archetypes, Śiva and Śakti, the male power of the great God Mahā Deva and the female power

15. The concept of liberation is a mystical and philosophical one that the student looks for as the ultimate goal of knowledge or realization. *Mokṣa* represents a state in which actions generated by *karma* of the past, present and future do not affect the spirit that dwells within man. This state is produced when he recognizes his own nature.

16. In *Kaula Rahasya*, a classic Tantra text, we find the following quote: "*Tantra* is constantly renewing itself, according to the needs of its disciples."

of the great goddess Mahā Devī, is projected in all the activities of his life. Of all these activities, two of them have greater importance: meditation and the sexual act[17].

The union of the three gods and the three goddesses is the concept of the sacred act of sexuality, paramaithuna[18], in which the God Śiva incarnates in the body of the man and the Goddess Śakti incarnates in the body of the woman. The God Viṣṇu incarnates in the mind of the man and the Goddess Lakṣmī incarnates in the mind of the woman. The god Brahmā incarnates in the spirit of the man and the Goddess Sarasvatī in the spirit of the woman. The gods are united in their dwellings, cakras, when a sexual encounter occurs.

The tāntric yogi is linked with all the beings found in his field of action and makes them part of his family. Because of this, he finds the inner strength to take care of the beings that are part of his family.

The sense of invocation

When a god is invoked, it is done with the objective of getting in touch with our higher selves in order to receive his profound energy, his śakti. This is basically done by two processes: meditation and the sexual act.

The sacred act of sexuality, paramaithuna, allows us to show our divinity and at the same time the divinity of our partner.

The basic sense of symbolism

The masculine strength of the god is principally represented in the liṅgam, the phallus, and the female energy of the godess is represented in the vulva, yoni.

Tantra considers the human body as a temple that should be purified by means of bathing, regulated diet, appropriate breathing and appropriate exercise. Besides this, the body should be strengthened as an essential requirement, by periods of austerity, through sexual abstention, appropriate diet, sleep and moderation of speech. The tāntrika, someone who practises tantra, is called a sacred warrior and has to be able to submerge himself in the most turbid of energies, and extract from them the nectar of immortality.

---

17. The *Tantra Rahasya* says: "The sexual union is a yoga full of blessings that brings serenity by implicating all the senses on the path of liberation."

18. *Maithuna* is the union of the masculine and feminine principles and is understood as a sexual relationship. *Paramaithuna* is the supreme and sacred *maithuna*

The concept of the masculine and feminine descends to the smallest, and ascends to the greatest, incarnating the destructive power and the creative power. People who practise Tantra venerate this divine force projecting themselves in its positive and negative aspects. The gods, in their iconographic representations, are a vehicle to bring the sense of divine powers to human understanding. We understand the existence of many gods by their power to control some aspect of the lives of other beings. We can prove that man may be a god to his friend the dog. In order for the concept of man to exist there must be relationship. All beings have their gods and all gods have their god.

In the Taittirīya Upaniṣad, it is narrated how the gods, after gathering to see which of them was the biggest, found out that Brahman was superior and as they were not able to explain his limits, they denominated him tat, which means 'that'.

From our understanding, the largest force in the Universe is expressed through three primary powers: to create, to preserve and to destroy: om tat sat. The letters a, u and m are contained in om. The a is creation, the u preservation and the m destruction. Om includes the three interrelated powers; tat encompasses and penetrates them; sat designates that what is real. So when we want to define the ultimate reality, underlying all others, we do it with *om tat sat*, "That which is in om is the reality".

The purpose of the invocation is to make the power of the three gods and the three goddesses present. It is done through the voice, with the mouth, the nose, ears and the articulated sound, or the non-articulated sound. If the sound is produced by the mouth, it can be articulated, if done through the nose, then it is not articulated. The non-articulated sounds for example, are those mantras that emit the vibration of the cakras, the root sounds, bīja mantras of the cakras. They can be done through releasing breaths, vāyukas.

The invocation is produced in the mind when the mantra is pronounced, expressing it together with the strength of the breath. A mantra that is repeated without adequate breathing does not have any effect.

THE SOUNDS OF *VYĀYĀMA YOGA*: THE MANTRIC FORCE

There are three types of sounds that produce different effects and are basic to the practice of Vyāyāma Yoga.

The sound 'a' is expansive, so during practice its use is recommended if you wish to perspire abundantly. It has to be observed with attention, as it produces a great combustion and alters the cardiac rhythm.

The sound 'ou' allows for energy exchange, facilitating the renewal of energy. The sound 'o' produces a relaxation effect by creating a 'plenitude void'[19]. When it is produced in an articulated way, the vibration is 'oooo....'. When it is not articulated through the nose, the vibration is 'mmmm.....'

The sound 'u' is used to obtain endurance and balances temperature.

The sound 'ie', takes out all the inert energy and prepares the body to mobilize the energy or to receive a great impact that goes directly to the core. The sound is cold and blocks the energy in the body creating an 'absence void'.[20]

The sound 'o-u' is linked to inhalation.

The sound 'i-e' is linked to retention.

The sound 'a' is linked to exhalation.

Vyāyāma practice with sound invocations is one hundred percent effective. As was previously stated, Vyāyāma practice has to be carried out with sonorous breathing, by means of bhrāmarī sounds to regulate the air that enters or exits through the nostrils. The bhrāmarī sounds produce the same effect as prāṇayamas in the static positions, regulating air ingestion through both nostrils.

The nature of mantras

"*mantrā varṇātmakāḥ sarve sarve varṇāḥ śivātmakāḥ*"

"All mantras are composed of syllables and each one of them makes up the nature of Śiva himself."

For the power of the mantra to be awakened, it must be transmitted by someone who has already awakened it, the master. It needs intense concentration and the breath or vāyu, so that ignition can be sustained.

Thanks to the ignition of the mantras, the seals that prevent the flow of śakti as Kuṇḍalinī in the different cakras are broken. In this way, the gods, the śakta devatās and the Goddesses, śakti devīs, are

19. This state of plentitude is produced when the mind is totally occupied by the vibration of the sound "o" without leaving space for anything else.

20. This state of absence is produced when the mind is emptied of everything except the vibration produced by the sound 'i-e'. When we want to get rid of an obsessive thought, we should emit a sound and slowly it begins to disappear.

awakened in the same cakras, providing the person who practises with different material powers, ṛddhis, and spiritual powers siddhis.[21]

The more people practise mantras, the more present the force of the gods will be in the world, as opposed to the force of inferior beings.

In Vyāyāma, the repitition of a mantra is included in magic Vyāyāma or Karaṇa Vyāyāma, forming an important part of daily practice. When physical force is no longer present in the body, then this is the essential practice.

There is a relationship between mantra and language. Mantra is the core of thought. Originally, the thought is a vibration that adopts the form of word and image in the mind, which is subsequently expressed through language. In Sanskrit, the alphabet is formed by fifty letters, each corresponding to a phoneme that is the articulated expression of a primary vibration. The combination of these fundamental vibrations, in its multiple forms, gives origin to the universe of shapes that are perceived by us. Each existent mantra is formed by the combination of these letters and expresses the most basic thoughts of the manifestation of śakti.

Words are rooted in thoughts. The form language takes will be manifested depending on the vibration of the thought and as the mantra affects the core of thought, an indirect relationship to language is established. The Sanskrit language is impregnated with mantras, as each letter of the alphabet is a mantra itself.

We might think of this mantra theory as something very esoteric and a question of faith, but it occupies the same importance as words in the language of our own lives. Without words there is no possible communication and without communication a collapse occurs. The meaning of words makes action and transformation in the environment around us possible. In the same way that the mantra expresses itself through articulated pronunciation, it also does through writing. Writing the mantra attracts its power.

The geometric way of expressing a mantra is known as yantra. A yantra is like a doorway to a determined level of consciousness because in it, the principles of this plane of consciousness are contained. With a picture, we are able to recall the beauty of a sunset

21. According to tantra, everything is gained and lost within ourselves, as all the gods dwell in the human beings in the seven planes of existence that coincide with the seven main cakras: Mūlādhāra, Svādhiṣṭhāna, Maṇipūra, Anāhata, Viśuddha, Ājñā and Sahasrāra.

and our mind is positively affected by structuring itself in a determined way. Thus, by visualizing a yantra, the mind structures itself in order to access a determined level of consciousness.

Just as the mantra contains the power of the god, the concept that the mantra expresses also contains the power of the god. The gods dwell on the very letters of the Sanskrit alphabet, called devanāgarī.

The mantra is written in the mind through the breath. As we can see, the breath is what maintains the power of the mantra. The breath is what moves the mind, determining the way something affects it according to its dynamics. The repetition of the mantra should be accompanied by a determined breathing that allows its installation in the mind. When this is accomplished, the mantra repeats itself automatically due to the inertia generated by the conscious repetition. This is called ajapā-japa, the highest stage of mantra repetition indicating that the power of the god has been awakened.

The Gods, Śakta Devas

The Creator God, Brahmā Deva/the Sun God, Surya Deva.

It is the god of masculine, essential and creative energy and represents the cycle of life in its birth phase. He is invoked in every creative process: to understand the knowledge of the Vedas, for protection before a journey, to obtain prosperous businesses and to have successful first relationships.

In the Taittirīya Upaniṣad we can find the following mantra "From Brahmā who is the highest I, space was born, from space air was born, from air fire was born and from fire, water. From water, the earth and from the earth vegetation arose, and from vegetation, food, and from food, the bodies of all creatures and humanity".

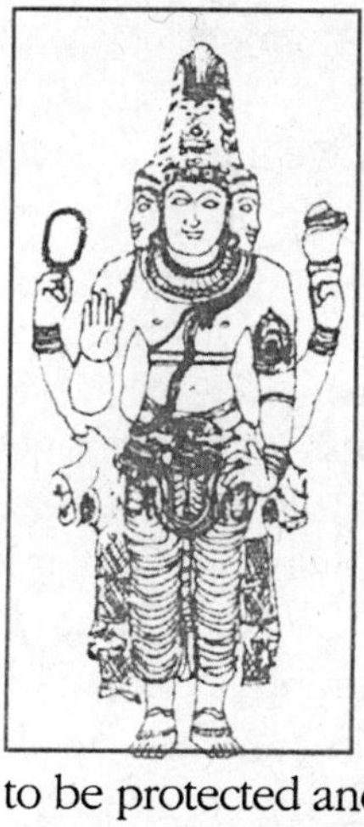

According to the Śiva Purāṇa, Brahmā initiated the process of creation, dividing himself into man and woman and like this divided all beings.

The force of the sun helps us control material elements, and the force of the moon helps us to penetrate our deepest intuitive states.

The God of Preservation, Viṣṇu Deva/ The God that removes obstacles, Gaṇeśa Deva.

He represents the masculine energy that allows life to be protected and regenerates it so the cycle of existence can continue.

The Viṣṇu Purāṇa says: "Viṣṇu is the preserver of all and has the power to be manifested in many different aspects. He is the great cosmic ocean who leans on the serpent of the infinite. He is the essential spirit of existence that has the power to rule the universe."

He is invoked to protect life, to recover and enhance ḥealth, to elevate spirituality, material prosperity, material happiness and good business.

Gaṇeśa is the force that removes all obstacles and eliminates all problems that arise during work.

The Pure Consciousness God, Śivadevatā/ The Lord of all creatures God, Īśa Devatā.

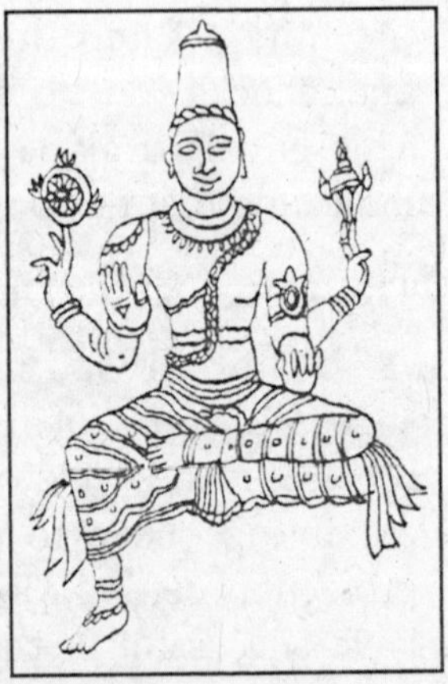

He is the power of the god that takes life to death and life from death. He is the complete power of the three gods together. By his power, our small 'I' is broken up and taken to the superior planes of consciousness. He is the power of transcendence. He gives liberation and allows us to say "śivo ham", which means, "I am Śiva", transforming human nature into divine nature.

The Śiva Purāṇa says: "Śiva is pure existence, is the divine immortal principle. He is pure, non-conditioned and transcendental consciousness. Śiva is the God of the night, the God of death, the Lord of yoga, the Ruler of the three worlds, the Winner over death. They call him the Boatman. The whole universe emerges from the seed that Śiva places on the egg of Brahma."

His invocation protects us from demons and negative internal forces that live inside or outside of us. He helps us to achieve our goals and blesses them, keeping our spirit free from perversion.

The Goddesses, Śakti Devīs

The Goddess of Wisdom, Sarasvatī Devī/The Goddess with the power of material nature, Umā Devī.

She is the spouse of Brahmā, the mother of creativity, fine arts and literature. The poem Sarasvatī Stotram says: "The body of Sarasvatī has a brightness which is more powerful than the shining of ten million moons. The energy that surrounds her has been purified by the

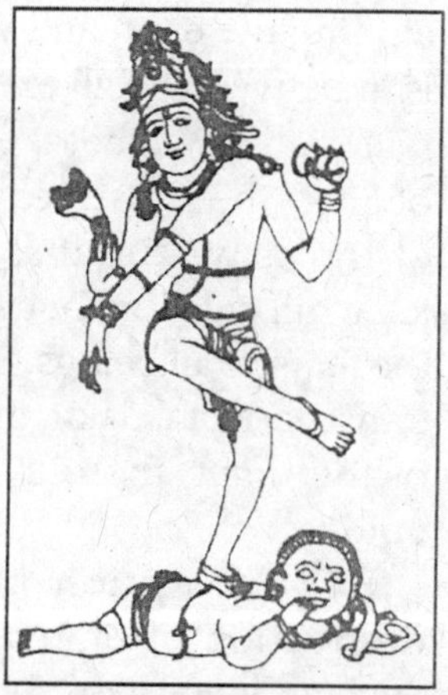

celestial fire. She is the mother of the Vedas, the true personification of sublime nature and is the patroness of all the arts and sciences. She always smiles and possesses extraordinary beauty. Her body is decorated with jewels and pearls, and when we merge with her we spontaneously reach the knowledge of the sixty-four arts."

Umā is the aspect of the goddess as the mother of the universe, Mother Nature.

The Goddess of Prosperity, Lakṣmī Devī/ The Protective Goddess, Durgā Devī.

The Lakṣmī Tantra says: "She is the consort of Viṣṇu and is as beautiful as the dawning of ten million suns. She is the incarnation of sensuality, with her garland-adorned body and her lotus-eyes she seduces everyone. She is the eternal lover of everybody. She lies on the thighs of Viṣṇu and is the patroness of prosperity."

Lakṣmī is invoked in order to obtain a healthy and beautiful body and a prosperous life.

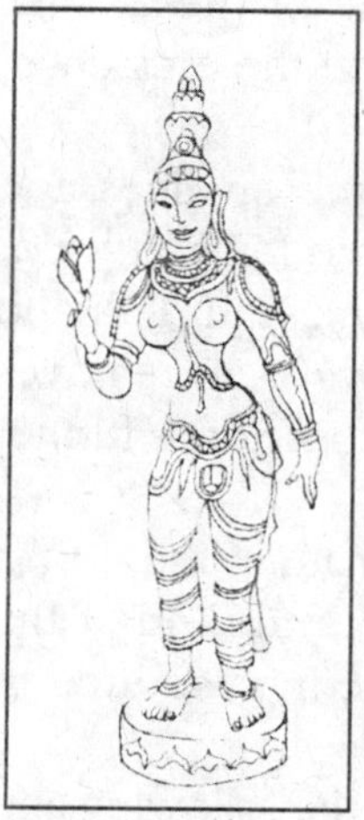

Durgā is the goddess who protects all beings with ferocity.

The Destructive Goddess, Kālī Devīmā/The Ferocious Goddess, Bhairavī Devīmā.

Kālī is the consort of Śiva. Her power extends through the channel by which life enters and exits, Suṣumṇā. Through her power the small 'I' dies, only to be reborn later in better conditions and prepared to meet Śiva. Kālī is the goddess of death and of all men who lack knowledge of Śiva, the one who ends all their hopes. However, for those who are inebriated with her knowledge, she is the gateway of life.

As an insatiable devourer, she is also known as Kālahārī. She is the beginning and where all things find their end. She is the cosmic dancer, the bloody dancer who performs her mortal dance over all beings and universes. In her dance, she waves her hands performing a cosmic turn.

In the scripture known as Kālikā Purāṇa it says: "Kālī is the liberator. She concedes her protection to the one who invokes her. She is space,

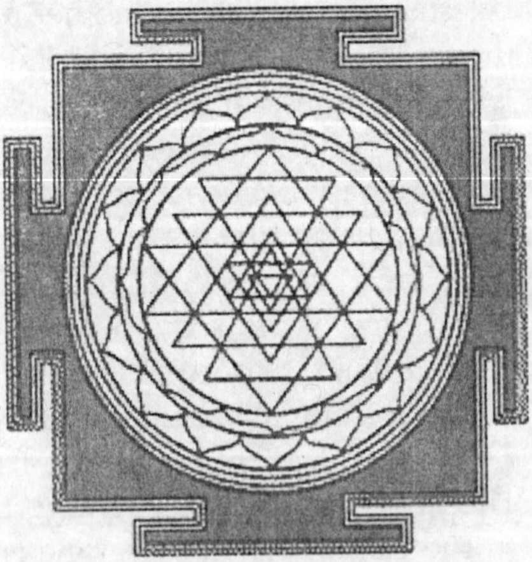

air, fire, the earth and what there is in between." Kālī executes and materialises activity, the karma of Śiva. She possesses the merits of the sixty-four arts; she gives joy to all creation, but also drinks the tears of all beings. She is pure transcendental Śakti, the shadow of the night, the only light and guide.

Her invocation brings the destruction of time and space. Such an invocation should never be done with bad feelings towards another person.

The most beautiful goddess who dwells in the three cities is Tripurasundarī. "The central triangle of the Shri Yantra has three angles, each one corresponds with one of these three cities. Tripurasundari dwells in the centre of the triangle in the Bindhu and for this reason it is said that she dwells in the triple city. Each one of these cities corresponds to a deity of the trimurti and one of the three essential aspects of Shakti which are Iccha, Kriya Y Jnyana".

Lalitā (who grants all wishes) lives in these three qualities and supports the activity of Brahmā, Viṣṇu and Śiva. She is Mūlā Vidyā or Śri Vidyā, the combination of the three powers: Kameśvarī, Kālī and Tārā. By Kāmeśvarī's will Kuṇḍalinī unite with Śiva. Kālī removes the fright of death and change and Tara drives the conscience further away from the modifications of the mind.

She is the gold-coloured goddess, the power of nature, the power of space and time. She is also known as Bhuvaneśvarī and at the same time she is Umā, Durgā and Kālī, protecting, seducing, transforming and destroying everything.

The mantric force of the letters or basic sounds is the following and should be kept in mind when pronouncing the mantras.

Non-articulated sounds, karṇāṭaka

'A' is the sound that prevails in the pronunciation of the prāṇava mantra Om, it is expansive, paternal, goes beyond matter and it is the beginning of everything.

'L' is the sound that prevails in the root sound, bīja mantra, lam. It is solid, earthly, heavy and voiceless.

'HA' prevails in the root sound, bīja mantra, ham. It is light, associated with air and the ether.

'R' prevails in the root sound, bīja mantra, ram. It is energetic and radiant.

Articulated sounds, varṇāṭak

The sound 'oh' prevails in the Mūlādhāra.
The sound 'ooo' prevails in the Svādhiṣṭhāna.
The sound 'ar' prevails in the Maṇipūra.
The sound 'eh' prevails in the Anāhata cakra.
The sound 'e' prevails in the Viśuddha cakra.
The sound 'ma/na' prevails in the Ājñā cakra.
The sound 'ṅg' prevails in the Sahasrāra cakra.

The breathing is vibrantly executed in the phonemes of the vowels in the following way:

'ar' phoneme

Vibrant breathing is produced with an expansive sound, stimulating the expansion of the inner energy. It is used to expand the force and at the same time to concentrate it, to respond to an aggression or a state of well being if needed. Expansive inhalations and long and strong exhalations should be done, by dragging the air through the throat. Louder and shorter exhalations can also be practised.

'ooo' phoneme

Vibrant breathing with "ooo" creates a very active endurance that blocks the interference of other threatening energies. By smoothly but quickly exhaling and ejecting air from the throat with a 'goo' like sound we impact and revitalize the heart. It improves resistance to fatigue and external concentration.

'e' phoneme

Vibrant breathing with the 'e' sound concentrates strength and generates a void. It is not expansive, so it creates an 'absence, void'. All the air is removed and at the same time the heart takes on an extraordinary force; it stops beating and causes the heart to immediately and powerfully expand. This way the body and the mind are condensed, isolating them from the exterior.

'e' phoneme

Vibrant breathing with 'e' adopts an aggressive position, protecting and focusing the mind in an offense attitude and high alert. It is not convenient to hold it for a long time as it activates adrenaline secretion.

'o' phoneme

Vibrant breathing with the 'o' sound leads to the adoption of an 'empty plenitude' state, prepares receptivity, inner concentration and isolates us from the exterior world in a very conscious way, with a profound sense of plenitude.

Protection mantra

The repetition of this mantra protects us in difficult moments by preparing the mind for a state of alertness when faced with the unexpected. It injects strength so the mind is able to submerge into its deepest layers directly contacting the consciousness of our being. It may be repeated everyday before going out of the house, before going on a journey, or before any activity that brings danger to us or to others. It can also be pronounced in the presence of one who has died.

Om Tryambakam yajāmahe
Sugandhim puṣṭivardhanam
Urvarukamiva bandhanāt
Mṛtyor mukṣīya māmṛtāt

"We worship the Supreme Consciousness that nourishes all beings, that frees us from death for the sake of reaching its reality."

Primary and essential invocation of all the bīja mantras

The root sounds, bījas, om, ah, hum along with the mantra "Om namaḥ Śivāya" are the symbolic mantras of Vyāyāma practice.

The root sound, bījas om, is the primary vibration from which everything that exists originated. It is composed of three letters a, u (both forming a diphthong which becomes o) and m and the vibrant sign, anusvāra, placed over the letter m. The a represents the God Vāyu,who brings sound and purifies the atmosphere, the letter u represents the king of gods, Indra, who transforms one thing into another. The letter m is the vibration that originates in the birth of something new and the sign anusvāra is the vibration itself. It is the fusion of the three previous letters and allows the condensation of matter giving origin to the vibration, structures and bodies.

The repetition of the root sound, bīja om, induces introspection and meditation. It establishes awareness of unity and aligns the tan of the body with the mind and spirit. It is the invocation of the absolute being, Brahman, through the three forces that manifest, preserve, and destroy the Universe.

The root sound, bīja ah

This bīja is formed by the letters a and h.

The letter h is the vibration that closes and invokes so that everything that is desired occurs. It is the vibration that starts tāntric action.

The repetition of aḥ purifies the mental atmosphere, preparing us prior to performing the gesture. It represents the ritual and is the sound of action

The root sound, bīja hum

Hum causes the body to become subtle if it is dense and *vice versa.*

The vibration of the bīja ah produces a balancing effect in the mind, allowing it to fall to the tan. It allows for the direction of energy to change by means of material and spiritual actions. The repetition of hum transforms the material into something essential and the essential into something material. Its projection prevents energy from being captured or utilized.

In Tantra "*Om Namaḥ Śivāya*" is the basic invocation mantra. It means: "In the search for om I surrender before Śiva."

When we pronounce *namaḥ* we are presenting ourselves to Śiva as we are, including both the good and bad things in us. When we pronounce *namaḥ*, it is our desire that Śiva does or does not do what he desires with us. It is sincerity, nakedness.

Śiva is pure consciousness that resides in everything and from where everything originates. He is our inner being. He welcomes everything, no matter what its characteristics are and because of this, Śiva moves everywhere, being hidden for the majority, but visible to those who pronounce *namaḥ*.

Complementary Knowledge

MUDRĀS, THE DRIVING GESTURES

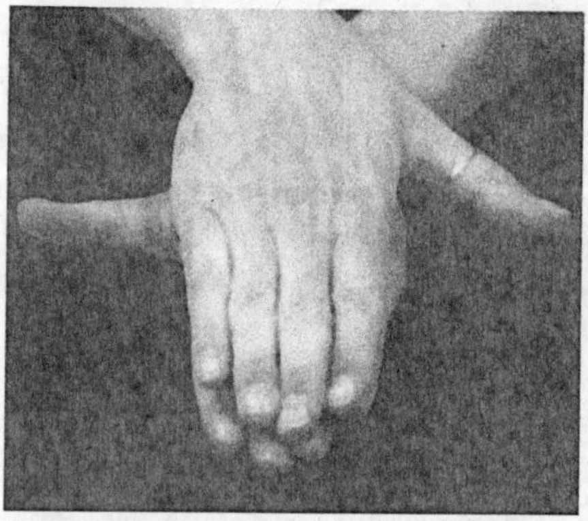

Our hands help us to reproduce our breathing and to balance the magnetic energy meridians. The gestures of the movements of the hands are called mudrās because they express our energy. There is no movement in Vyāyāma Yoga that is not directed by the hands.

When moving our hands, we are magnetically setting the coordinates of the many meridians and talas, the energy distribution centres of the body. Prāṇa flows through the fingers in its five basic forms: breathing, Prāṇa; excretion, apāna; digestion, samāna; swallowing, udāna; and the movement of all body fluids, vyāna. Moving the hands means moving the joints and all of our energy.

Control of the breath and control of the mind are directed by the movement of the hands. The mastery of a person who practises Vyāyāma Yoga can be determined by the expression of the movement of his hands at any moment of his daily life.

The index, middle and thumb fingers have a main role in the movement of the hands. The thumb stabilizes the movement, the index finger focuses the movement and the middle finger regulates it.

There is a whole philosophy and esoteric science about the hands in tantra. There are five subtle channels, nāḍīs that run through our hands and that carry the energy of the five essential elements which connect with the fundamental vital organs. Because of this, when we move them, we are stimulating the functioning of these energies and the organs that depend on them.

The hands represent gestures, words and on many occasions the power of communication of the hands is superior to the word itself. With them, agreements are sealed, prayers and salutations are made and a whole specific communication is transmitted. It is the main symbol of what man is, as no animal has developed this sense in the way we have. We build the whole world with our hands and we are grasped, pushed and touched by them. That is why the human symbol of tantra is the hand. The hands help us to capture and transmit energy.

In Vyāyāma Yoga, when we move our hands, we obtain a stable temperature in them. When they are cold, it is a clear sign that the ***tan*** is losing energy, the energy goes in and goes out, but its essence is not retained. A balanced tan produces warmth in the hands.

VYĀYĀMA YOGA APPLICATIONS

Vyāyāma Yoga is a healthy gymnastics that is an ideal complement to the practices of yoga, bio dance, belly dancing, aerobics, rehabilitation therapies, massage therapies, psycho-dynamic therapies, psycho-energetic therapies, passive gymnastics for the elderly, pre-and post-natal therapies, and many others.

There are two ways of executing the practice of Vyāyāma Yoga, each with a different style and results.

1. Similar to yoga exercises, with deep stretches, called Yogasthya
2. Similar to combat or martial art exercises, called Kangasthya

Yogasthya, is the Vyāyāma Yoga that regulates energy and physical, psychic and spiritual health.

Kanga Vyāyāma, kangasthya is the original Vyāyāma Yoga, which can be practised either with metal or wooden swords or with the hands. It helps us to project the energy. We call this the original style because the initial movements came from those who used the sword.

Āyurveda Vyāyāma is the Vyāyāma of health. By means of massage and knowledge of the 108 vital points and the work done on them through the hands, energy is developed in the talas and helps us to restore our health.

Nāṭya Vyāyāma is the Vyāyāma of dance and theatre.

These styles of Vyāyāma emerged as primitive movements with the purpose of acquiring strength and releasing tensions accumulated before moments of combat. As time went by, they continued acquiring various shapes and styles. The source of Vyāyāma can also be traced back to the narrations of a dynamic practice in the life of great warriors like Prince Śri Rāma.

The practice of Vyāyāma teaches the foundations for the expression of body energy, awakens internal energy and teaches how to express it with strength, balance and harmony, making us graceful and subtle. It allows the hands, the eyes and the movement of the feet and the whole body to become powerful. It makes us capable of easily expressing our inner feelings.

Inside the tantric tradition, different types of dance are known by the generic term *tāṇḍava*. They are gestural and gymnastic movements of Vyāyāma applied to dance, among which the following are the most noteworthy: mystic turns, the tan dance, the energetic dance, the primitive warriors dance and the God Śiva dance. They are of a vigorous and joyful nature and move towards the immediate mobilization of energy to purify and to reach cathartic levels. It is the dance of the spirit, removing miseries and mental depressions by regenerating the body and keeping it alive.

ADVICE ABOUT PRACTICE

Vyāyāma Yoga can be practised at any time of the day, but it is highly advisable to do it in the morning before starting one's daily activity, in order to vitalize energies that have been dormant during the night, making them positive.

It is advisable to wear comfortable cotton clothes. It can be done barefoot or with shoes that have a good grip but still allow flexibility. 'Tabis' or japanese shoes are perfect.

It is very pleasant to practice in the open air or in a well-ventilated room. We should keep in mind that in Vyāyāma Yoga we work a hundred per cent with the breath, so a poorly ventilated room could be harmful. Working with the breath means acquiring great amounts of the energy that surrounds us and transforming it inside us.

One of the secrets of Vyāyāma Yoga, to know whether we are breathing and practising correctly is perspiration. To sweat abundantly is a sign of a good and effective practice. On the contrary, a difficulty in the perspiration indicates certain difficulty or a non-effective practice.

Most of the movements are executed while flexing the legs, because it causes the tan to descend between the knees, guaranteeing a stable posture.

The movements of the hands or mudrās are fundamental. There must not be any movement of the body direction from the gestures of the hands.

It is absolutely fundamental to keep perfect alignment of the talas in the body; otherwise the movement will be produced in a clumsy way and will lack balance.

There are no special conditions required to practise Vyāyāma Yoga. It can be practised by anyone and in any physical condition. It adapts itself to any circumstances and is even possible to practise by only moving the hands.

TEN MOVEMENTS THAT STRENGTHEN THE ESSENTIAL ENERGY IN THE NUCLEUS

Daśa Śakti-Vikāsaka Vyaṅga tan-sthānam abhyāsa-krama

FIRST MOVEMENT

Vyaṅga pictures: C-1-2-3-4

The inverted mountain

TADA ŚAKTI-VIKĀSAKA

Although this is a dense movement, sthūla, it can become an energetic movement, sūkṣma. It is one of the most important and can be considered the king of all vyaṅgas. It executes its main benefits on the shoulders, elbows and hands, giving them strength. It also unblocks tension and releases inert energy in these areas.

It tones the central nervous system, drains the lungs, expands and enhances the volume of the thoracic cavity, strengthens the pleura, increases breathing capacity, protects the heart and renews the blood stream and lymphatic flow. The back and chest are enlarged and the pectorals and muscles of the neck are strengthened.

In general, this Vyaṅga is highly revitalizing, provides physical and energetic balance and a great mental force.

This is the equivalent to the head stand posture in Yoga, Śīrṣāsana. It works on the vital energy cores and the cordial axis of the maṇipūra and anāhata cakras.

Execution

It begins with the feet together. Both hands are brought to the tan and from here the arms and hands are spread to the sides, inhaling until they are parallel to the ground. Exhaling, the arms go down and back to the tan. After performing this movement several times, the arms are finally kept parallel to the ground and at the same time we exhale. We should visualize how the energy projects along the arm and exits through the middle finger. We perfectly align the arms so that shoulder, wrist and hand are at the same level. In order to do so, we look to the right side while exhaling to check the alignment and inhaling we turn our head back to the centre and then repeat this movement on the left side. Inhaling, we take the breath to the base of the throat, vāyu kanda, while the trunk stretches to the sky. After this, we let the breath fall down to the tan with a breath of concentration, vāyuka. Some tension is held in the knees and buttocks and we breathe in the lower tan area, projecting downwards with short inhalations and exhalations.

This vyaṅga is completed by inhaling while raising the hands upwards from the middle fingers and exhaling while taking the arms and hands back to the tan.

SECOND MOVEMENT

Vyaṅga pictures: C-5-6-7-8-9-10

Building and raising the dome of the temple

MANDAR-PRATIṢĀ ŚAKTI-VIKĀSAKA

This vyaṅga is an energetic Vyāyāma, sūkṣma Vyāyāma. Warriors frequently used this figure as a preparation for martial arts practice.

By raising our hands we visualize that we are raising the dome of a temple. It strengthens and releases tension in the shoulders, arms, wrists and neck. It also releases muscular tension in the chest by opening the thymus gland and unblocks emotional tension. It drains the kidneys and the lungs and helps to correct back problems by spreading Prāṇa, vital energy, along the spine. By separating each vertebra from its cradle, it liberates the nerve impulses of the principal nodules that tone the vital organs of the body. It works on the cordial axis core, on the vital force seat and the three great vital rivers, āhata cakra, nābhi āditala and the Brahma, Iḍā and Piṅgalā nāḍīs.

Execution

Standing, the hands are raised projecting out from the tan until the arms are completely parallel to the ground. Exhaling, the arms are bent from the elbows, still parallel to the ground and inhaling the hands are united in the centre of the chest, performing a greeting gesture. Exhaling, the hands are pressed together with strength and inhaling, the hands are raised along with the arms above the head and the elbows are pulled backwards. While exhaling, the arms are raised in their full length, stretching completely. Inhaling, the hands turn outwards so they join on the other side. Exhaling, they separate and laterally descend with the arms until they are parallel to the ground. Inhaling, the arms are again bent to the chest.

To end this movement, the hands which are united at the chest, are projected forwards along with the arms and are separated at the level of the tan.

THIRD MOVEMENT

Vyaṅga pictures: C-11-12-13-14-15-16-17-18

The lighting of the lamp that illuminates the heart

HṚDJYOTI DĪPIKĀ ŚAKTI-VIKĀSAKA

This is an energy giving vyaṅga, sūkṣma Vyāyāma. It represents the heart and essential wisdom. It awakens feelings such as love and compassion. In ancient India, when the masters were prepared to teach, they performed the mudrā that this figure demonstrates. It provides physical and emotional balance, nourishing us with balanced and upright thoughts. It opens the heart energy centre bringing mental serenity and purifies the core of external awareness. It works on the heart core and the core of external awareness, Anāhata cakra and nāsāgra aditala. It also strengthens the wrists.

Execution

We start in a standing position, and with the indication and help of the right hand, the right foot is bent next to the left foot, supporting the toes of the right foot on the ground and its heel over the ankle of the left foot. In this way, the right leg is bent from the knee, pointing outwards to the right. With the hands on the tan, inhaling, the left arm is raised laterally until it is parallel to the ground and exhaling this arm is bent at the elbow, placing the wrist at the centre of the chest, with the hand in a vertical position. The thumb touches the chest and the little finger points to the front. Inhaling, the left arm is laterally raised until it is parallel to the ground and exhaling, this arm is bent at the elbow, placing the left wrist under the right wrist, so the left hand is just below the right arm. In this way, the arms represent the shape of a lamp. After inhaling and exhaling, this vyaṅga is undone by inhaling while raising the arms up to the forehead and exhaling while lowering them again and taking the hands back to the tan.

FOURTH MOVEMENT
Vyaṅga pictures: C-19-20-21-22-23-24-25-26-27-28-29-30-31-32-33-34

The figure of the archer that shoots the big bow

DHANURATA ŚAKTI-VIKĀSAKA

This vyaṅga is an energetic Vyāyāma, sūkṣma Vyāyāma. It is performed by holding the bow with the hands, focusing the mind on a fixed point and shooting the arrow toward that point. It is a warrior's posture and symbolizes the process of yoga; the bow is the body, the arrow is the mind, and the bull's eye is the target of concentration. The bowstring is the discipline of the method.

It expands the chest and strengthens the arms and torso, giving us a healthly appearance, strength and security. It regulates accumulated energy, balances the thymus gland and reinstalls self-esteem. It works on the breath and the inner attention projection core, Viśuddha cakra and bhrūmadhya aditala.

Execution

From a standing position, the legs are separated a distance slightly larger than the width of the shoulders and the hips are pushed inward. Inhaling, both the arms extend upwards in front of the body, keeping them at the same level and exhaling when they reach a position parallel to the ground, we stand on tiptoes. This first part is called 'to pull the bow out of the tan'. Once the bow is secure we inhale and the left foot rotates to the left together with the arms and torso. Next, the trunk and arms are projected forward while exhaling. Then we go back to the upright position while the arm goes to the right shoulder blade, as if picking out an arrow and then, exhaling, the right hand moves towards the left hand, putting the arrow on the bowstring that the left hand is holding. The right hand draws the bowstring back while concentrating the breath and visualizing the target. With an exhalation, in which we pronounce "ishu", we shoot the arrow and we finalize with a discharge breath in "kha". Following this, we perform the same movements with the right foot. The vyaṅga ends by taking śakti from the ground and drawing it to the tan.

FIFTH MOVEMENT

Vyaṅga pictures: C-35-36-37-38

The step of the mighty lion or tantric dragon

BHAIRAVAYĀNA ŚAKTI-VIKĀSAKA

This vyaṅga is an energetic Vyāyāma, sūkṣma Vyāyāma. These are the steps that are applied to martial arts, the steps of the fight, which give great confidence to the warrior. It provides great strength to muscles and legs and stimulates the functioning of the heart and regulates its beat. It is a great physical exercise and its habitual practice may be the equivalent to jogging. It enhances breathing capacity and actively works on the kidneys and on the regulation of body temperature, thus regulating the metabolism. It helps the peristaltic movement by alleviating inflammation of the intestines and activates sexual performance by stimulating adrenaline secretion. It works the heart axis, the axis of strength in the body, creative sexual energy and the three great rivers, Anāhata cakra, Maṇipūra cakra, Svādhiṣṭhāna cakra, nābhi āditala and the Brahma, Iḍā and Piṅgalā nāḍis.

In this vyaṅga, the hands should accompany the movement of the legs, making gestures as if they were picking rice from the hip and releasing it toward the knees.

Execution

From a standing position with the hands placed on the tan, the legs are separated a distance similar to the width of the shoulders. From here, directing the movement with the right hand, a step forward is taken with the right leg. The same is performed with the left hand and the left leg and then the right leg moves back and then to the centre. All these movements are repeated, but this time starting with the left leg.

SIXTH MOVEMENT

Vyaṅga pictures: C-39-40-41-42-43-44-45-46

The eagle that extends its wings looking for its prey

GARUḌA ŚAKTI-VIKĀSAKA

This vyaṅga is a dense Vyāyāma. It is a sthūla Vyāyāma. The eagle represents the active concentration capacity of the yogi, the external concentration. It is preformed by firstly projecting to the right and afterwards to the left. The head is projected forwards and the eyes are kept wide open, fixed, and still. In this position mental work is very important as we should visualize and introduce ourselves into the nature of the eagle. This posture may also be performed in movement, as if the eagle were flying. It empowers the alert state of the mind and directly influences the balance of the spine by releasing energy blockages. It invigorates the kidneys and improves the opening of the energy centres in the hands and the feet.

Execution

From a standing position with the hands on the tan, the left foot is rotated to the left. The hands and arms flap smoothly as if they were wings, inhaling as they ascend and exhaling when they descend. From below and with the arms crossed, the hands are taken to the energy distribution centres of each shoulder, talas. The eyes are wide-open and fixed on the ground, as if they were observing their prey. From here, the left leg projects to the left while the arms are half-bent as if they were wings, with the scapulas pulled back and the hips pushed forward.

This Vyaṅga ends by taking the arms to the left leg and from there they rise above the head completely extended while the legs come together. The arms move down to the tan by forming a circle.

SEVENTH MOVEMENT

Vyaṅga pictures: C-47-48-49-50

The reed (the sevenholed flute)

MURALĪ ŚAKTI-VIKĀSAKA

This vyaṅga is a dense Vyāyāma, sthūla vyāyāma. It is one of the most stimulating positions of the set. If it is done properly and maintained for some time, it completely regenerates the energy of the body by turning it into a channel through which the most sublime and dense energies pass. After the execution of this position, our Vyāyāma changes, becoming more harmonious and balanced.

It is very good to practise this when there is anger, aggressiveness and lack of sleep. It works on the basic energy core and the psychic axis, Mūlādhāra cakra,and śiraākāśa tantala.

Execution

Standing with the feet together, the whole body is squeezed, tensing the abdomen to achieve an erect posture. The head is held high and the body resembles a reed that comes out of the water. Afterwards, the buttocks and abdomen are released and relaxed and an absolutely still posture is maintained with minimal tension. The body moves only if the inner energy sways it. The eyes are kept closed and the attention is focused on the tan. This vyaṅga finishes with an exhalation and relaxation of the body.

EIGHTH MOVEMENT

Vyaṅga pictures: C-51-52-53-54-55-56-57-58-59

The mystic tree that has its roots in the sky and fall to the earth

AŚVATTHA ŚAKTHI-VIKĀSAKA

This vyaṅga is a magical and dense Vyāyāma, sthūla and karaṇa vyāyāma. The aśvattha is the sacred tree of India, where yogis used to live. From its branches, other branches are projected to the ground and take root, forming small caves. It is very important to perform the identification process or saṁyama in order to absorb the energy of the tree.

It is a meditation posture and can be held for a long time. The knees are flexed and the fingers are loose, positioning the hands at the same level as the talas, the energy distribution centres of the shoulders. It improves the sleep state, introverts and sedates. The kidneys rest and the spine is freed, allowing energy to rise to the head. It is recommended for meditation and its objective is to capture energy from the earth (which is why we keep our knees bent) and from heaven (the head is stretched from the back of the neck). It activates the flow of energy on the main meridians and works with balance on the centres of consciousness and on basic energy, harmonizing them with the three great rivers of vital energy, Ājñā cakra, Mūlādhāra cakra and the Brahma, Iḍā and Piṅgalā ṅāḍis.

Execution

From a standing position with the feet together, the left foot is rotated to the left. The body is bent downwards to a crouching position with the arms bent. From here the body is projected to the left, by opening the legs similar to the width of the shoulders, the knees are flexed and the hips are pushed forward. The arms are flexed upwards, with the hands completely relaxed at the same level as the shoulders and facing each other. The vyaṅga is completed by extending the arms above the head, then to both lateral sides completely elongated and from here they descend, moving the fingers slightly and finishing in the tan.

NINTH MOVEMENT

Vyaṅga pictures: C-60-61-62-63-64-65-66-67-68

The fortified tower

VARMA VIRĀTA ŚAKTI-VIKĀSAKA

This vyaṅga is a dense Vyāyāma, a sthūla Vyāyāma. It is one of the positions of the "Master chess board series". Great density is created in the body because it is completely compacted, giving inner strength and eliminating inert energy. It strengthens the structure of the skeleton and the whole body, making the mind stronger and giving the person great powers of observation and alertness. Sciatic tension is drained and it also strengthens the kidneys and activates the diaphragm. It works to strengthen energy in the body, maṇipūra cakra.

Execution

Standing with the feet together, the left foot is rotated to the left. With the hands and the arms, the energy is gathered from outside towards the tan. Once this is performed a number of times, the body crouches with clenched fists and the arms cross in tension. From here, the body is projected to the left by separating the legs. When the left leg is placed on the ground, the right hand grabs the left arm near the elbow and the left hand is extended over the right forearm near the elbow. In this way, a padlock is made with the arms.

The hips are pushed forward and the body contains some tension. The vyaṅga ends by taking the fists to the left knee and from here the arms are completely elongated above the head while the legs come together. Exhaling and applying force to the arms, they are lowered to the tan.

TENTH MOVEMENT

Vyaṅga pictures: C-69-70-71-72-73-74-75-76-77-78

The figure of the lookout that marks the four cardinal points

SĀKṢĪ ŚAKTI-VIKĀSAKA

This vyaṅga is a sūkṣma Vyāyāma. It massages the spinal column and stimulates the functioning of the internal organs. It invigorates the nervous system and brain circulation and allows better concentration of the mind, awakening many intellectual faculties. It works on the vital breath centre and the main nodes of vital energy condensation, Viśuddha cakra and Suṣumṇā nāḍī.

Execution

From a standing position with the feet together, the right arm is raised, stretching the middle, index and thumb fingers. The sight is fixed on them and follows them as they move up. When the arm is parallel to the ground and completely elongated, we exhale. Next, we turn the arm 90 degrees to the right while inhaling and staring at the fingers all the time. Then we exhale and further stretch the arm by turning it along with the torso and the hips 90 degrees more to the right. Then inhaling, we turn the body back to the centre and exhaling the arm goes forward with the torso and the head, exhaling once again. Next, we inhale and while exhaling the arm moves down while the sight follows it. The same process is done with the left arm.

The assiduous practice of this routine strengthens the energy in the tan, allowing it to be distributed by the subtle channels, nāḍīs and to be balanced in the condensation and distribution centres.

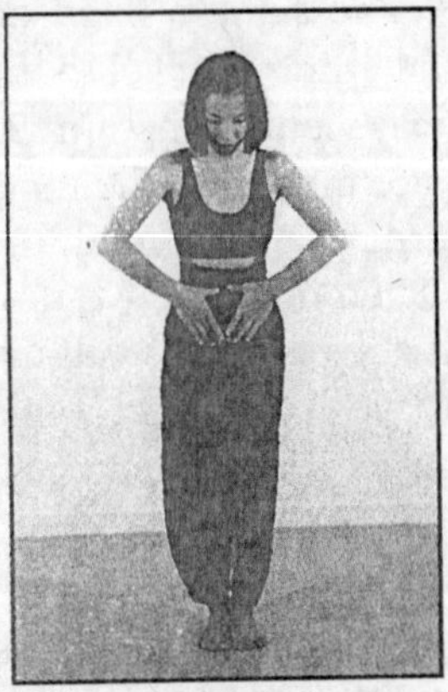

C-1

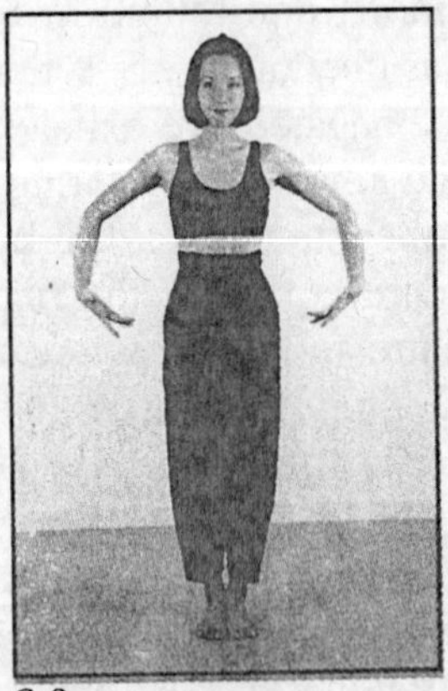

C-2

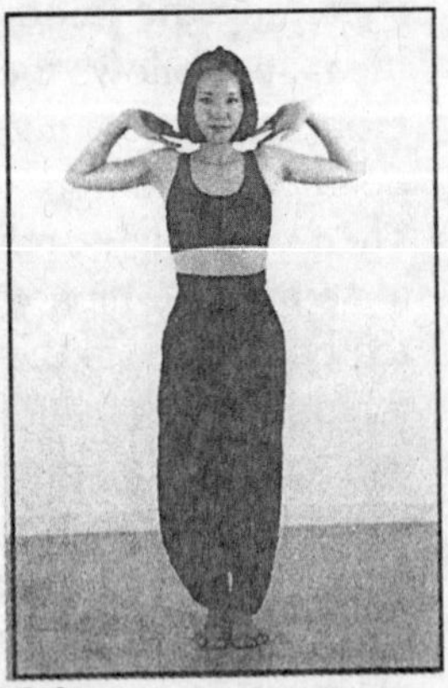

C-3

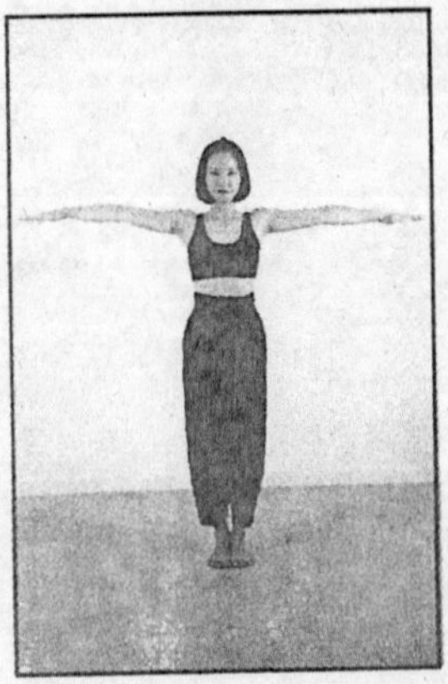

C-4

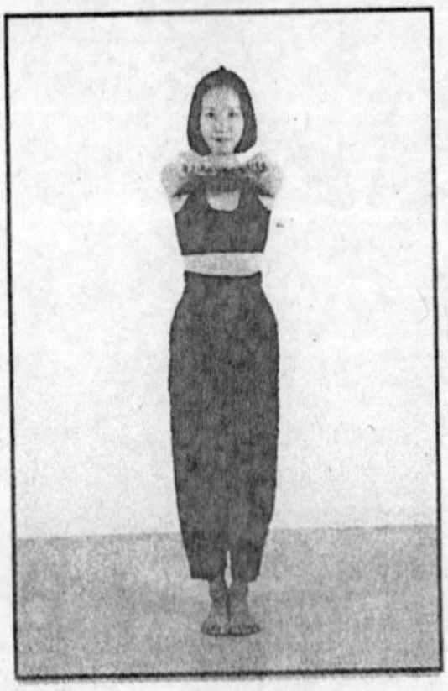

C-5

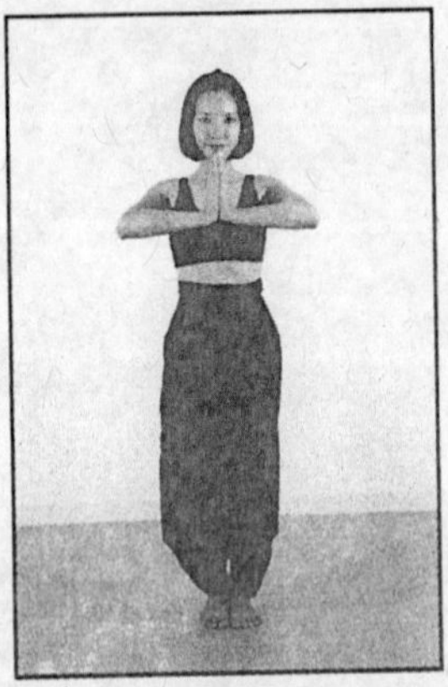

C-6

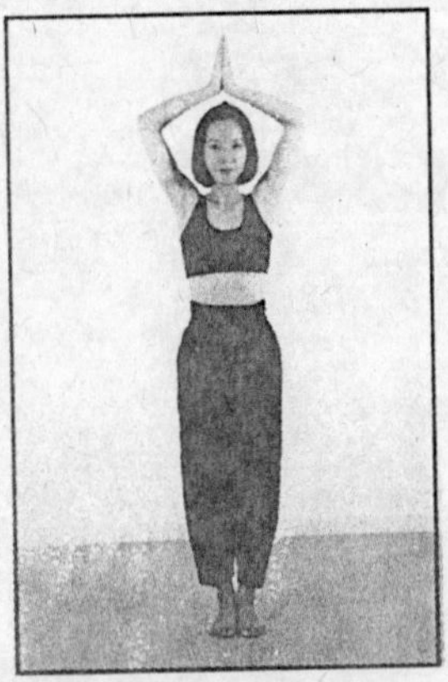

C-7

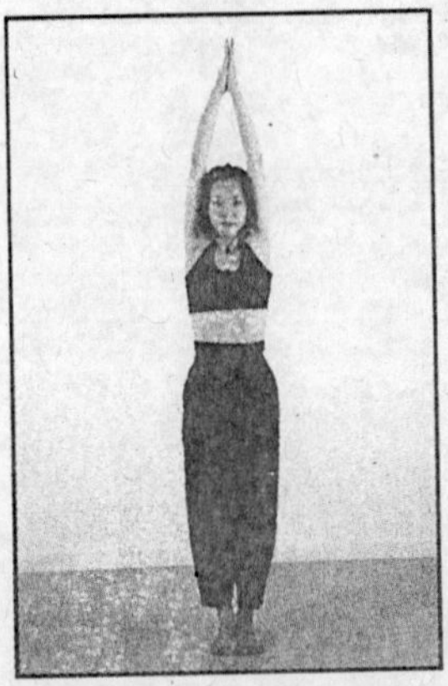

C-8

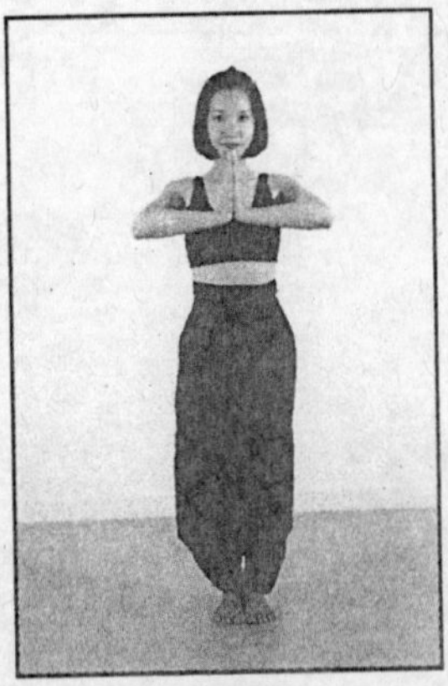

C-9

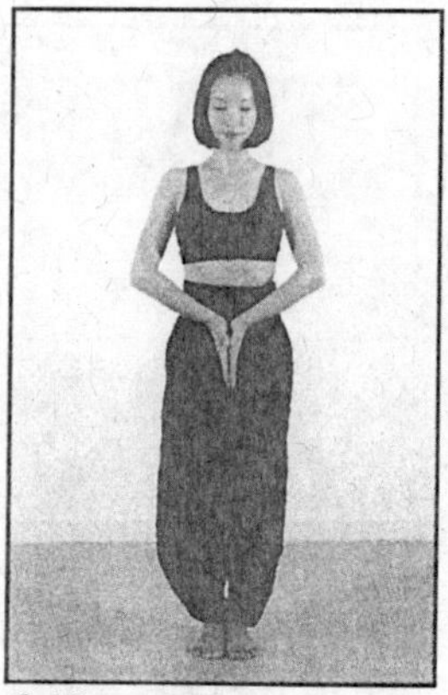
C-10

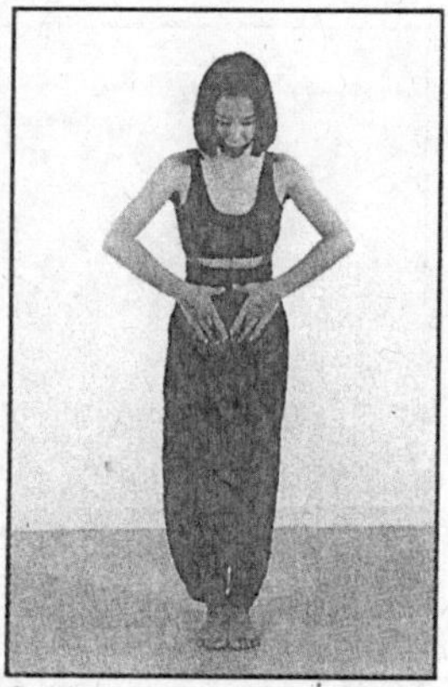
C-11

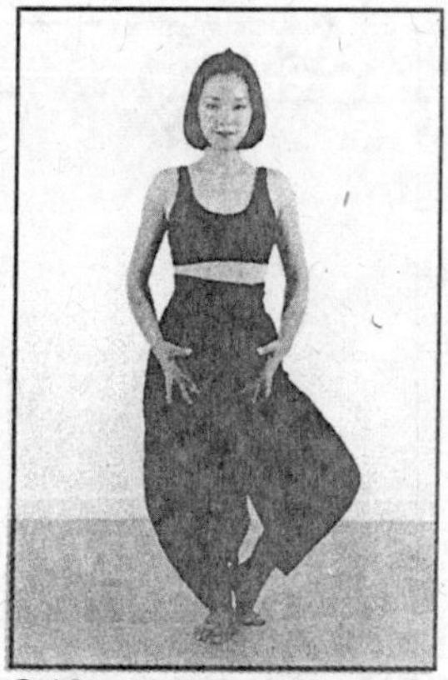
C-12

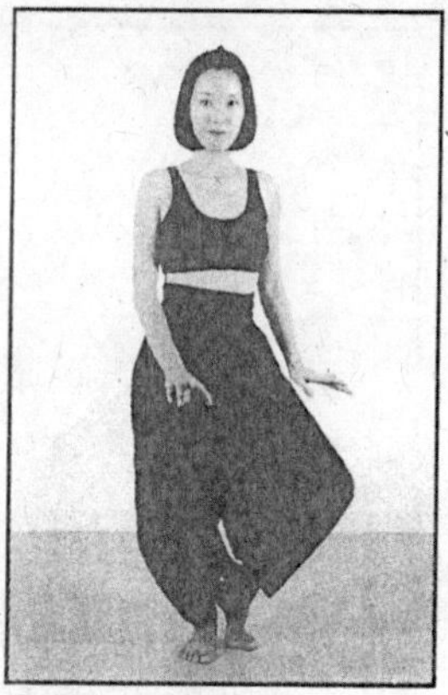
C-13

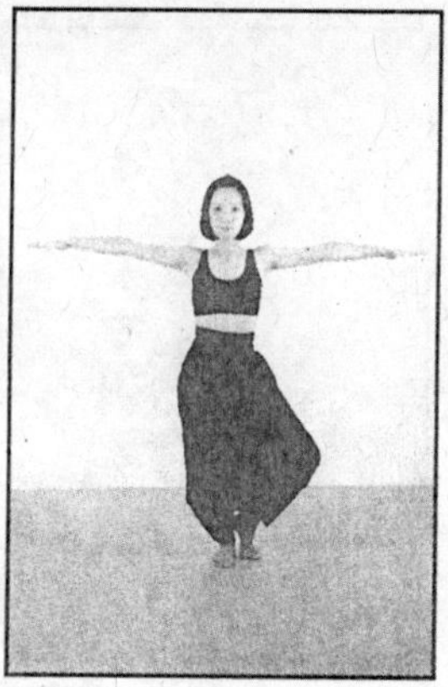
C-14

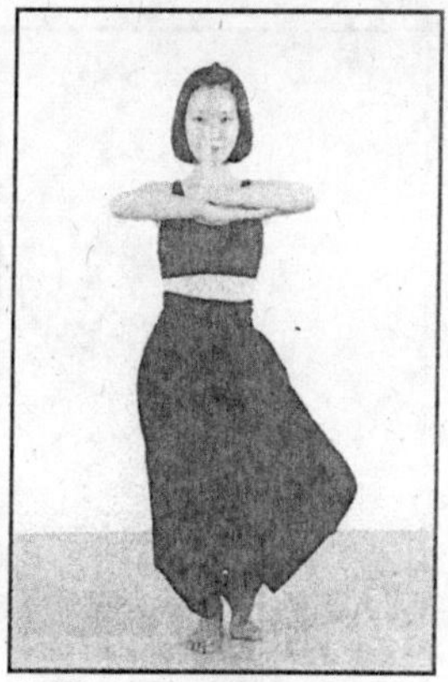
C-15

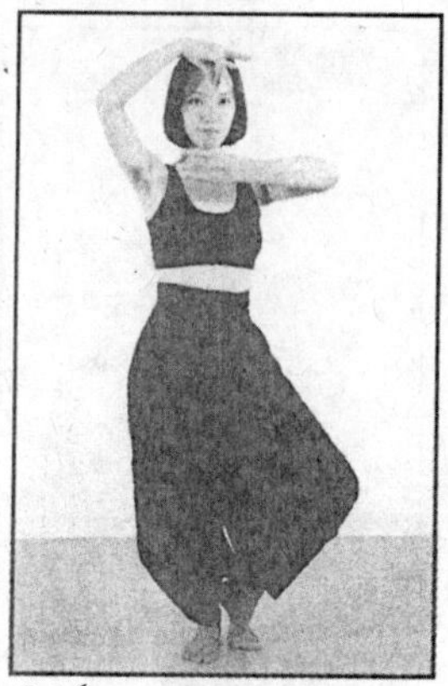
C-16

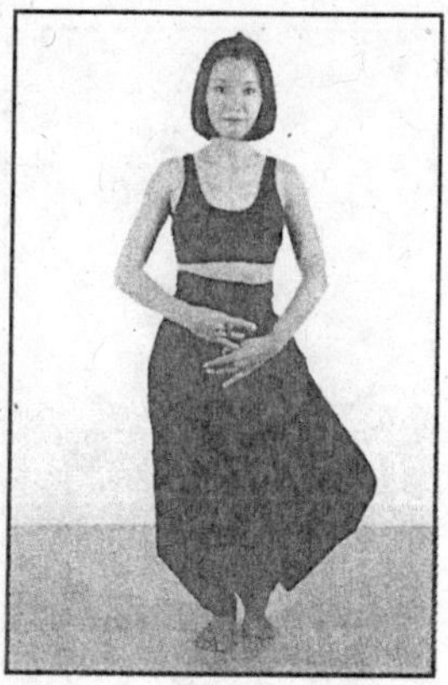
C-17

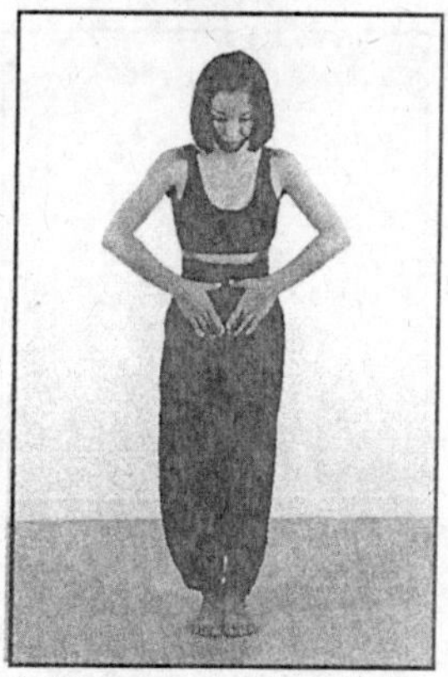
C-18

The movements from C-11 to C-18 are repeated on the other foot.

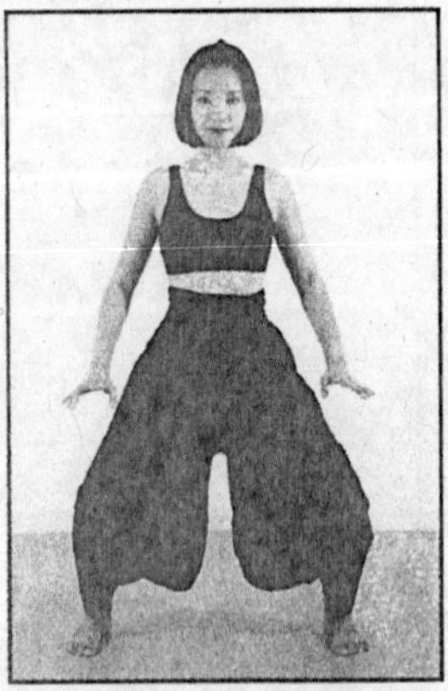
C-19

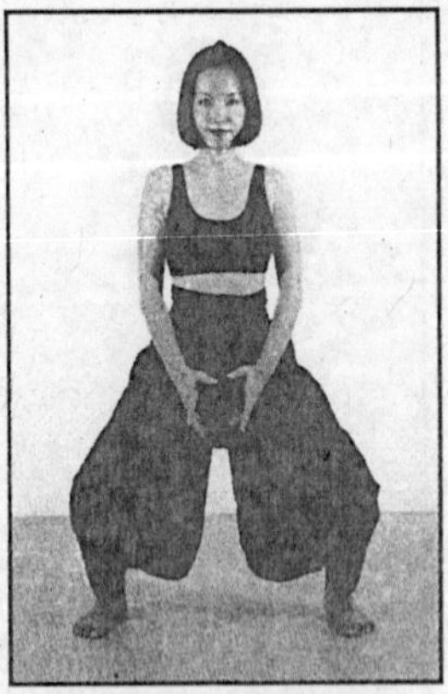
C-20

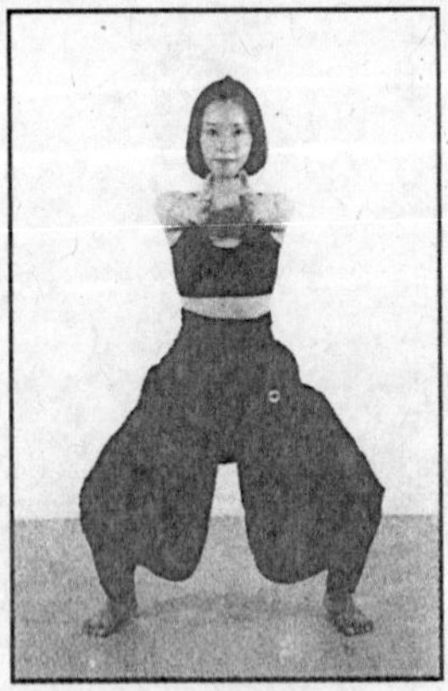
C-21

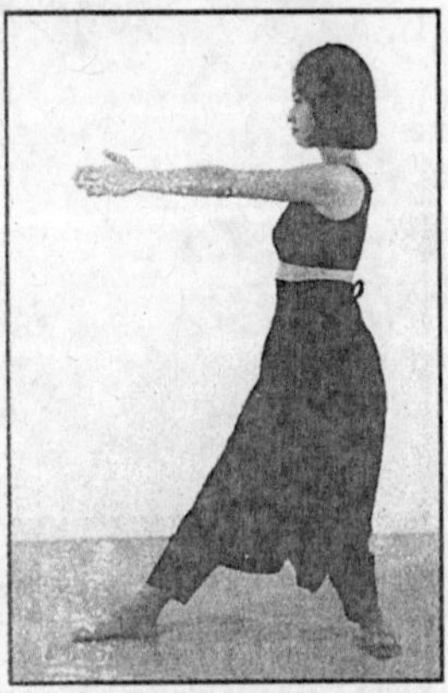
C-22

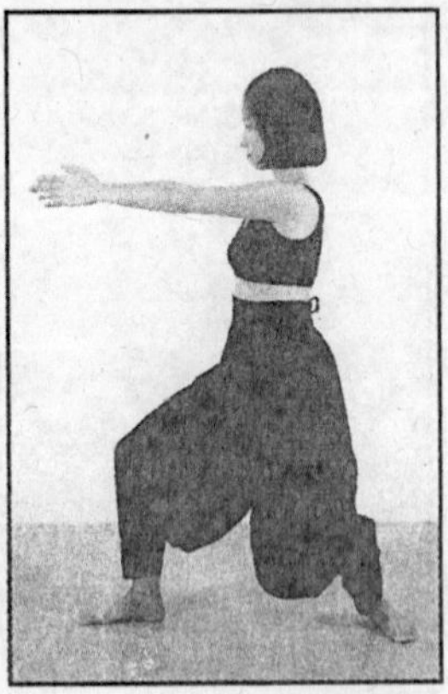
C-23

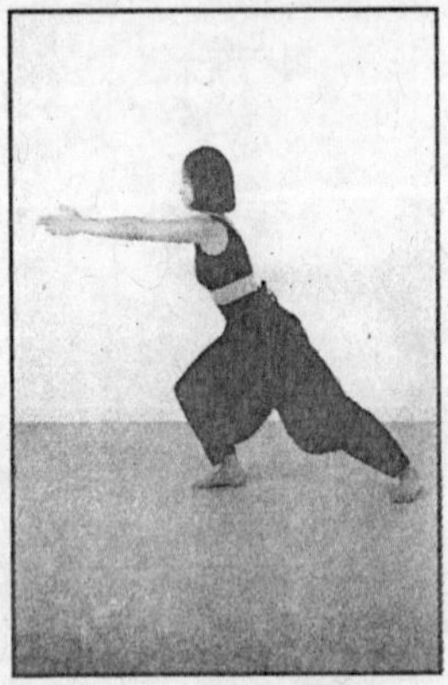
C-24

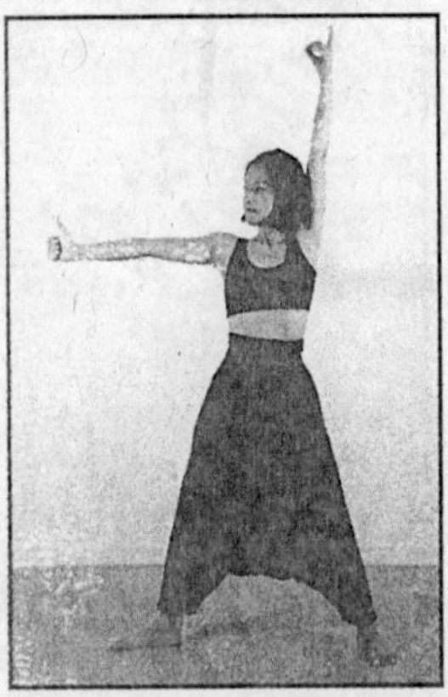
C-25

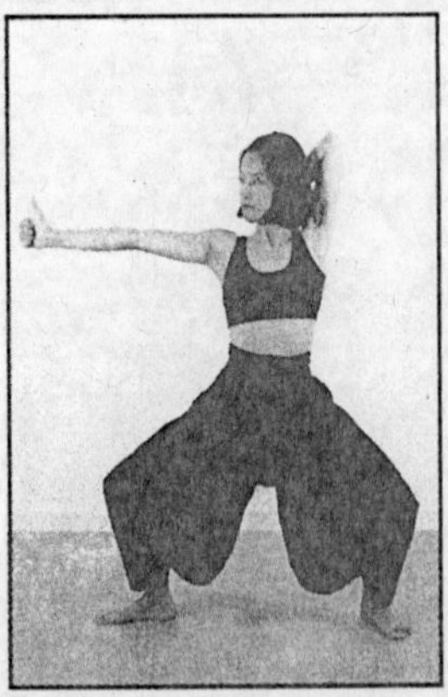
C-26

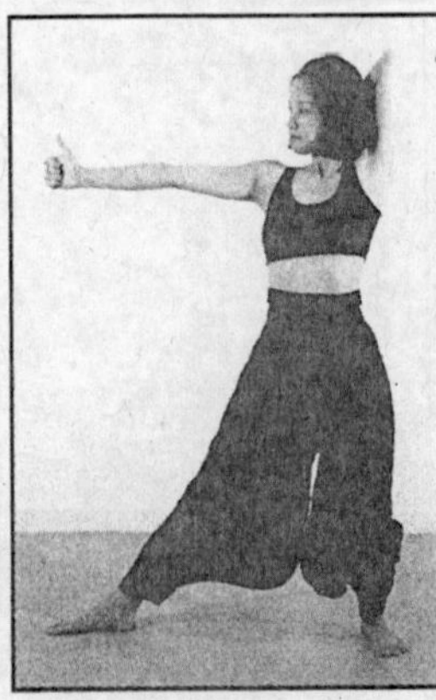
C-27

The movements from C-19 to C-32 are repeated on the other side.

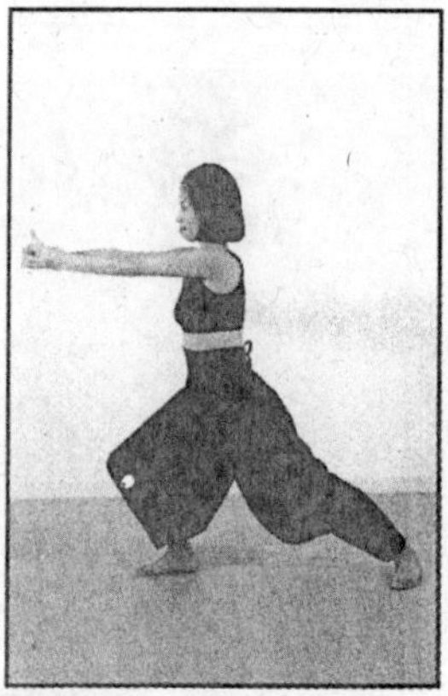
C-28

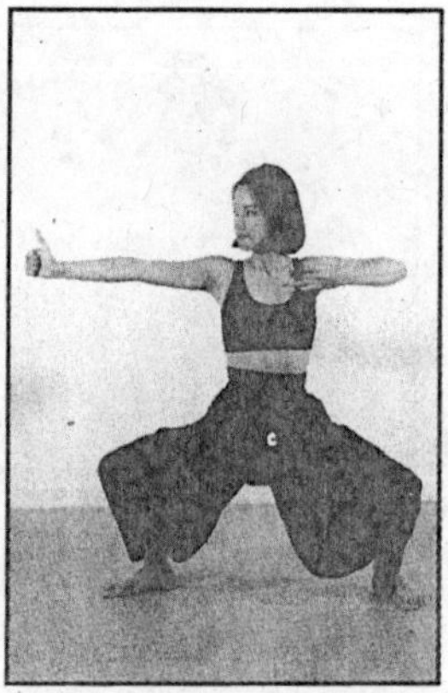
C-29

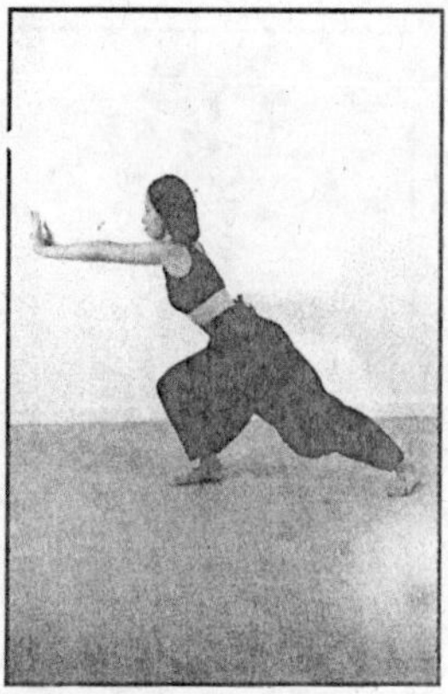
C-30

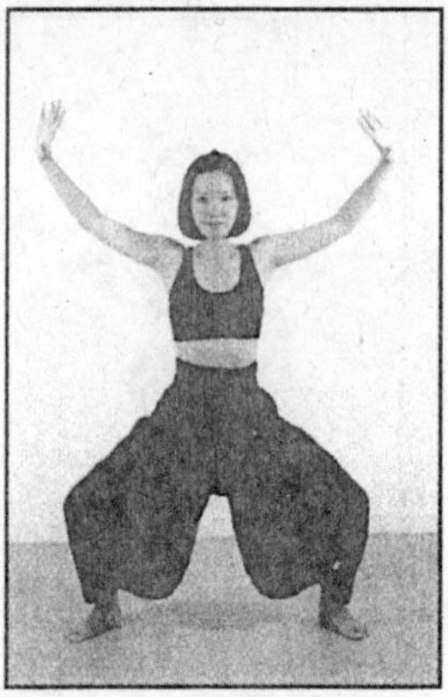
C-31

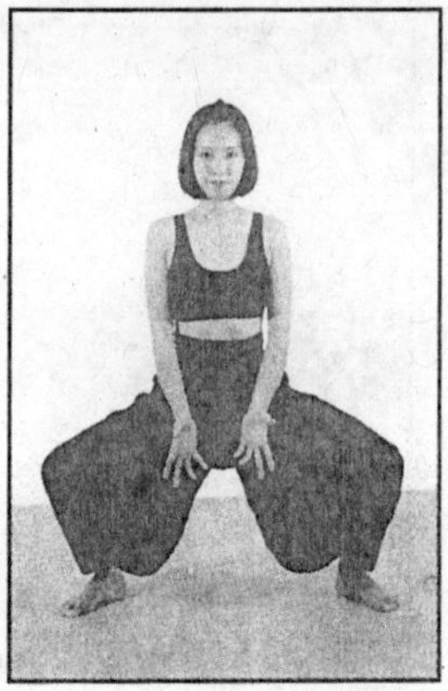
C-32

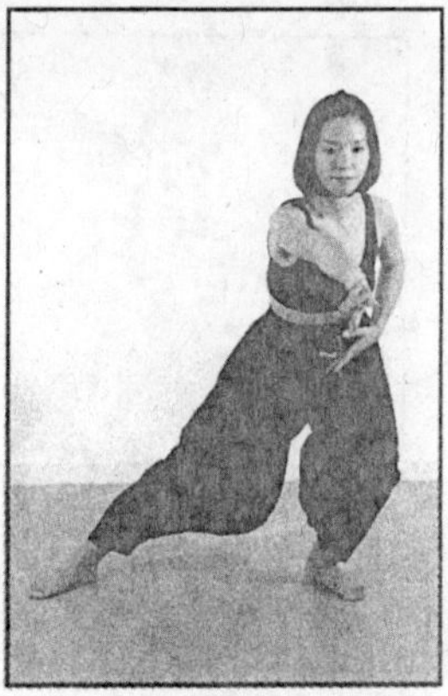
C-33

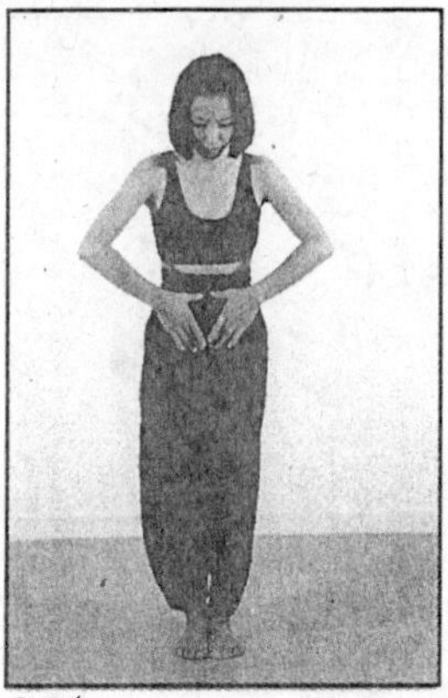
C-34

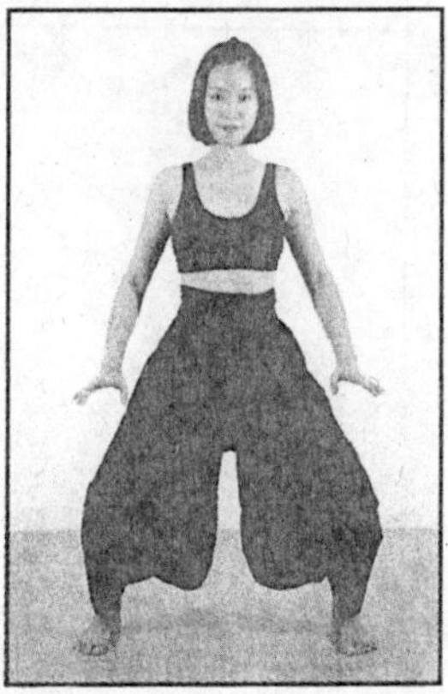
C-35

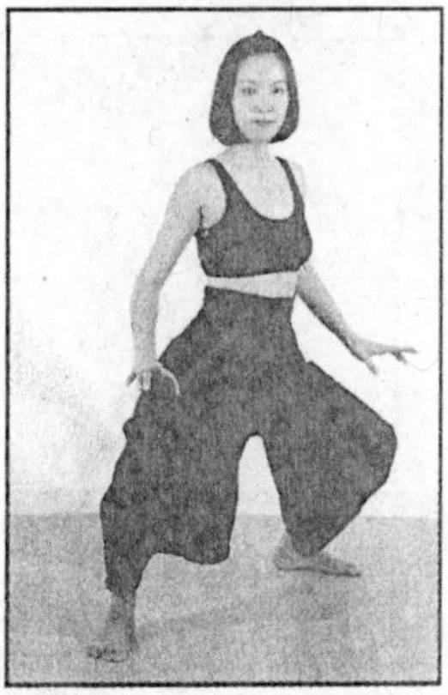
C-36

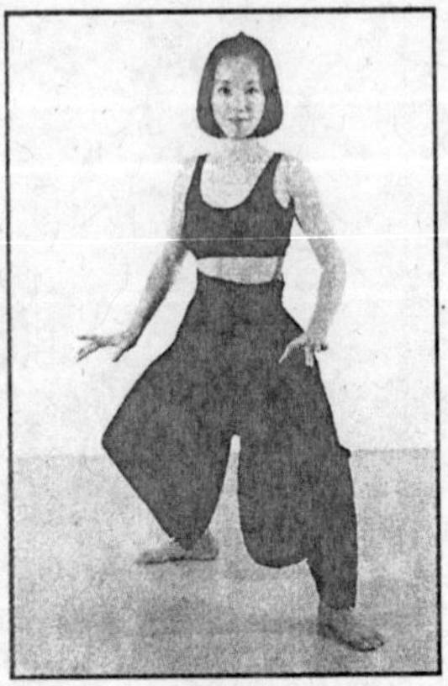
C-37

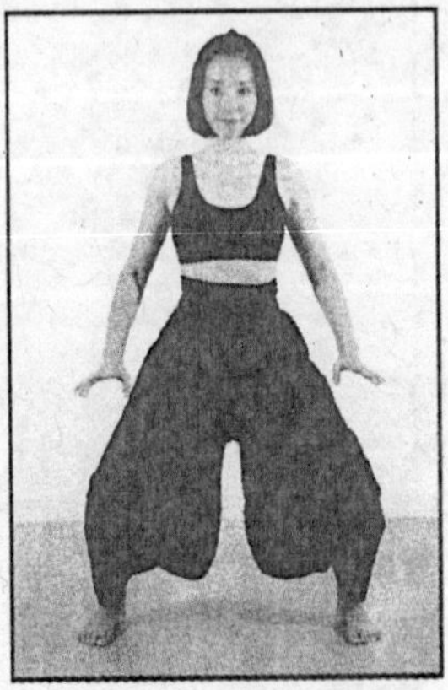
C-38

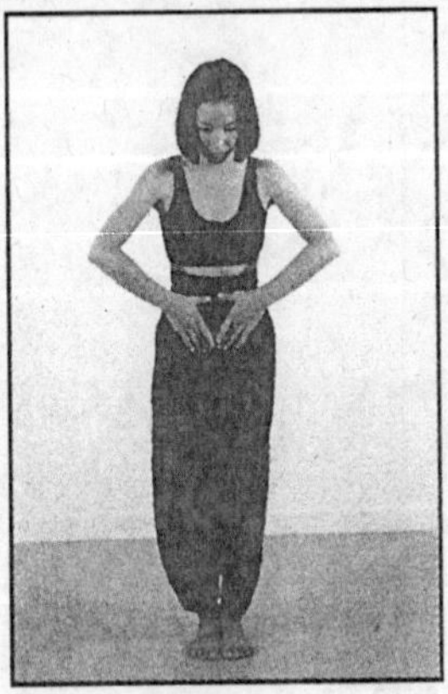
C-39

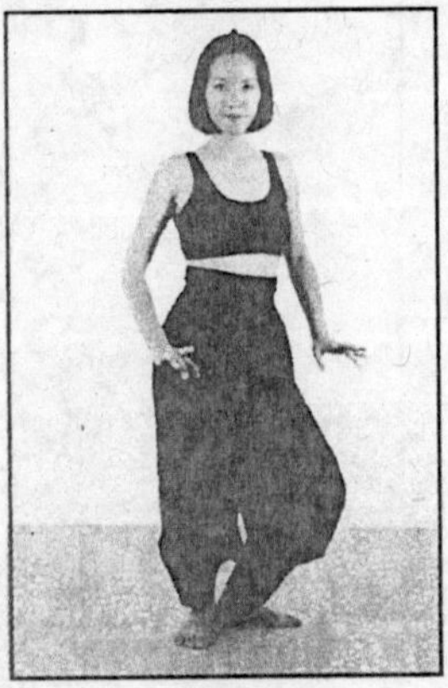
C-40

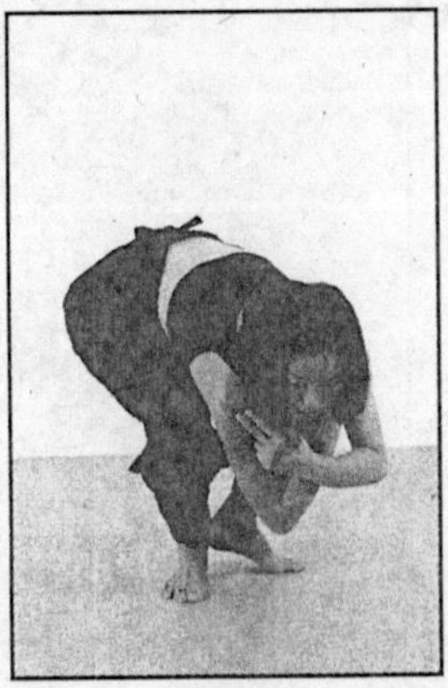
C-41

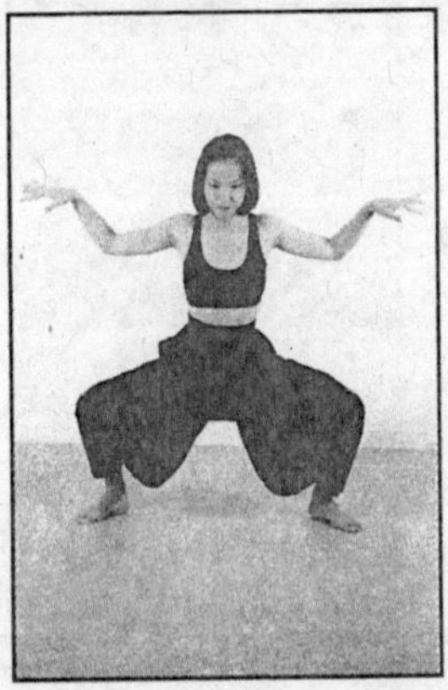
C-42

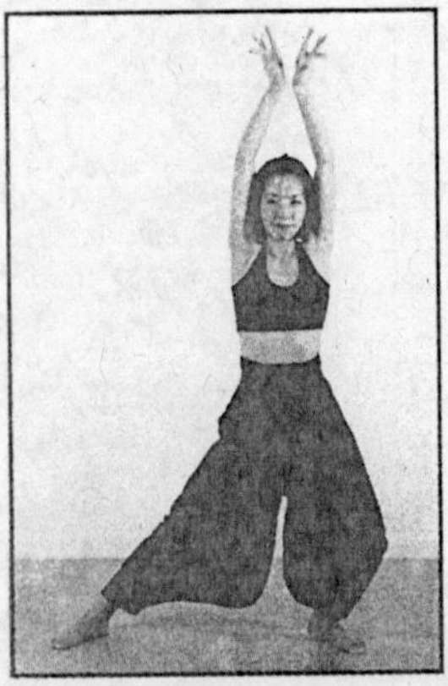
C-43

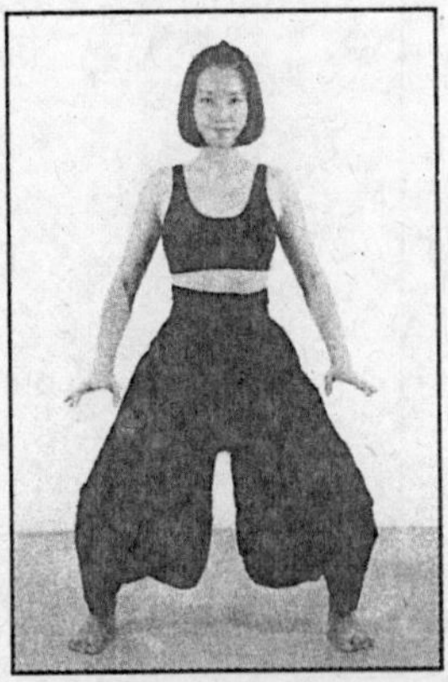
C-44

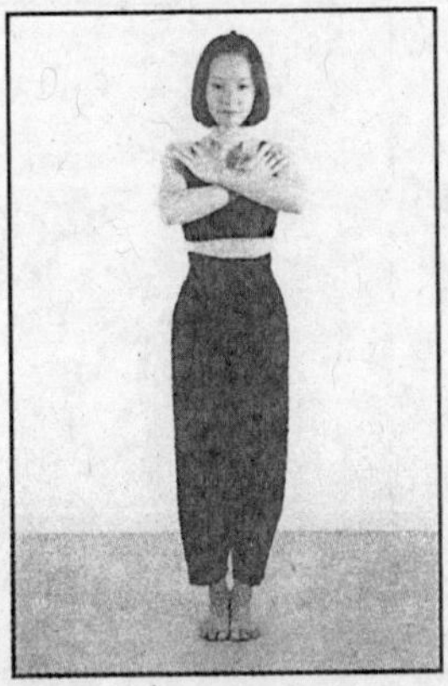
C-45

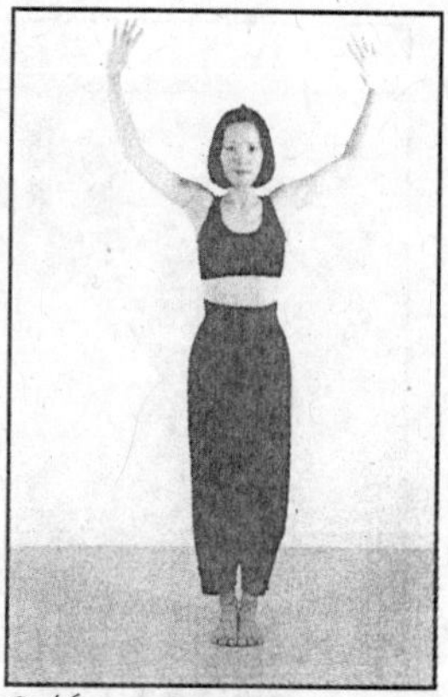
C-46

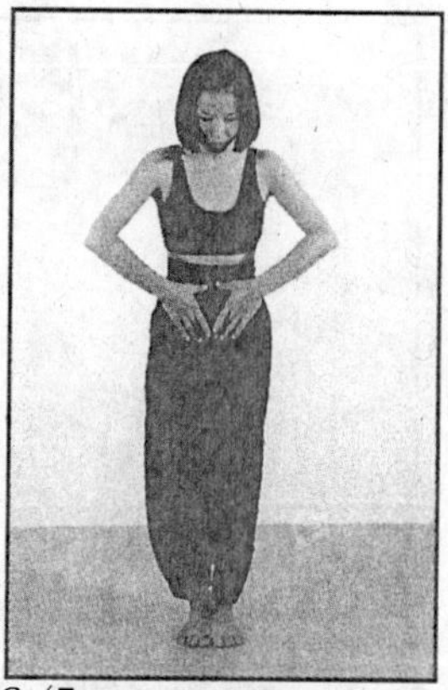
C-47

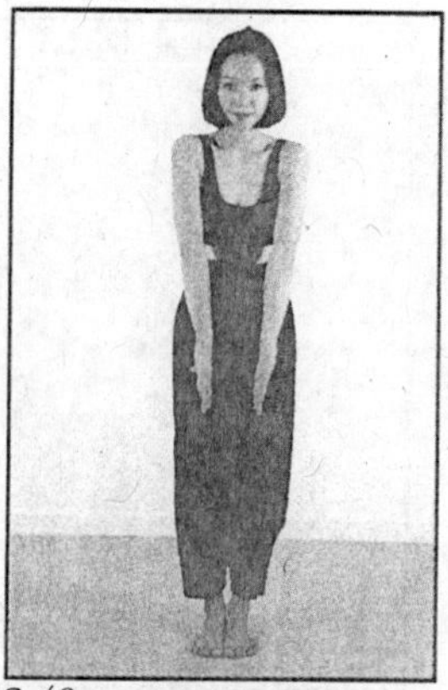
C-48

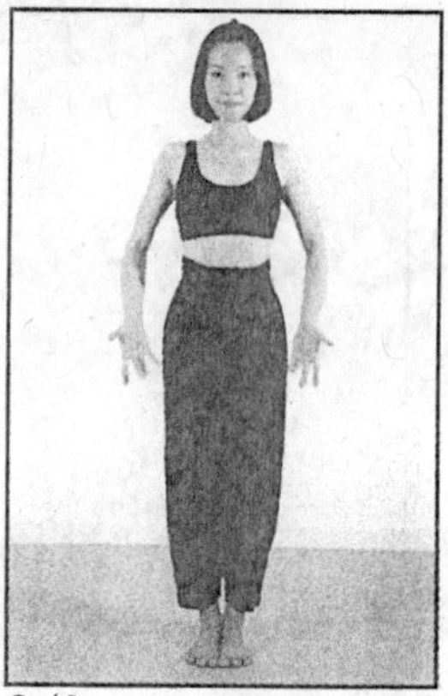
C-49

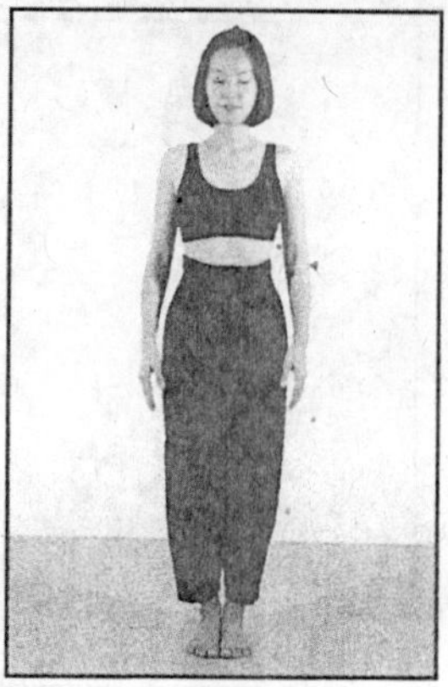
C-50

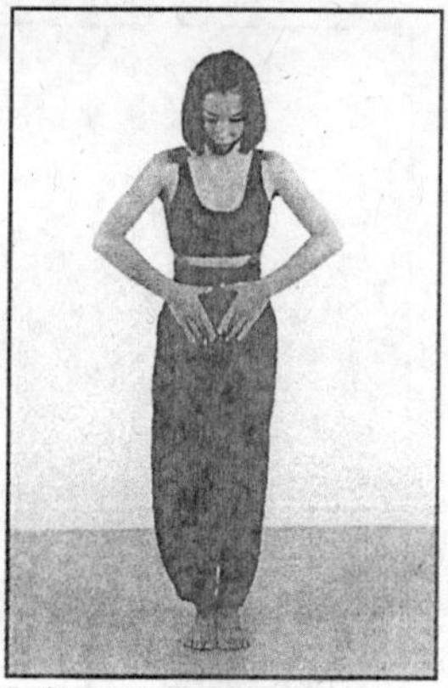
C-51

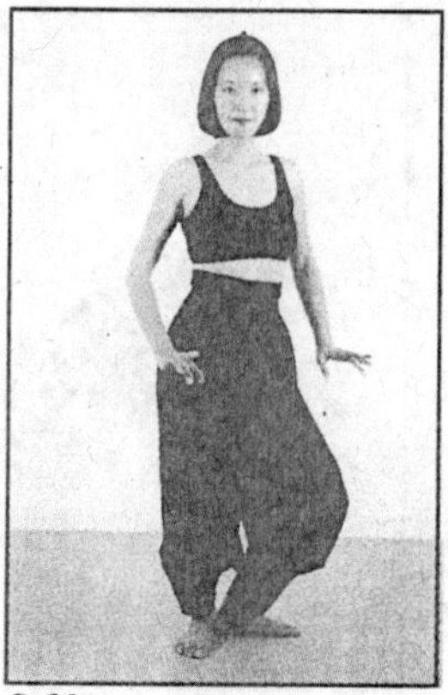
C-52

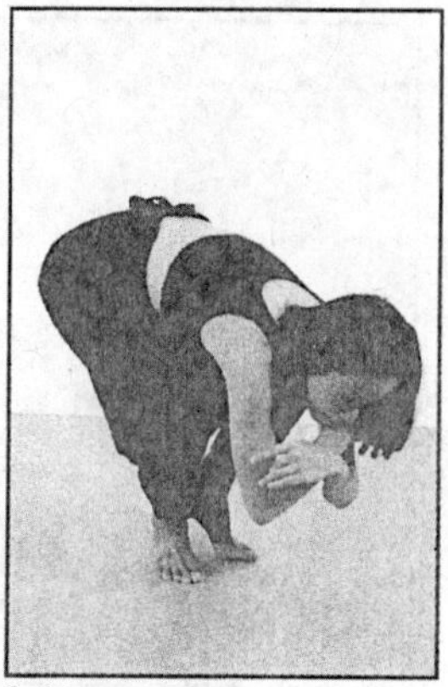
C-53

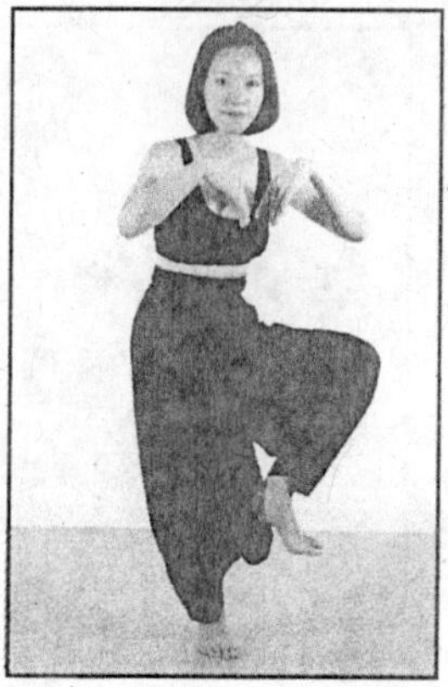
C-54

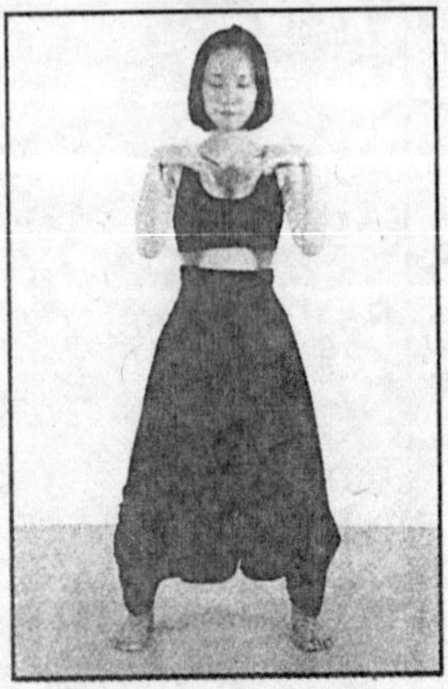
C-55

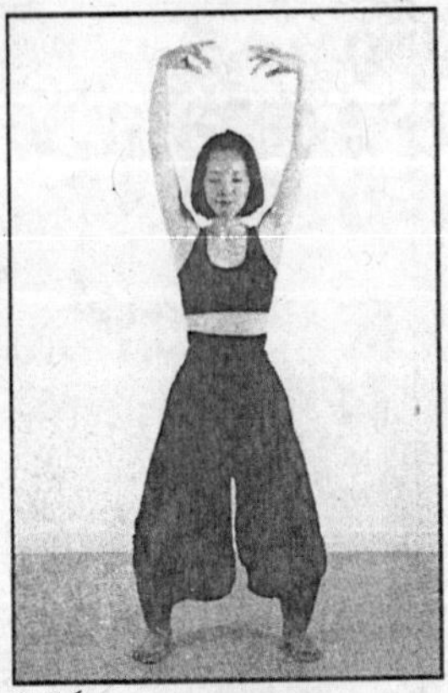
C-56

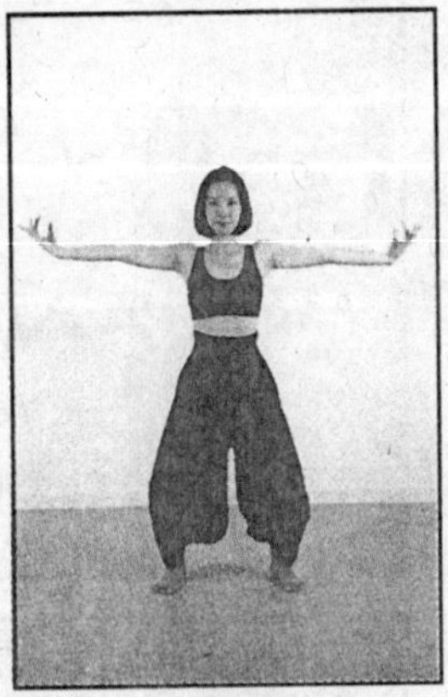
C-57

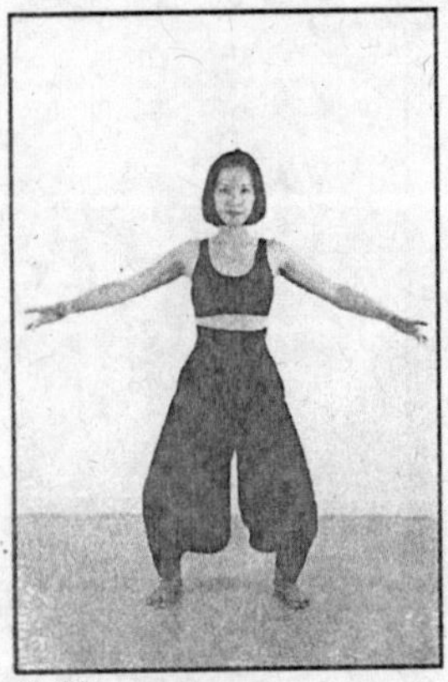
C-58

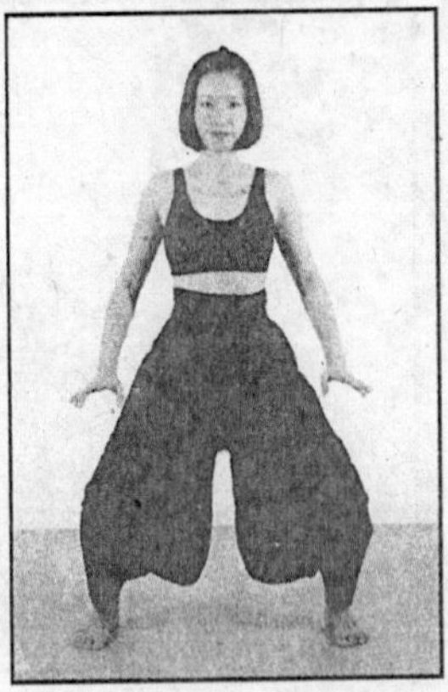
C-59

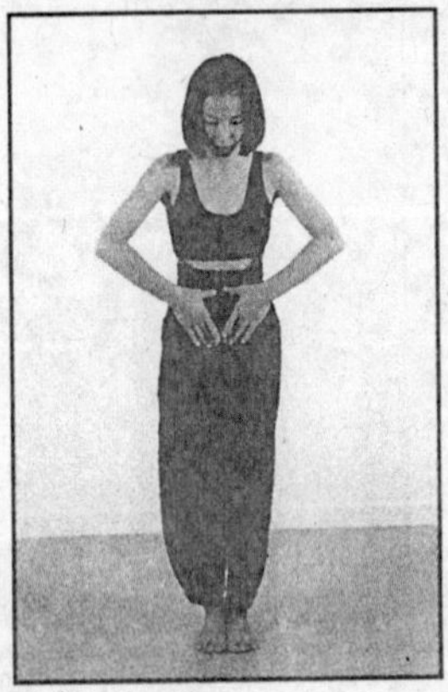
C-60

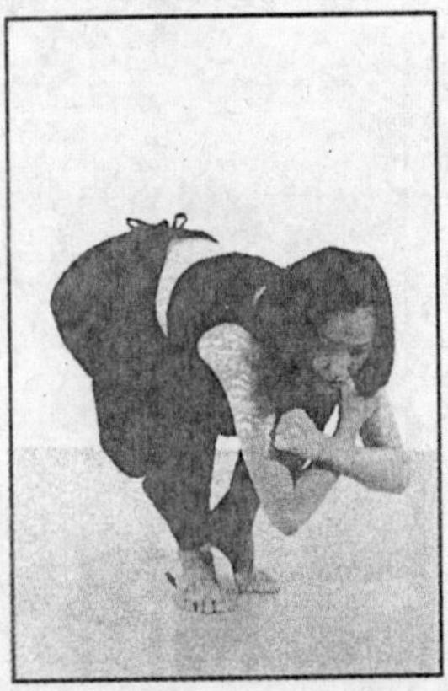
C-61

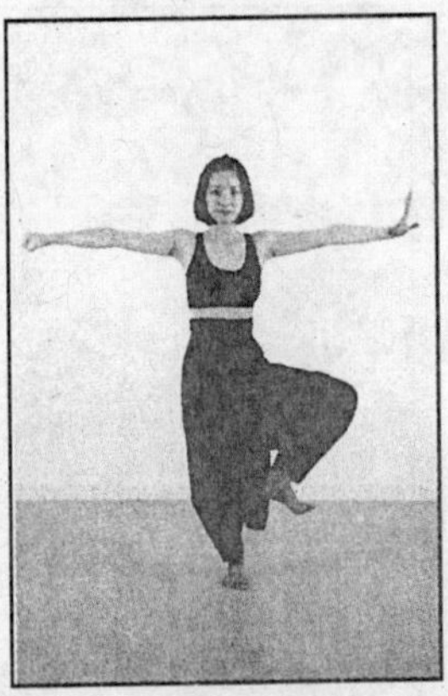
C-62

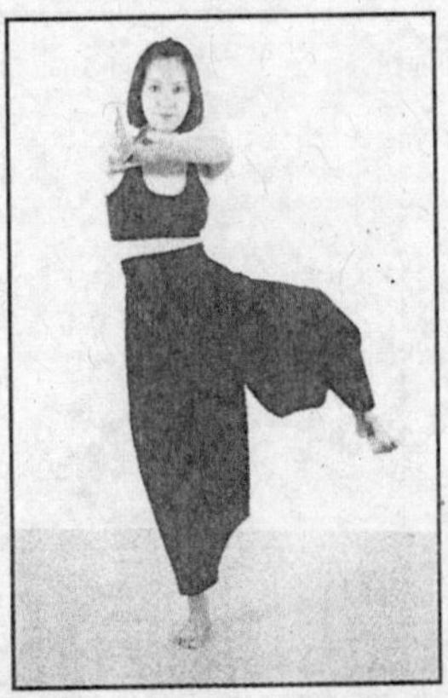
C-63

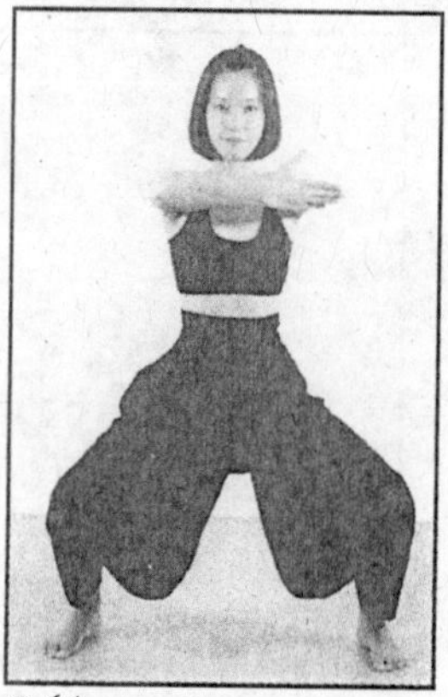
C-64

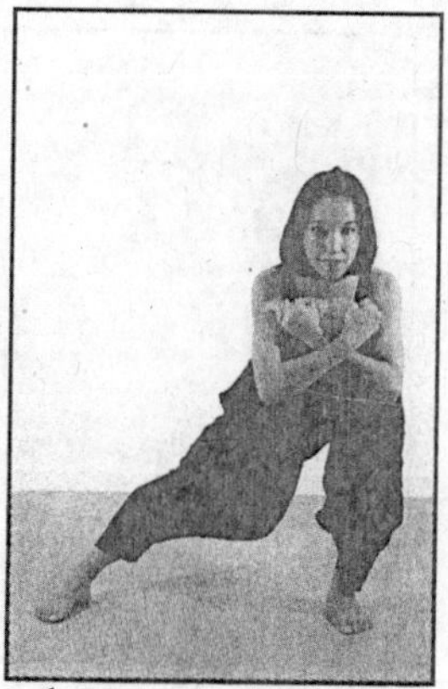
C-65

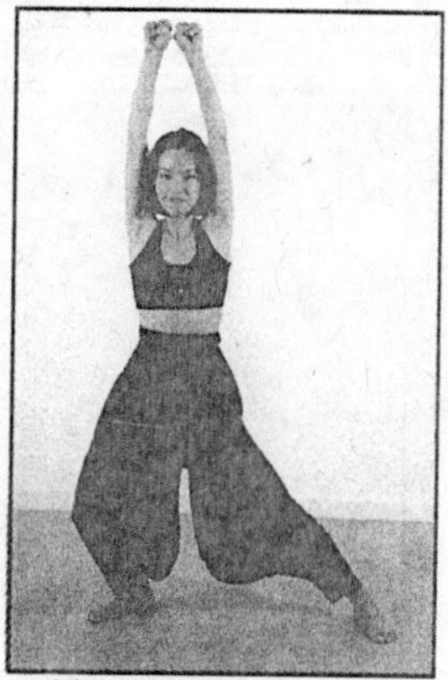
C-66

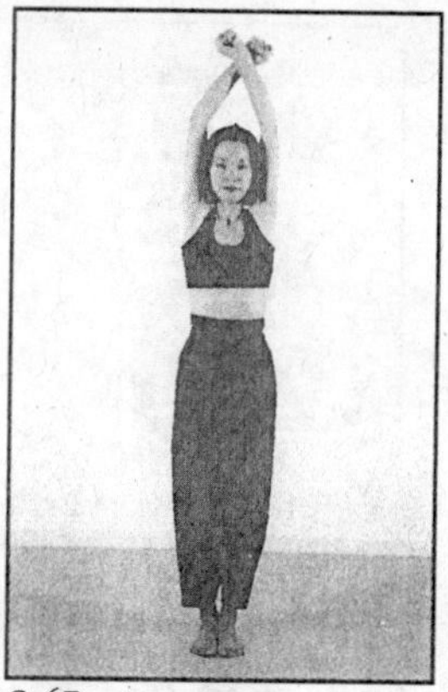
C-67

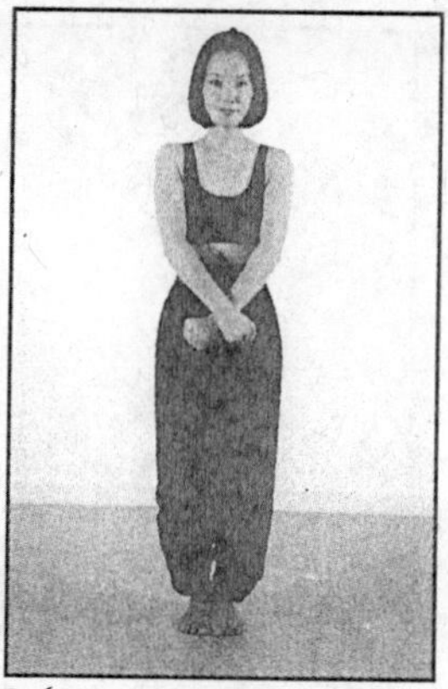
C-68

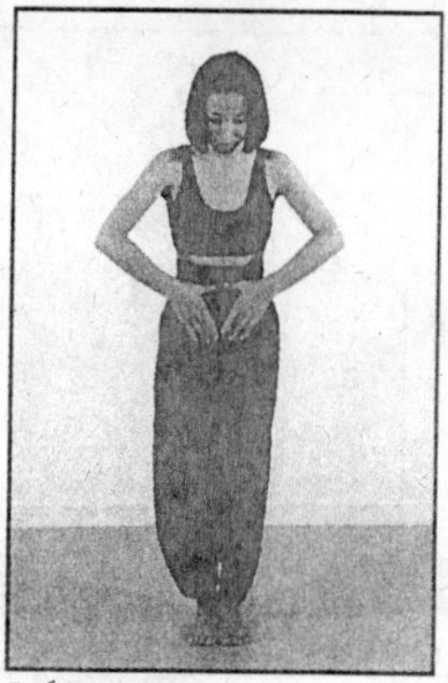
C-69

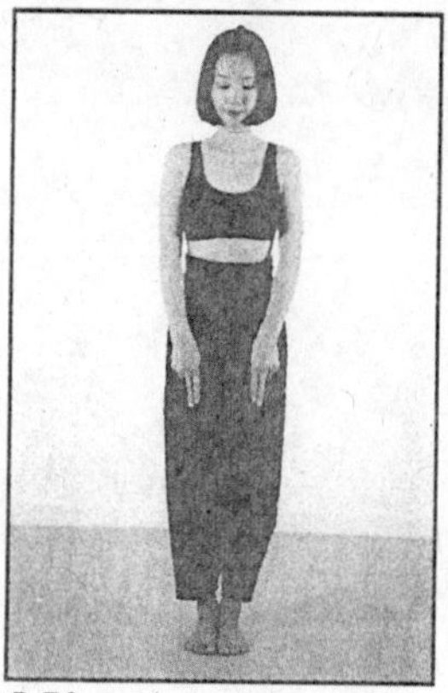
C-70

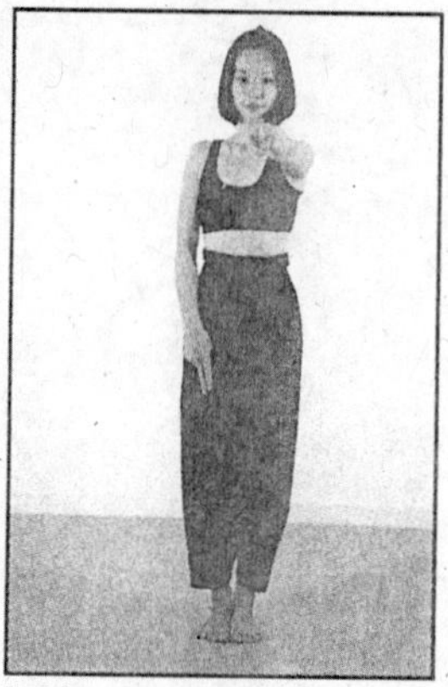
C-71

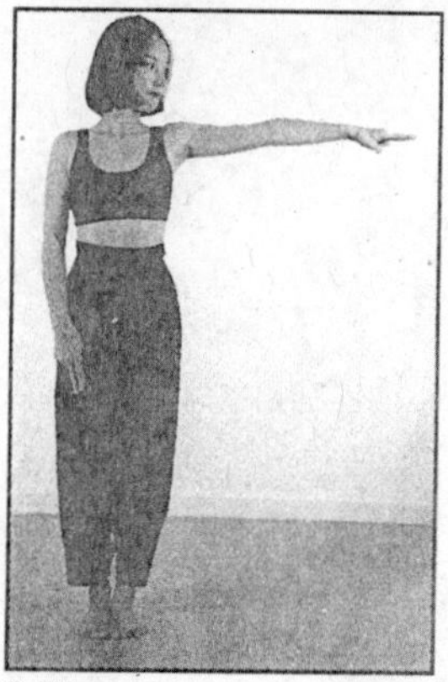
C-72

The movements from C-69 to C-78 are repeated with the other arm.

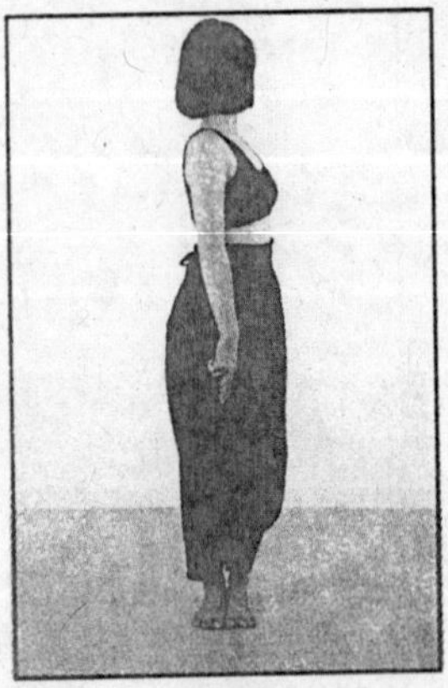
C-73

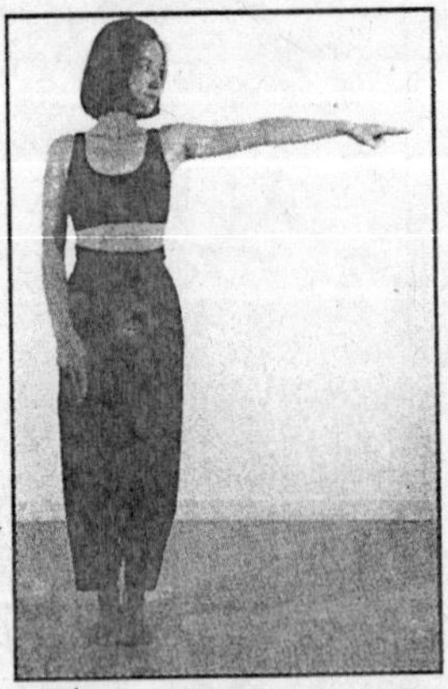
C-74

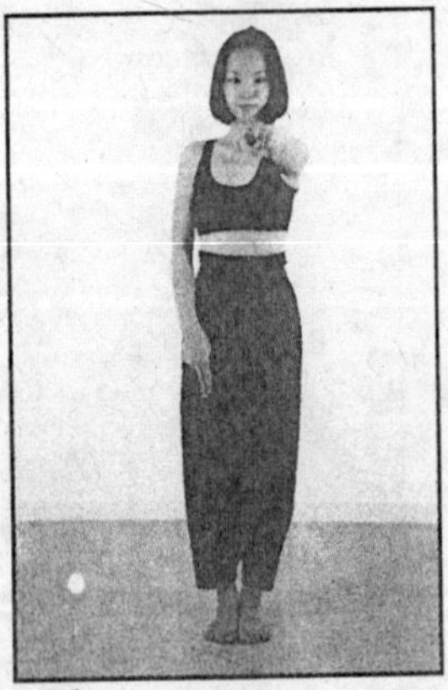
C-75

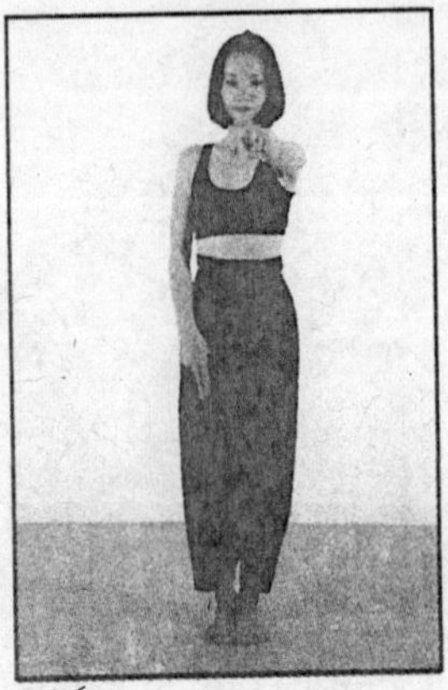
C-76

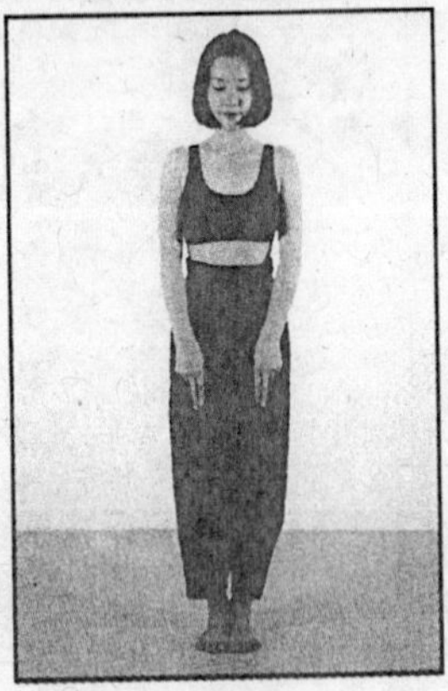
C-77

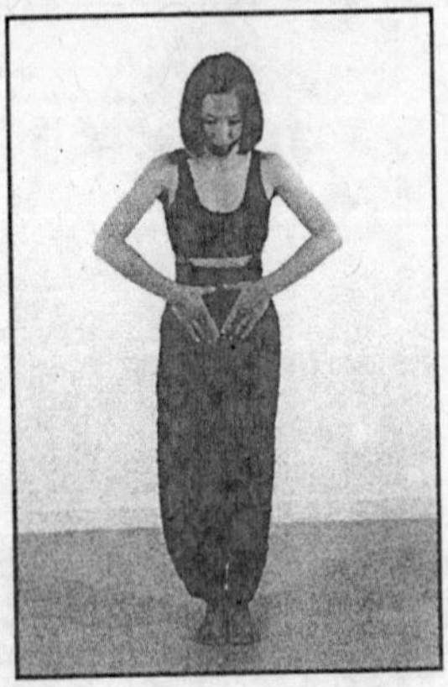
C-78

THREE SERENITIES SERIES (JAPANESE SERIES OF THE THREE PIECES OF KUMAHARA SHORI)

Śama Traya Krama Vyāyāma

As a whole, this series of movements provides very important stretching for the back muscles and the vertebral articulations. It enhances flexibility, rejuvenates the spine and keeps the blood and lymph nerves healthy.

It is appropriate for people who have great physical and mental rigidity.

FIRST MOVEMENT

Vyaṅga pictures: D-1-2-3-4

The inverted mountain

Execution

This movement has already been explained in the *ten* movements that strengthen the essential energy at the core.

SECOND MOVEMENT

Vyaṅga pictures: D-5-6-7-8-9-10-11-12

Linking ha and ṭha

This vyaṅga is performed by keeping the hips and the body firmly placed. The abdomen is pulled in and the chest projected forwards with the spine upright and the vertebras well placed one over the other. Thorough breaths are performed, using the three areas of the lungs, balancing the entrance of air to the higher, middle and lower areas of the lung, providing them with greater capacity. This movement strengthens the talas of the shoulders, the muscles of the arms and makes the joints of the elbows and shoulders more flexible.

Execution

With the legs and feet together, inhaling and raising the hands, we clench the fists with strength until shoulder level. Here the air is retained and the fists are turned, moving to the centre of the chest and with a bhrā marī exhalation we release the tension in the fists, lowering them to the ground in front of the chest.

THIRD MOVEMENT

Vyaṅga pictures: D-13-14-15-16-17

The step of the powerful dragon

This movement has already been explained in the Ten movements that strengthen the essential energy at the core.

FOURTH MOVEMENT

Vyaṅga pictures: D-18-19-20-21-22-23-24-25-26-27

Scalding the cotton

This movement is appropriate for improving mind-body coordination.

The exercise of opening and closing the fingers activates and helps to regulate the functioning of diverse internal organs due to the connection that exists between them through the nāḍī channels.

It strengthens the muscles of the arms and legs and provides flexibility to the wrists and hands, preventing degenerative osteoarthritis.

The hand and its finger distribution is one of the organs that allows for the faculty of intelligence and this is why the execution of this vyaṅga helps to maintain mental activity agile. The movement of the hands is very important for the mental development of children.

Execution

With the legs open and the feet parallel, raise the arms in front of the body and separate them at shoulder width until parallel to the ground. Once here, the hands are crossed, closing and opening the fingers and turning the wrists.

FIFTH MOVEMENT

Vyaṅga pictures: D-28-29-30-31-32-33-34

The Itorsion of the fish prince

This movement produces a very important effect on the articulations of the spine, especially at the lumbar and sacral levels. It stimulates the nerves that go through the vertebrae of these areas and the organs they connect with. It unblocks the vertebral articulations and allows the elimination of negative and already utilized energy through the feet when the body is turned to the back. It compresses the inner organs from both sides, especially the intestines, by influencing the peristalsis.

The movement of the hands results in the elimination of excess heat. It provides tranquility in relation to disturbing mental emotions such as anger, excessive happiness, fear, anguish, obsession, sadness and fright.

Execution

Starting with the legs and the feet parallel, we inhale moving the hands towards the tan. We then exhale while turning the trunk towards the back accompanied by one hand. The other hand remains in front, in the same line as the other hand. The palms are facing down and the knees are bent and opened to the sides. The movement is then repeated on the other side.

SIXTH MOVEMENT

Vyaṅga pictures: D-35-36-37-38-39-40-41-42-43-44

The mystic tree

This movement has been explained in the Ten movements that strengthen the essential energy at the core.

SEVENTH MOVEMENT

Vyaṅga pictures: D-45-46-47-48

The dancer

This movement strengthens the muscles of the legs and keeps the spinal joints flexible on both sides. It widens the pelvic region and one side of the abdomen is extended while the other side is laterally bent, keeping the abdominal muscles in good condition. The lateral movement of the spine may alleviate suffering for people with lumbar stiffness.

Execution

The starting position is with the feet together and the hands on the tan, one over the other with the palms facing opposite sides. The left leg is moved with the right hand, which virtually pushes the left leg by performing an opening. The right arm keeps going up dragging the left arm with it. The left leg stays on the ground while the left arm is extended parallel to the ground, flexed in a 90-degree angle next to the head. From here, the trunk is laterally flexed to the right while the left arm is placed above the head and the right arm goes down to be placed parallel to the trunk. The middle fingers of each hand are united by a virtual cord and the arms are held as if they were holding a sphere between them.

This position is undone by moving the trunk back to the centre with the arms opened at the same level of the shoulders and lowering them, reintegrating the left leg to its starting point. Then the posture is repeated on the other side.

EIGHTH MOVEMENT

Vyaṅga pictures: D-49

Sustaining the heavy mountain

This movement strengthens the muscles of the legs and lungs and expands them.

Execution

With the legs separated and the arms laterally extended at shoulder height and parallel to the ground, the legs are flexed projecting the direction of the knees to the sides of the body.

NINTH MOVEMENT

Vyaṅga pictures: D-50-51-52-53-54-55-56-57-58

The turtle

This movement keeps the lumbar-sacral articulation and other joints of the spinal column very flexible because the whole body bends when descending.

It descends all the back muscles, eliminating possible pain. It compresses all the internal organs improving their functioning and stretches and relaxes the entire upper body area.

Execution

Starting from the sustained mountain vyaṅga, the trunk is bent by taking the arms and the head to the space between the legs and from there they return to where they started from, taking the arms above and behind the back, and while exhaling we place the hands at the same level as the hips. Extending the arms forward we stretch the back and we return by bringing the hands back to the tan.

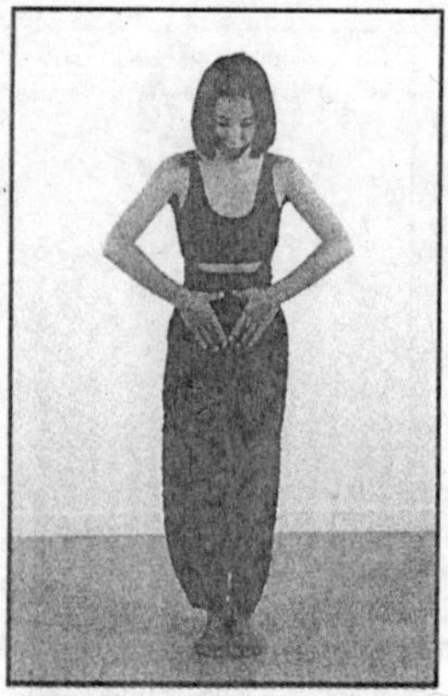
D-1

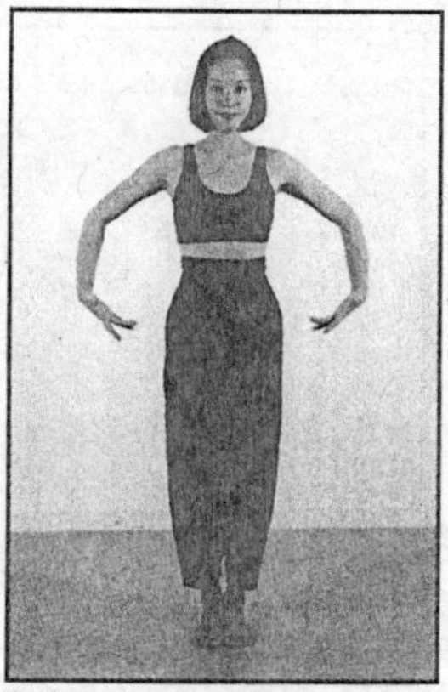
D-2

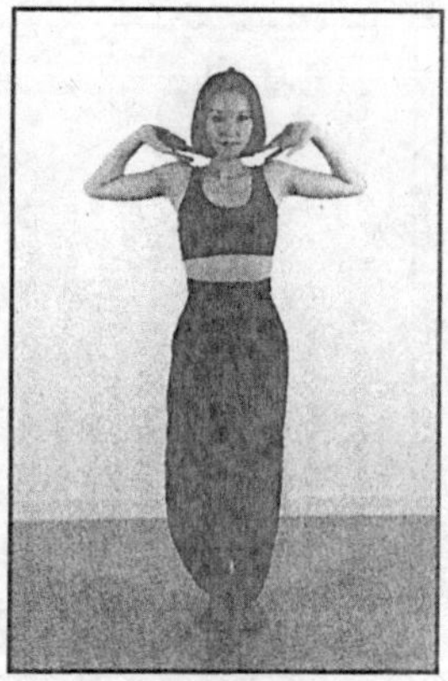
D-3

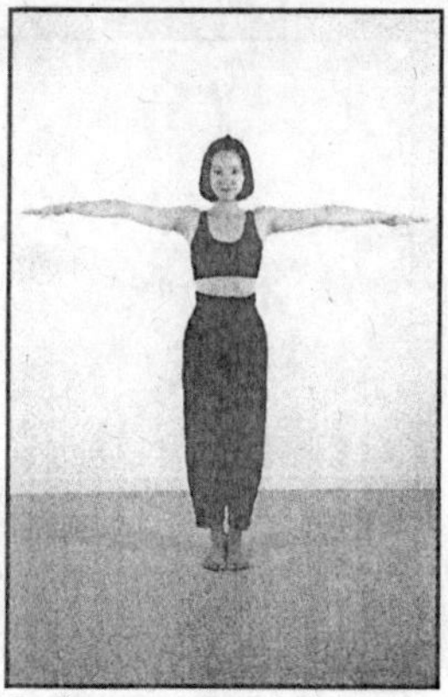
D-4

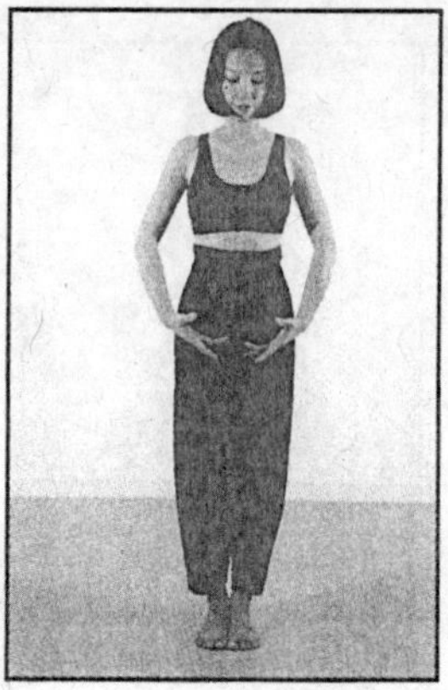
D-5

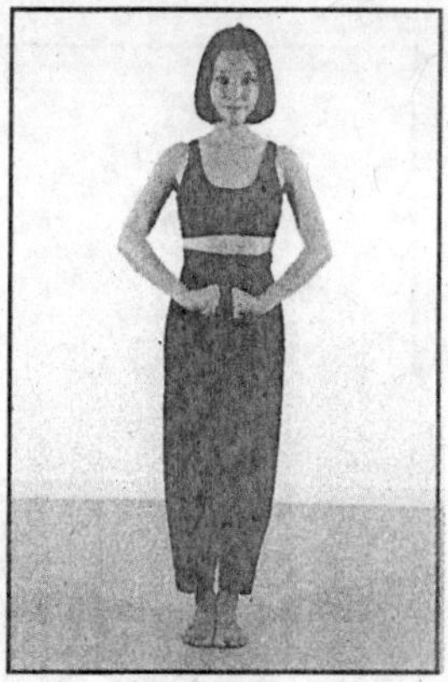
D-6

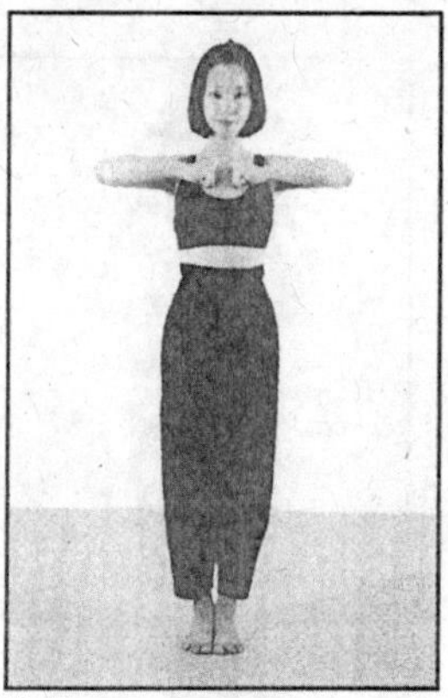
D-7

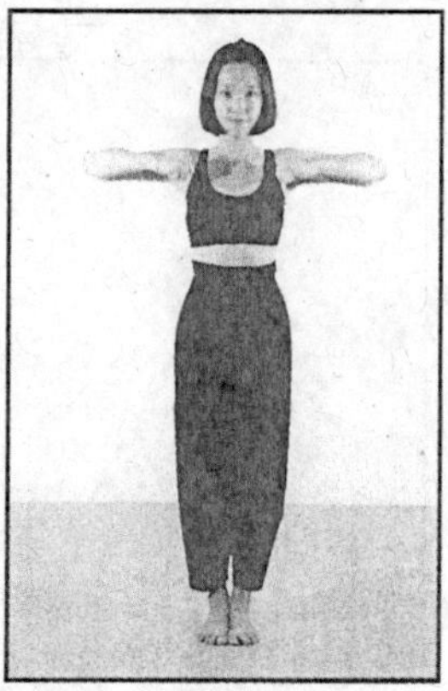
D-8

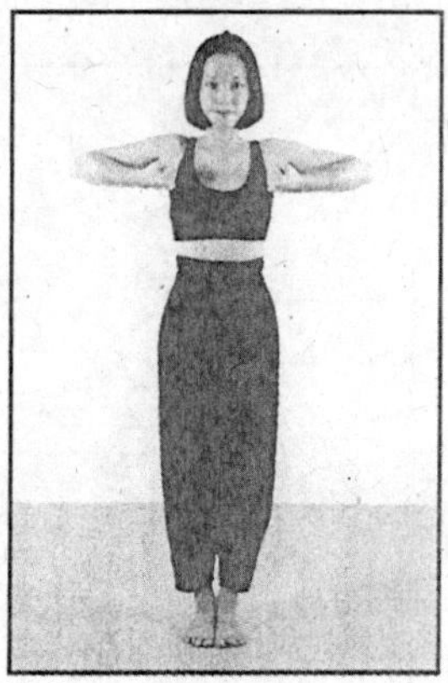
D-9

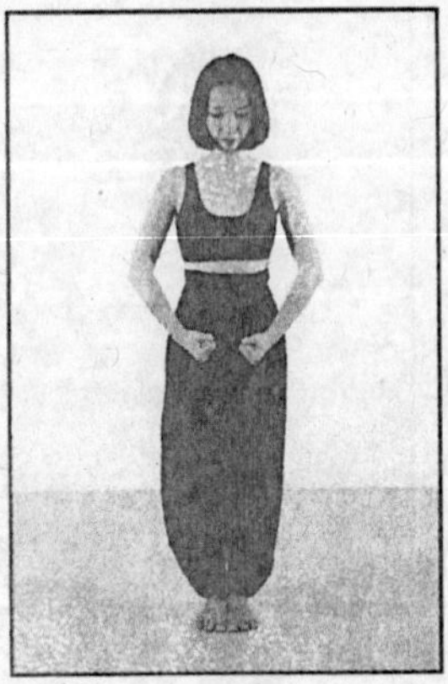
D-10

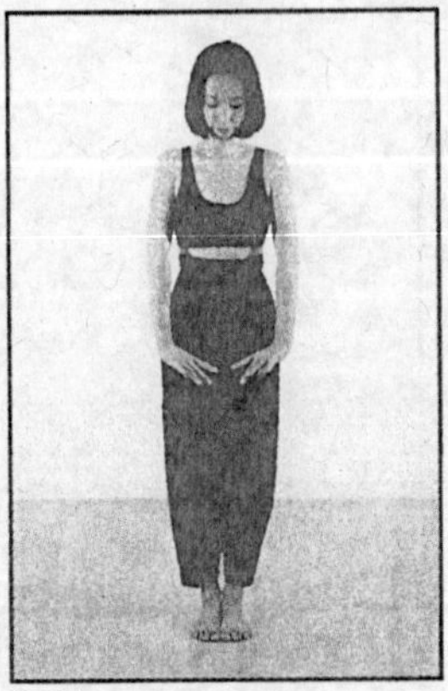
D-11

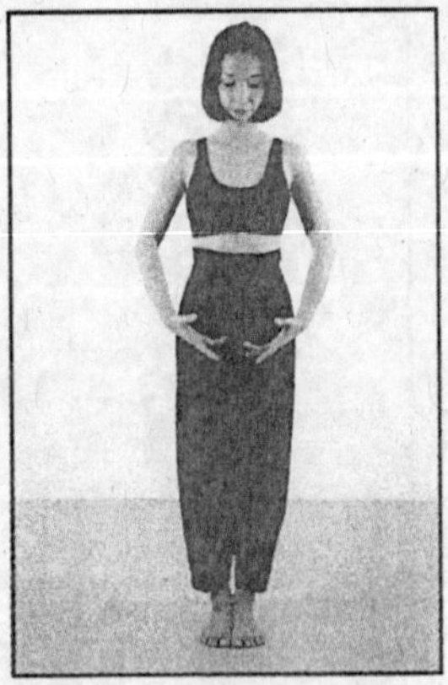
D-12

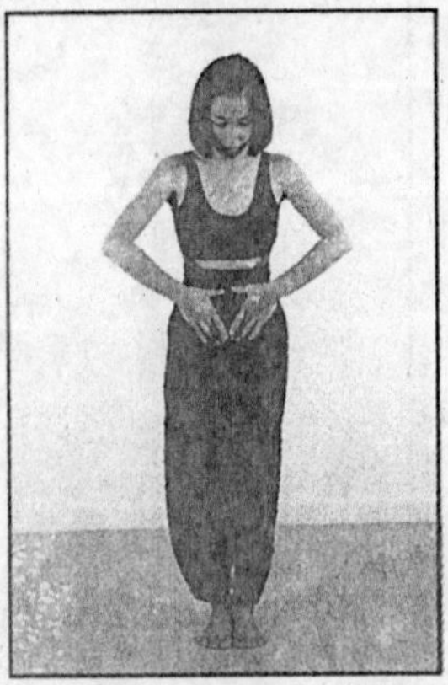
D-13

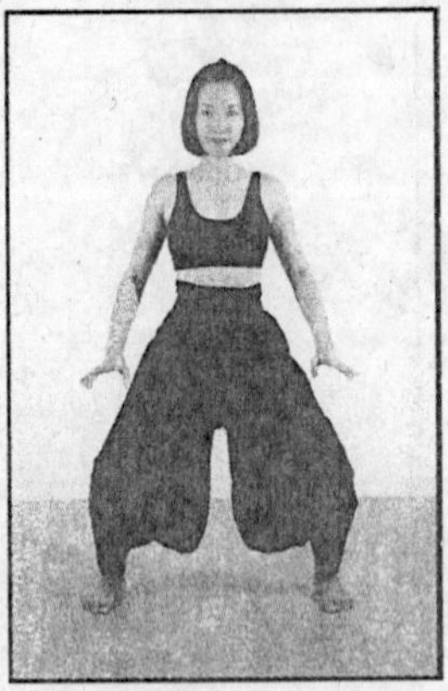
D-14

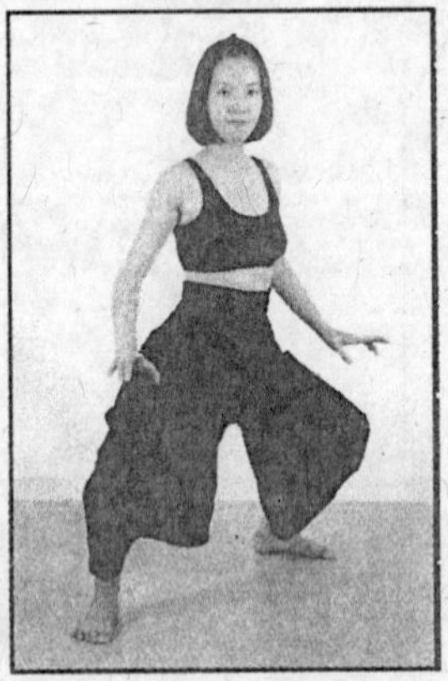
D-15

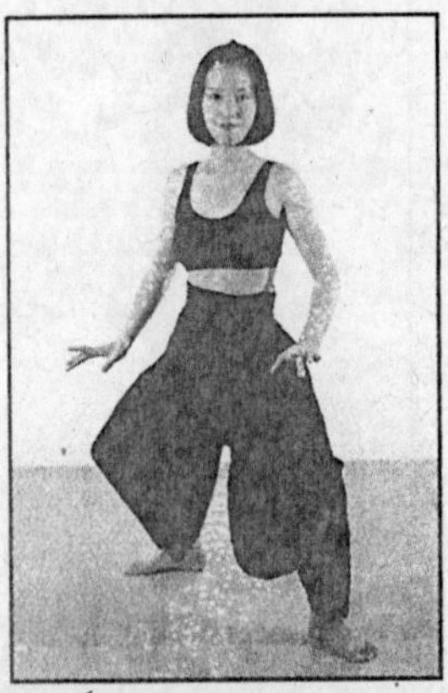
D-16

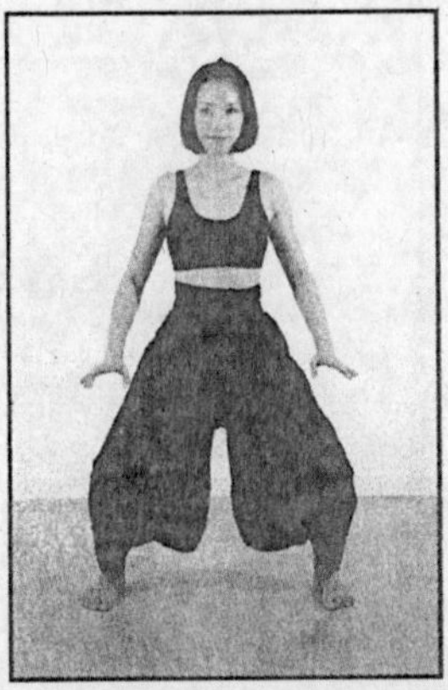
D-17

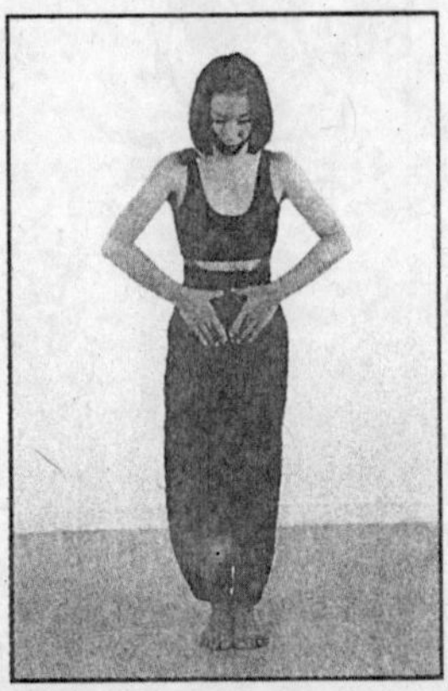
D-18

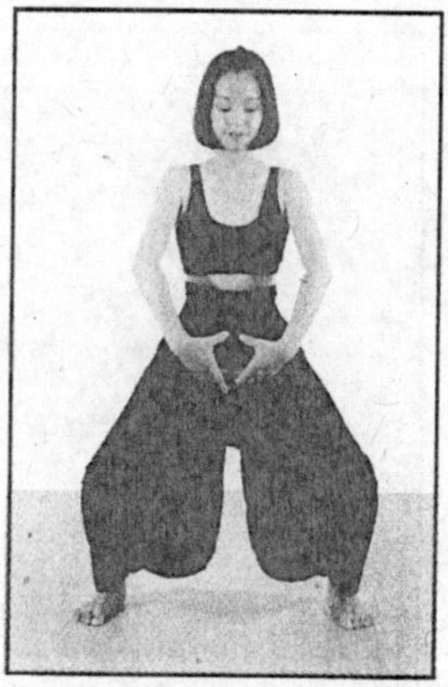
D-19

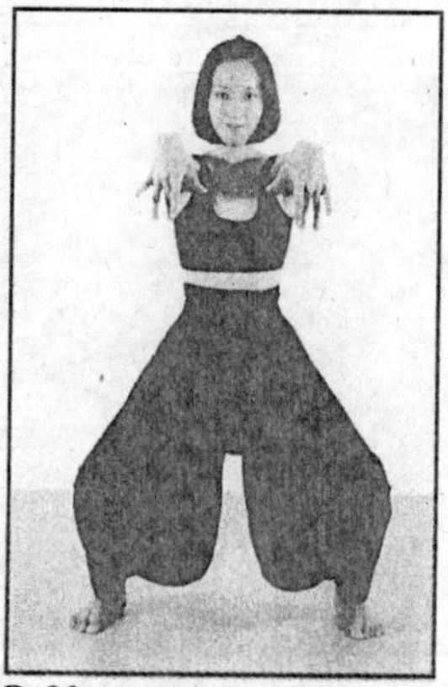
D-20

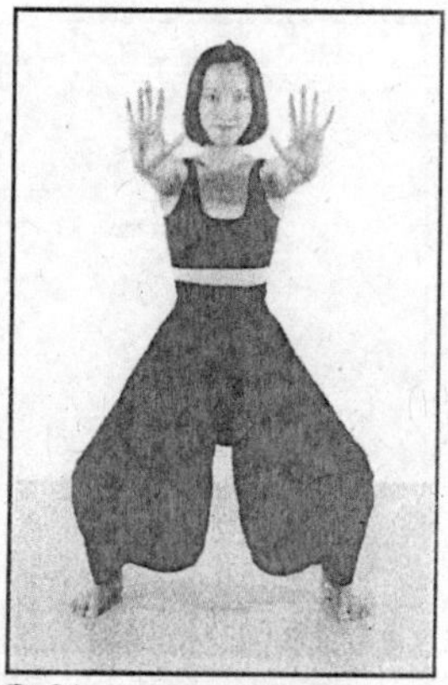
D-21

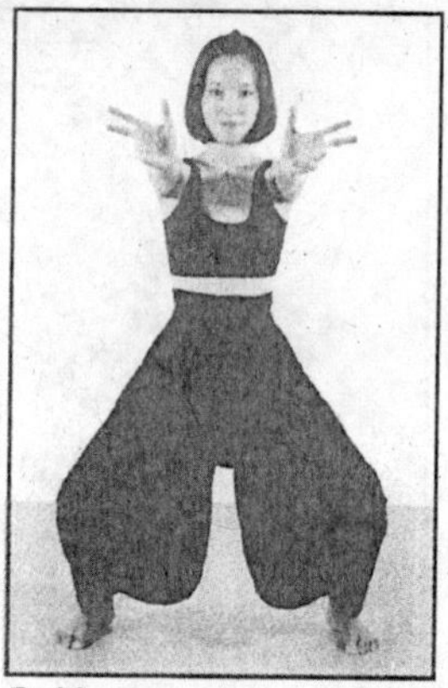
D-22

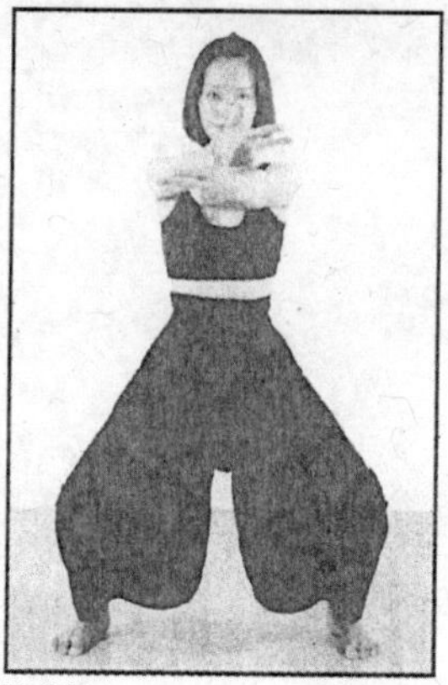
D-23

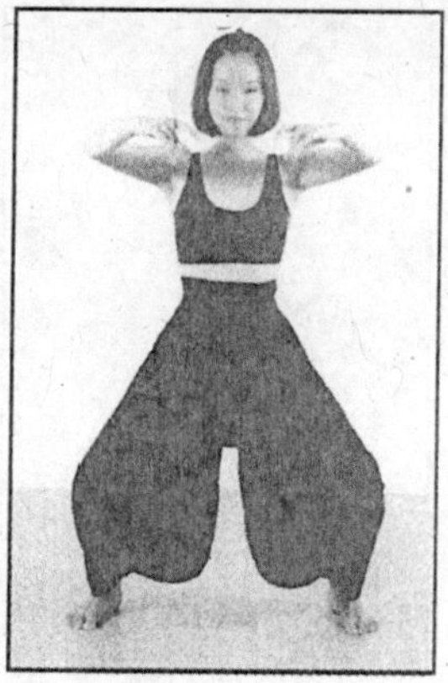
D-24

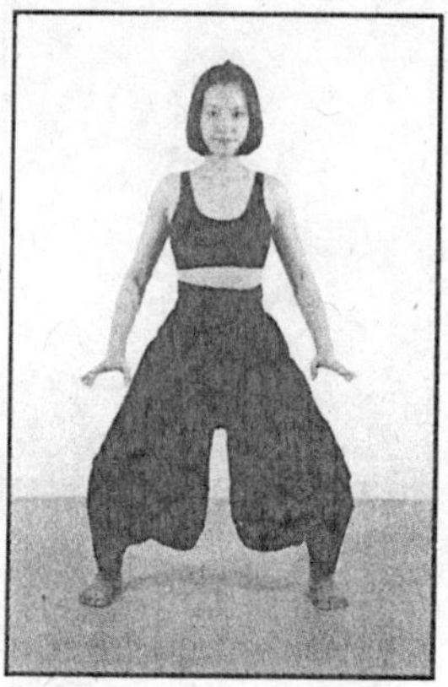
D-25

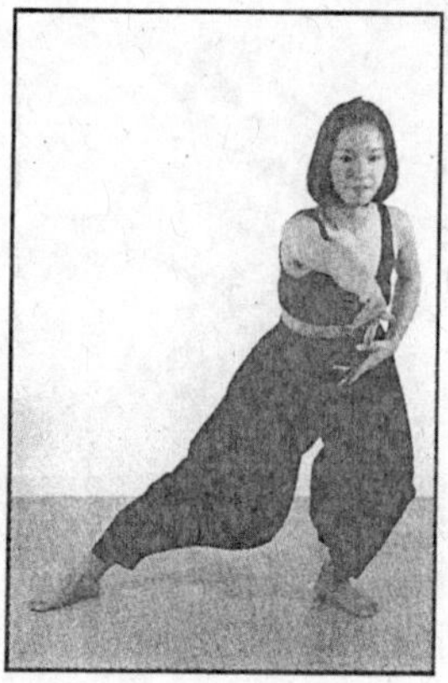
D-26

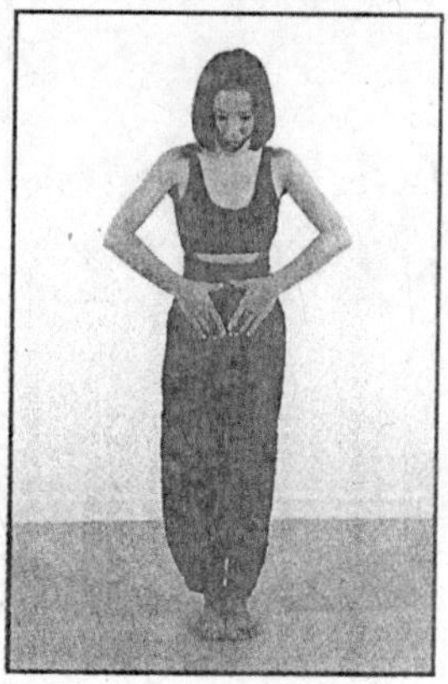
D-27

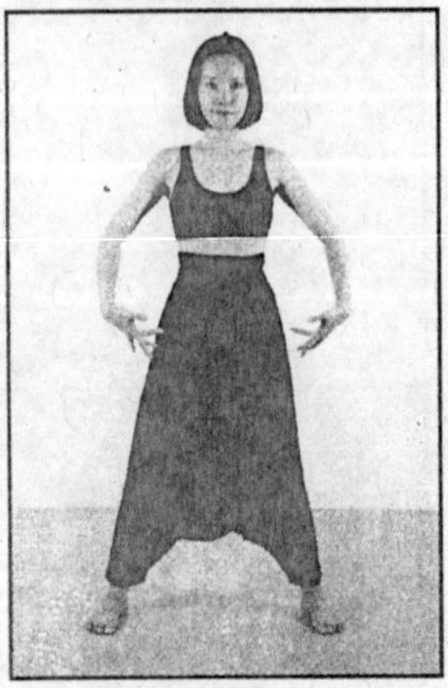
D-28

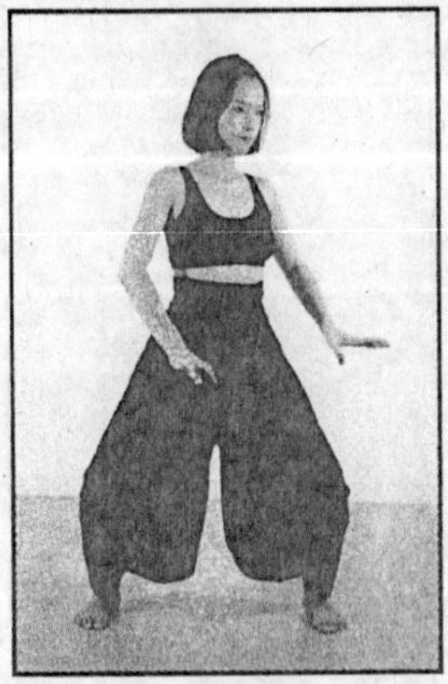
D-29

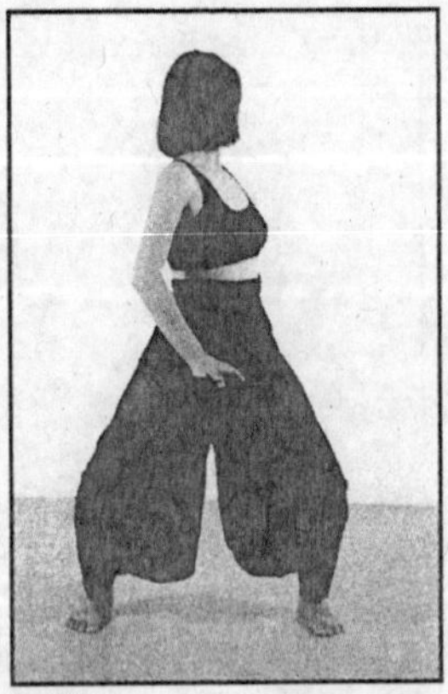
D-30

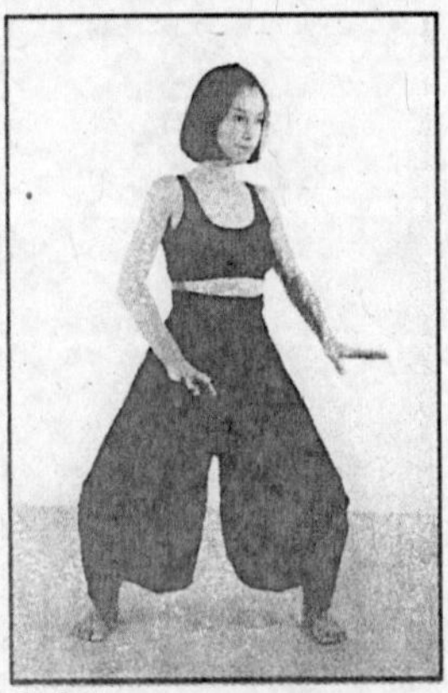
D-31

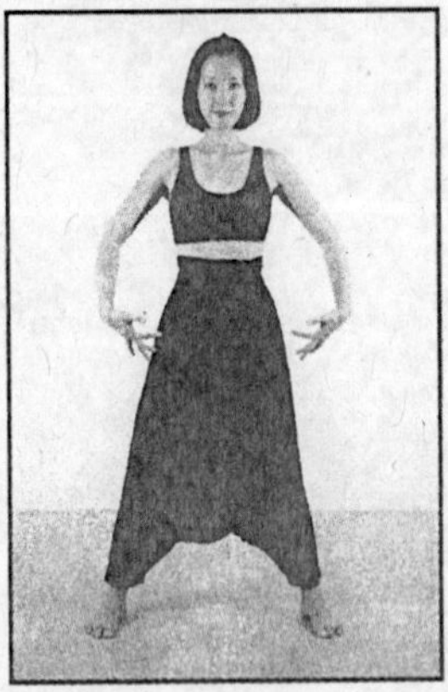
D-32

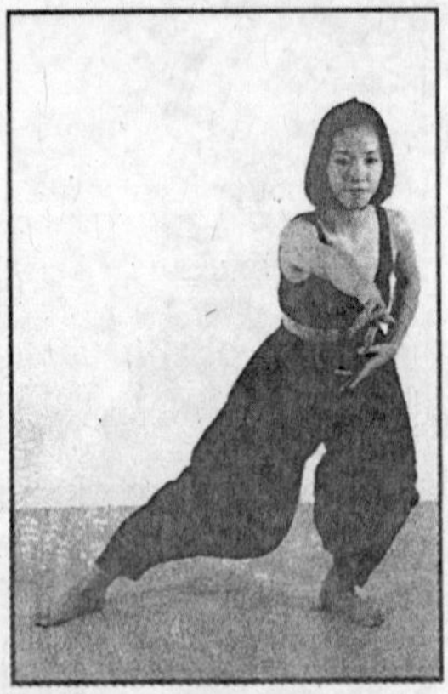
D-33

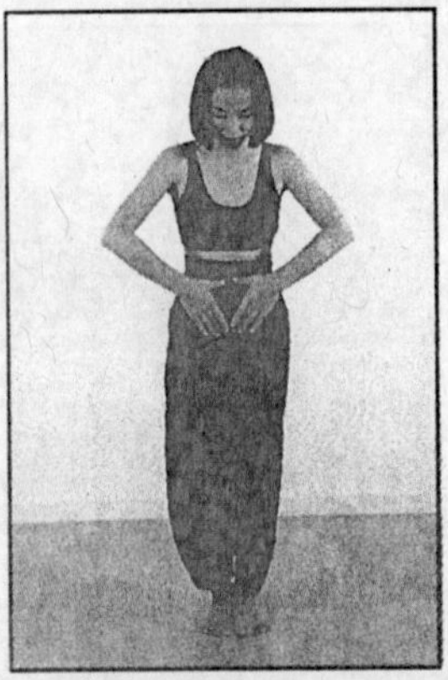
D-34

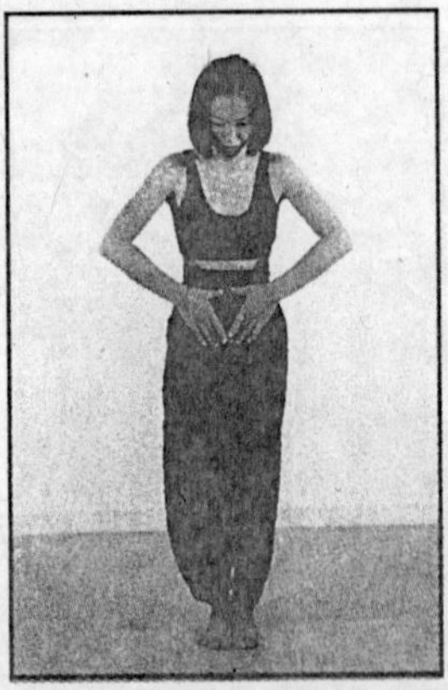
D-35

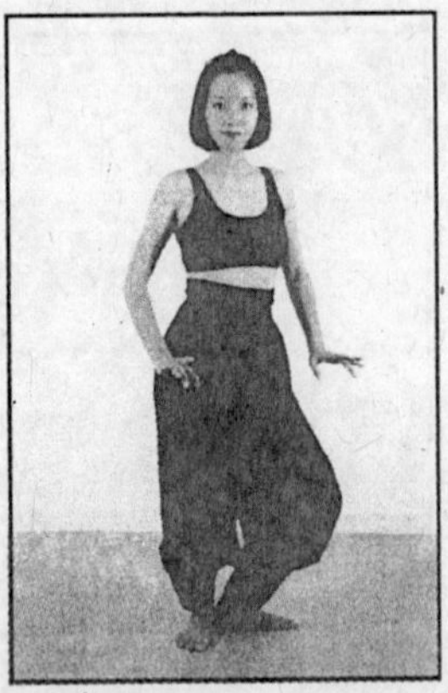
D-36

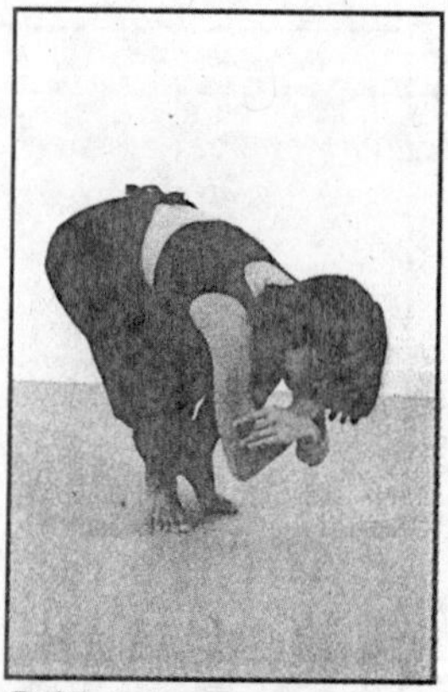
D-37

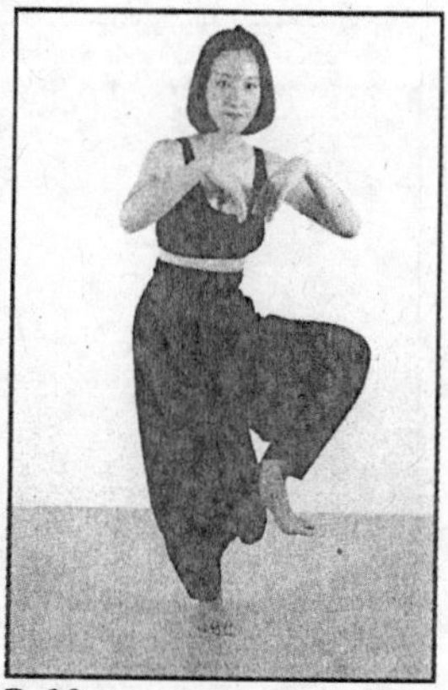
D-38

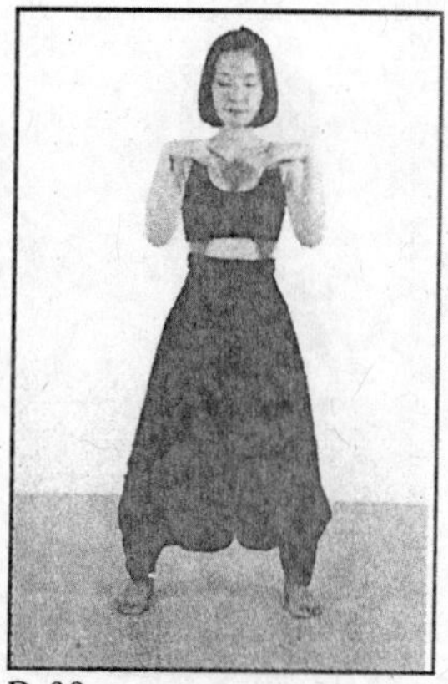
D-39

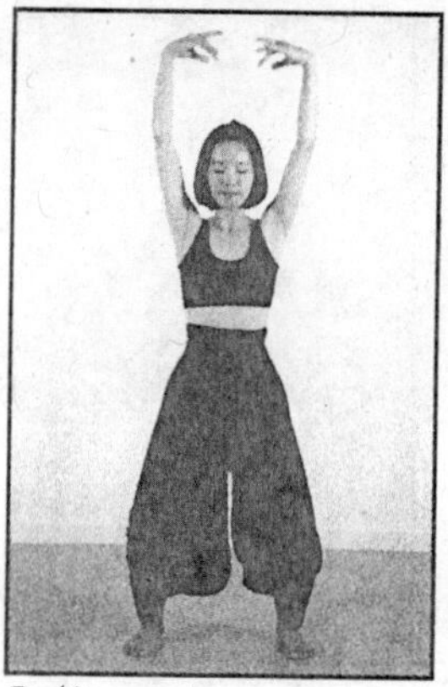
D-40

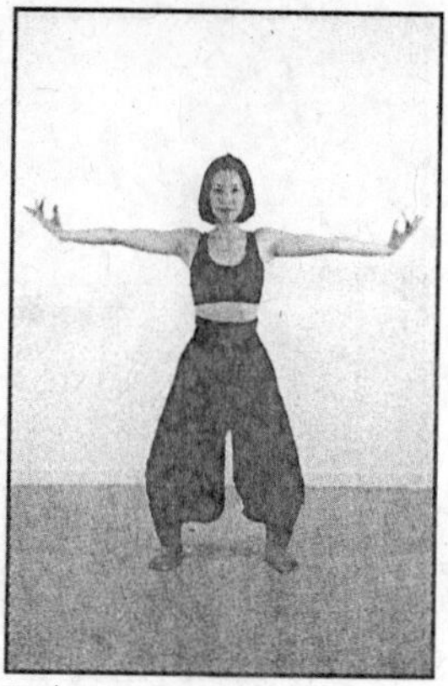
D-41

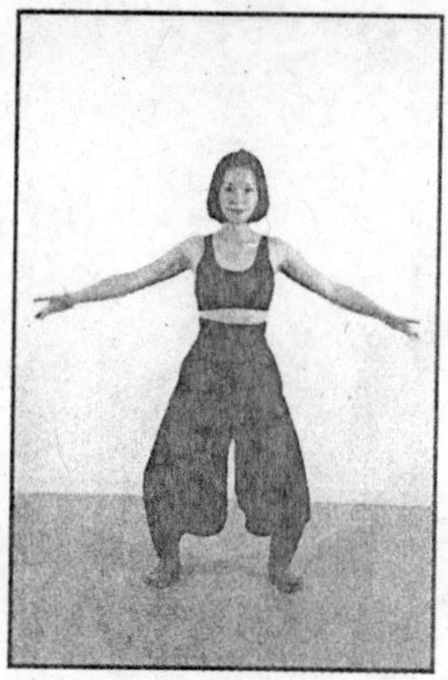
D-42

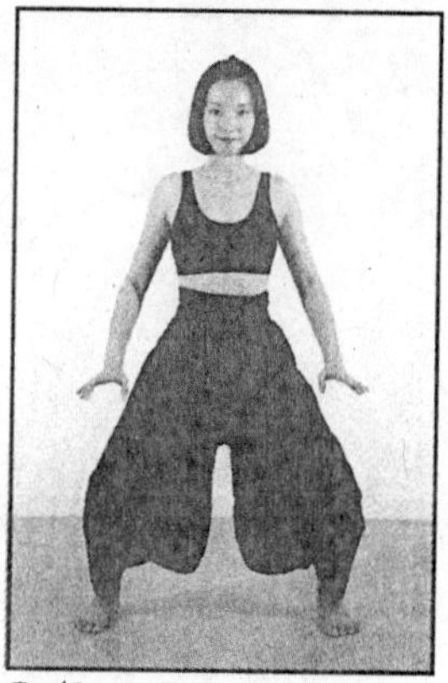
D-43

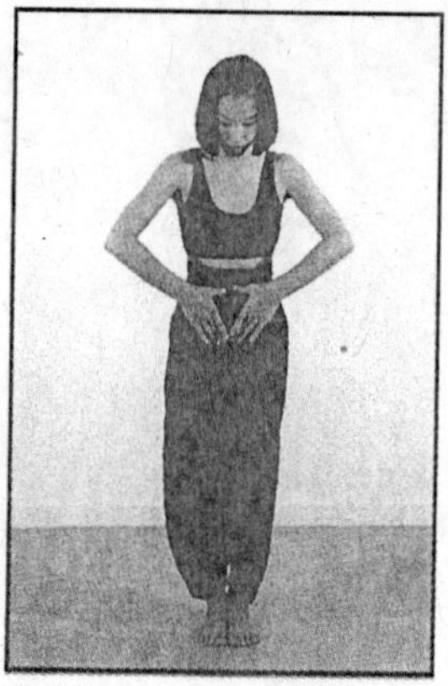
D-44

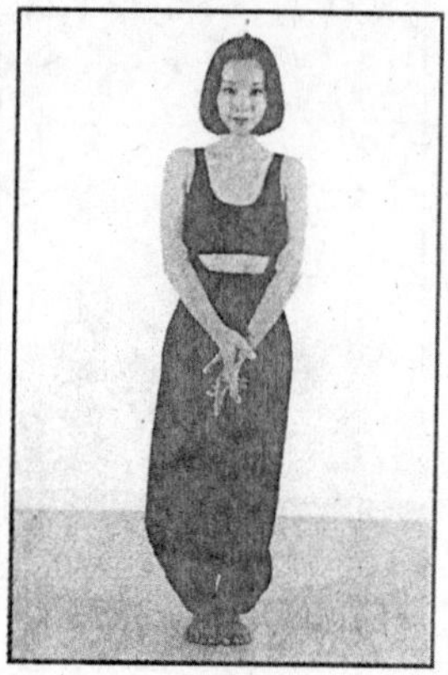
D-45

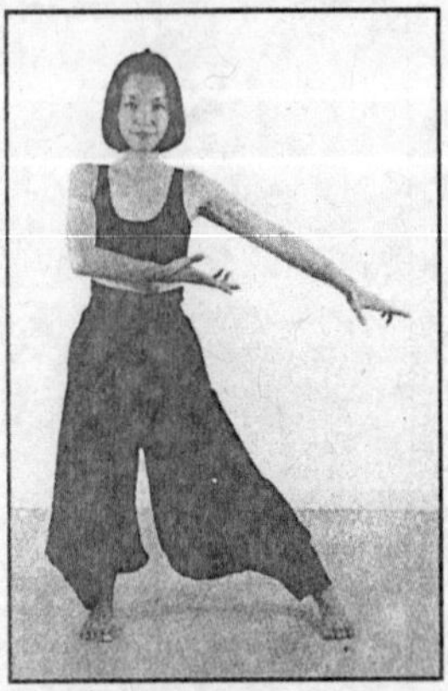
D-46

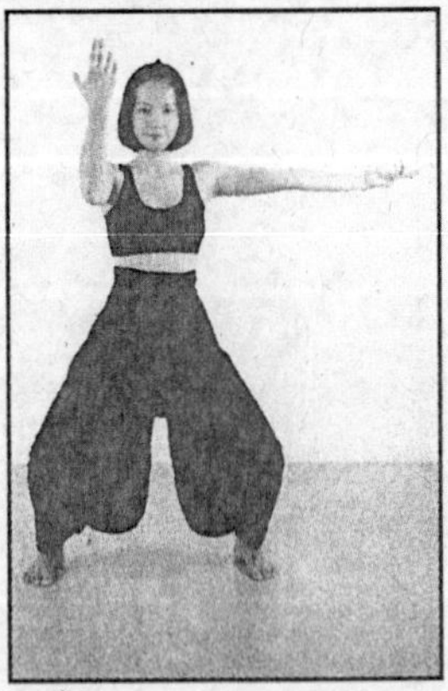
D-47

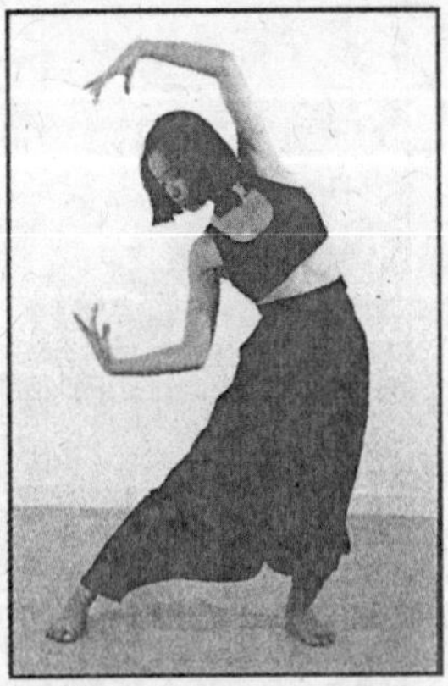
D-48

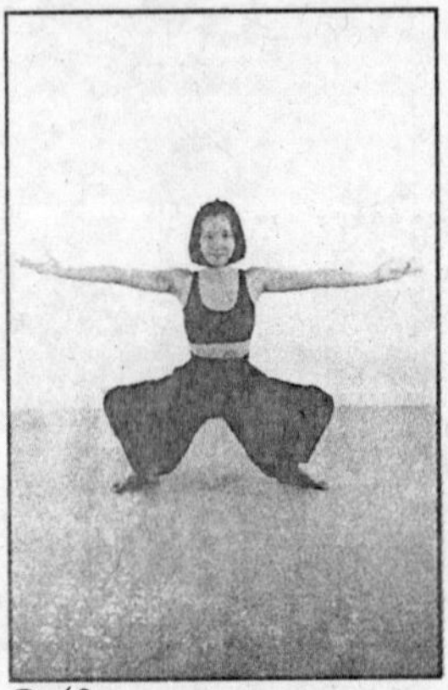
D-49

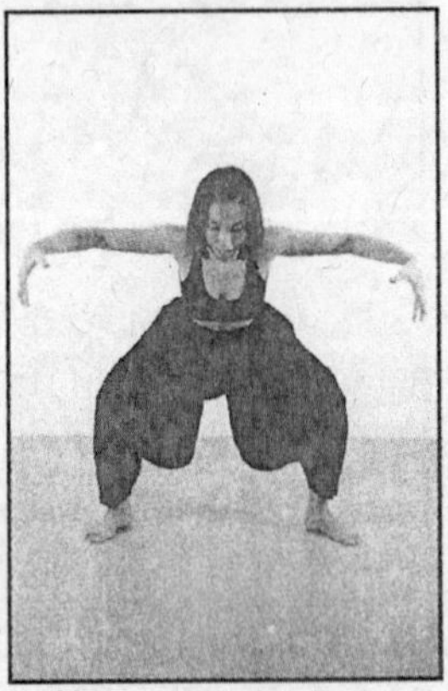
D-50

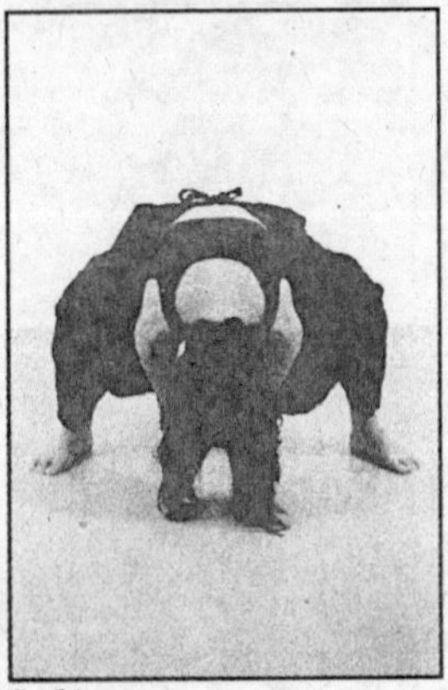
D-51

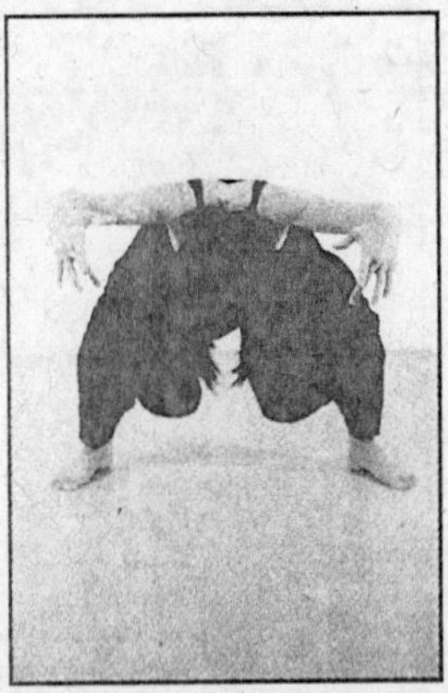
D-52

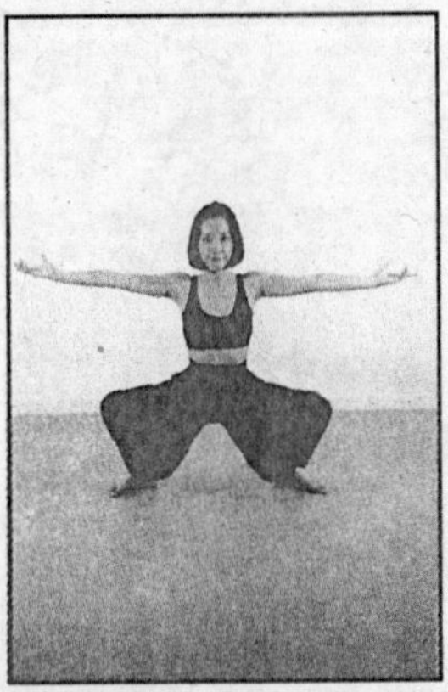
D-53

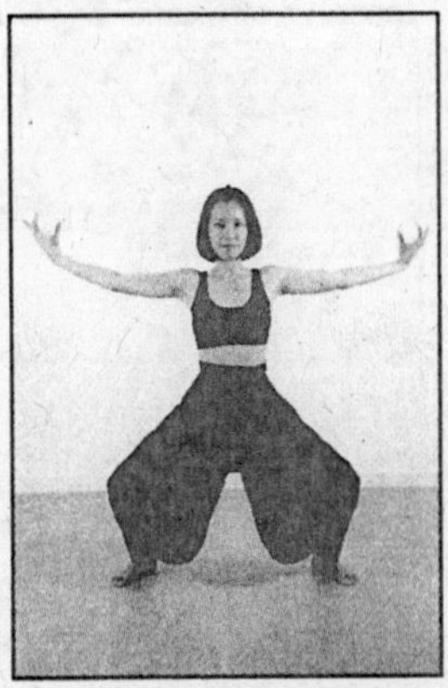
D-54

The movements from D-45 to D54 are repeated, flexing the trunk to the other side.

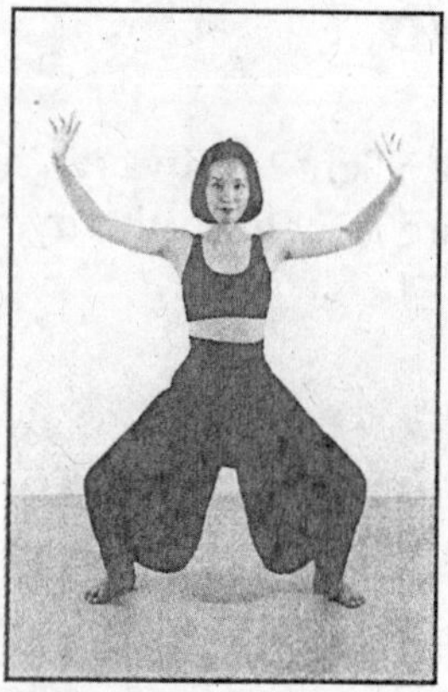
D-55

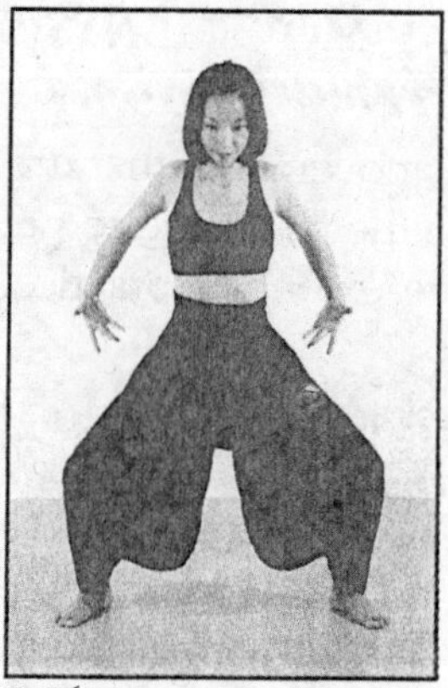
D-56

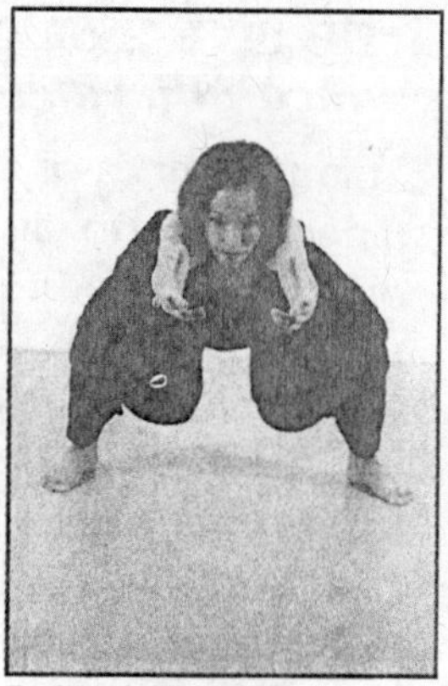
D-57

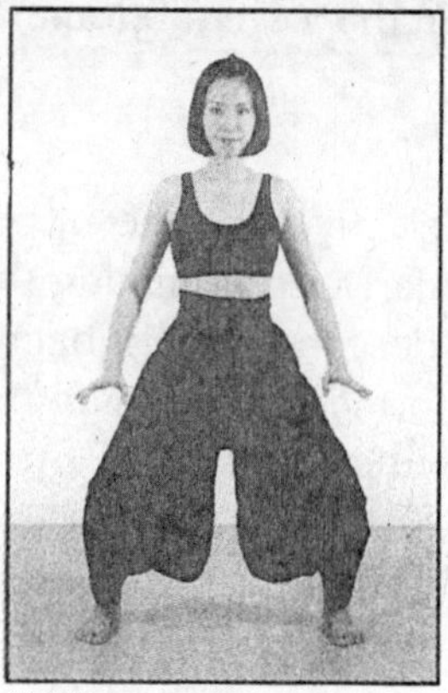
D-58

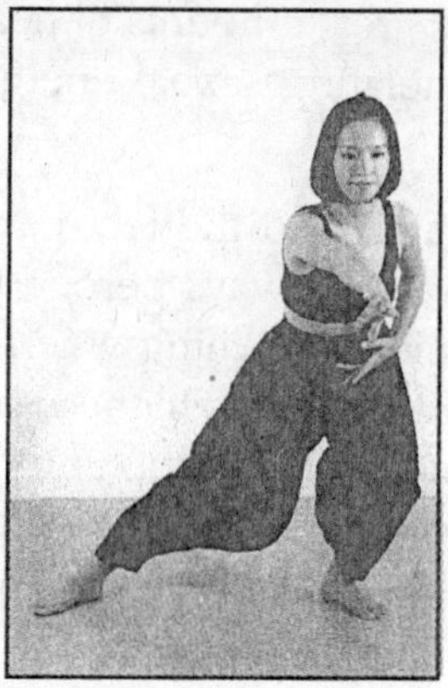
D-59

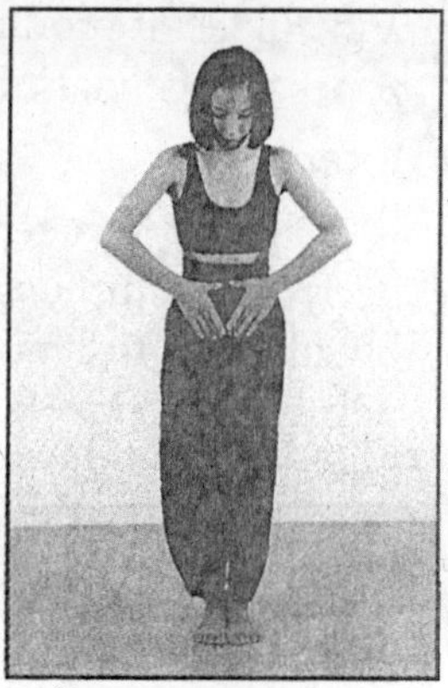
D-60

THE FIVE ESSENTIAL MOVEMENTS SERIES
Pañca adivyaṅga krama Vyāyāma

This is a series of five movements that are excellent for awakening inner energy, to vitalize the body and to prepare it for any other type of activity or for a more extensive practice.

FIRST MOVEMENT

Vyaṅga pictures: E-1-2-3-4-5-6-7-8-9-10-11-12

The locomotion of the Śakti that unwinds the serpent (the power that preserves and supports the universe)

ŚEṢA ŚAKTI GATI VYAṄGA

This movement mobilizes energy in the tan.

It strengthens the muscles of the legs, the articulations of the knees and ankles. It produces great amounts of heat in the lower abdominal zone and genitals, stimulating sexual energy.

Execution

With the legs separated and the feet parallel, niyudha, the upper body moves up and down, always perpendicularly, coordinating the breath with the movement, exhaling when it descends and inhaling when it ascends. Firstly, the movement is performed by keeping the feet parallel and moving the hands up and down in front of the trunk area. Afterwards, the feet are turned outwards and the hands descend parallel to the legs.

SECOND MOVEMENT

Vyaṅga pictures: E-13-14-15-16-17-18-19

The locomotion that stretches and rounds the Śakti

NAUKĀSAÑCĀLANA ŚAKTI GATI VYAṄGA

This movement stimulates and improves the quality of energy in the kidneys, especially if it is done standing, as it can also be done sitting by leaving the hands resting on the knees. It stimulates the flow of energy to the hands and produces a deep and internal stretch of the hip and the articulations of the lumbar-sacral area. The muscles of the back are stretched and strengthened and it smoothly compresses the internal organs, helping to alleviate intestinal peristaltic problems.

Execution

While standing, the body is bent forward at the hips until the trunk reaches a horizontal position parallel to the ground. This is done with the arms separated from the body, turning and lowering the hands and the trunk at the same time. From here, the trunk and the body are lifted while turning the hands. It is also performed on each side of the other hip, projecting the chin forward.

THIRD MOVEMENT

Vyaṅga pictures: E-20-21-22-23-24-25-26-27-28

Beating the ocean of energy

SĀGARA CŪRṆA ŚAKTI GATI VYAṄGA

This movement provides balance and strength and improves the posture of the back.

It activates and stretches the nāḍīs of the bladder, kidney and liver (it works on the back, especially the lumbar area). By performing very energetic breathing, it eliminates waste in the lungs and strengthens them. It stimulates the circulation of body fluids and the activity of the organism in general.

In the second part of this movement, the nāḍīs of the arms, the large intestine, the tridoṣa, the small intestine and the heart are stimulated. It opens and makes the wrists more flexible. It opens the shoulders and shoulders, stretching their joints and making them more flexible.

Execution

With the legs flexed and separated, the upper body is bent forward. The arms and hands are projected to the ground as if they were digging in the earth. Little by little the movement of the arms becomes quicker, and the trunk, the head and the neck become even looser. The movement finishes by inhaling while stretching the arms, with the hands bent at the wrists, raising them to the sky. Then when exhaling the arms are lowered.

FOURTH MOVEMENT

Vyaṅga pictures: E-29

The mountain lashed by the winds

TIRYAKADATA ŚAKTI VIKĀSAKA

It strengthens the energy by re-establishing the emotional, physical and psychic balance. It tones the muscles of the legs and brings a relaxing sensation. It awakens the psychic powers at the core of the mind and gives strength to overcome the desire for compulsive eating, sex and other unbalanced needs.

Execution

With the body standing upright, one of the legs is bent so that the foot rests against the inner thigh of the other leg. The arms are then raised until they are parallel to the ground. The leg that stays down may be either bent or stretched and our glance remains fixed on a point and remains calm.

FIFTH MOVEMENT

Vyaṅgas pictures: E-30-31-32-33-34-35

Rotating the wheel on its axis

KAṬICAKRA ŚAKTI VIKĀSAKA

This movement helps the mind control the different parts of the body. It generates great amounts of heat, activates the energy of the Mūlādhāra and Svādhiṣṭhāna cakras, mobilizes the hips and awakens the energy of the organs in the lower area of the abdomen, like the genitals. It stimulates sexual energy and the movement of the contents of the intestine.

Execution

With the body standing upright with both feet on the floor, the arms are raised in front of the body until they are at the same height as the shoulders, with the palms of the hands facing each other. In this posture, a twist of the hip is performed on its axis, trying not to move the shoulders or any other part of the body.

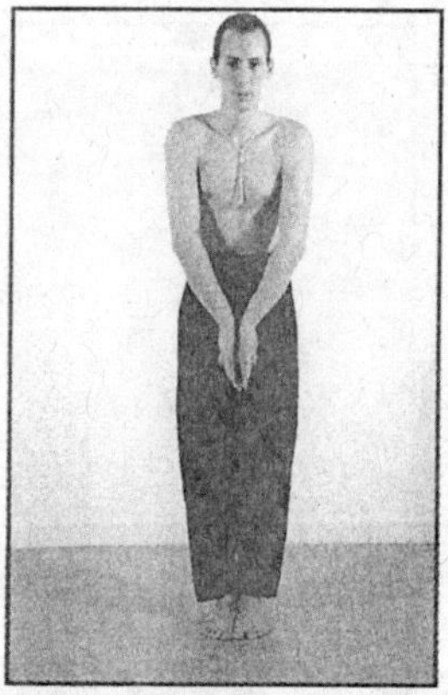
E-1

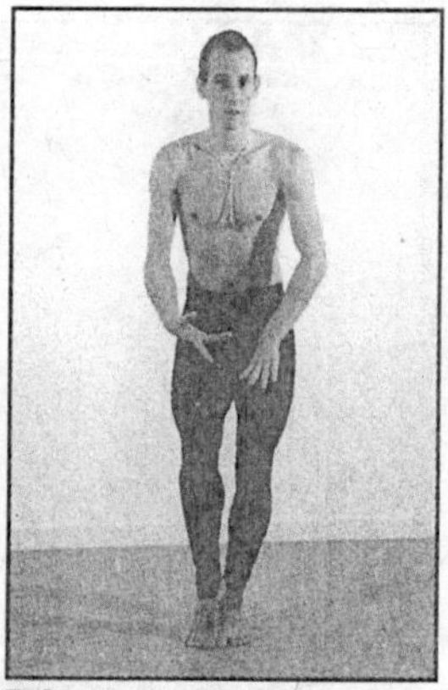
E-2

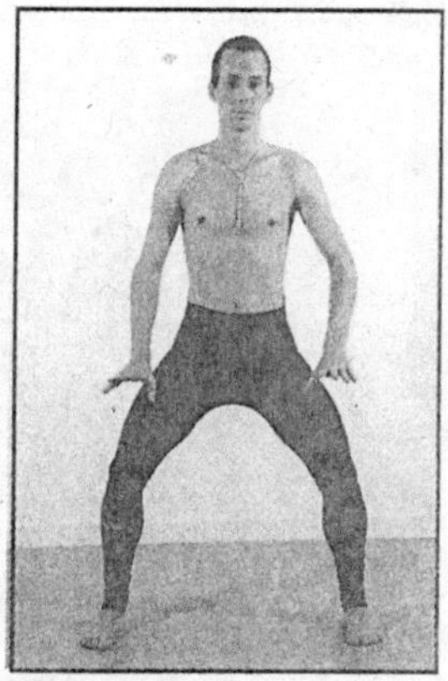
E-3

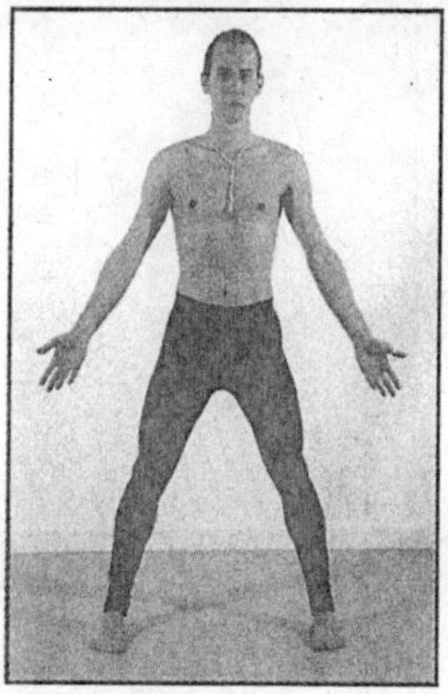
E-4

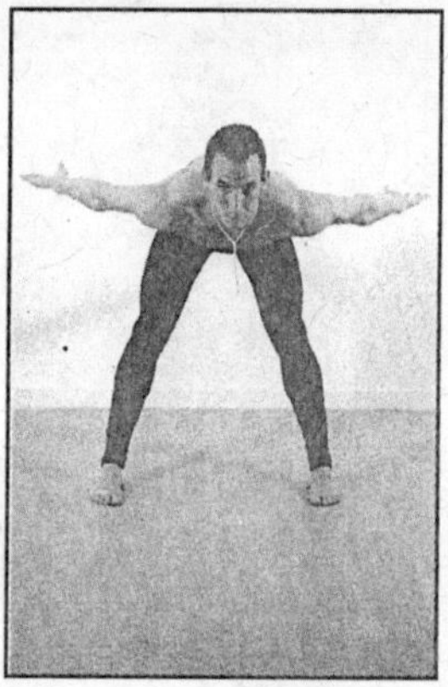
E-5

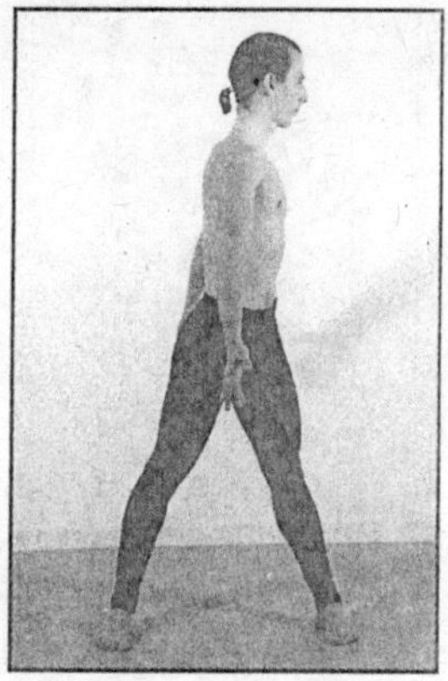
E-6

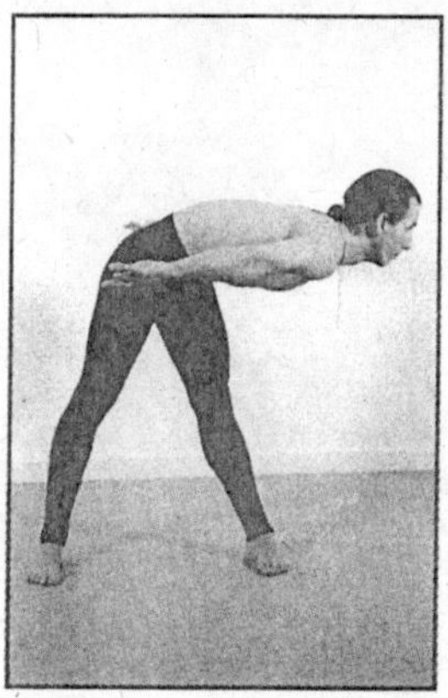
E-7

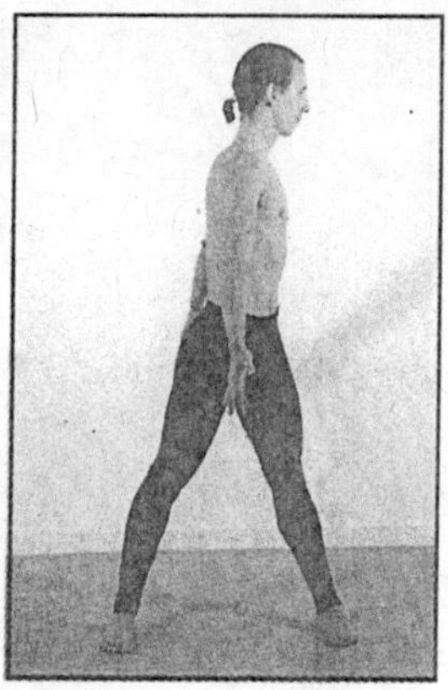
E-8

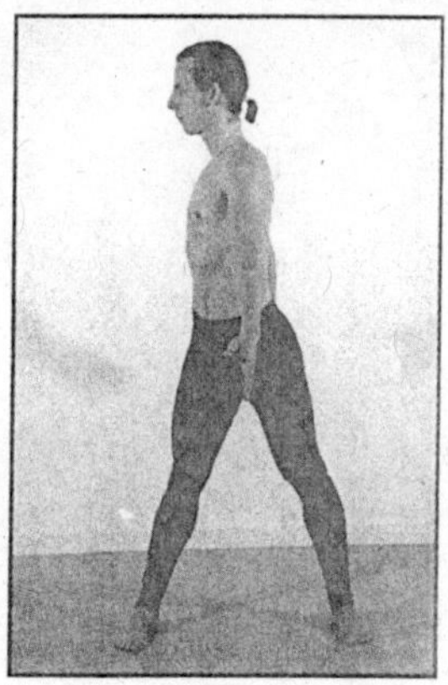
E-9

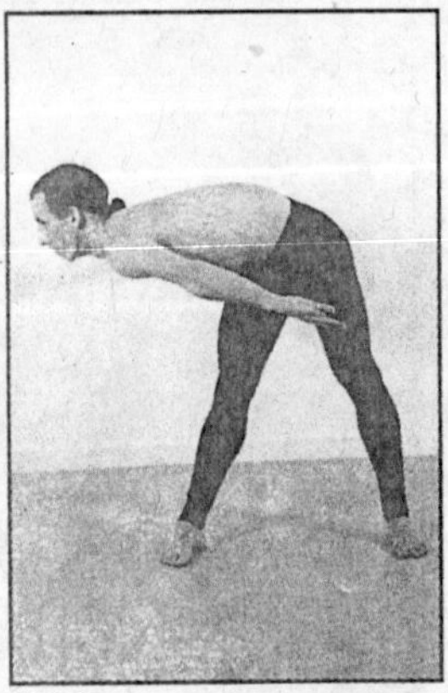
E-10

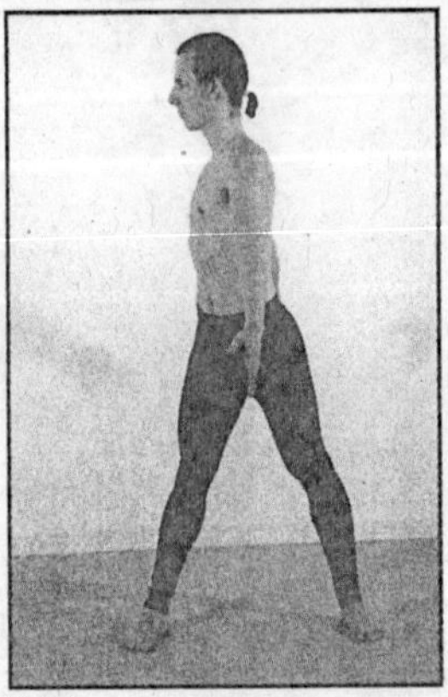
E-11

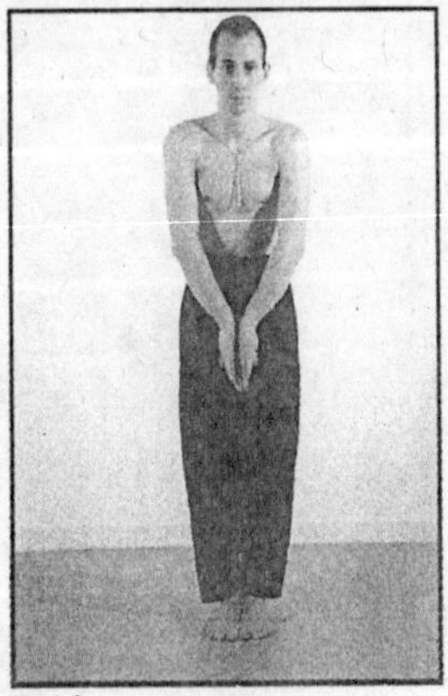
E-12

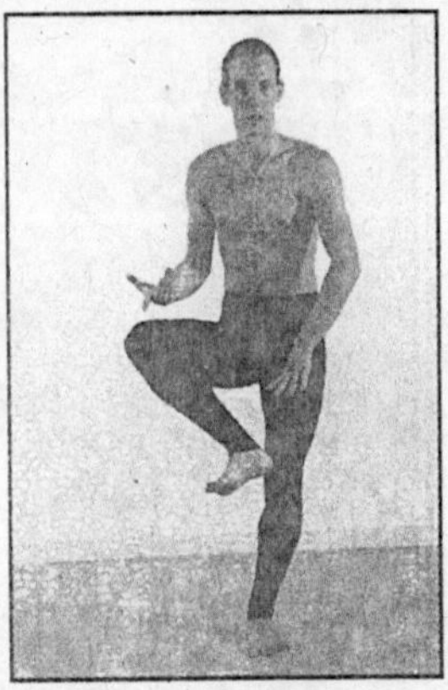
E-13

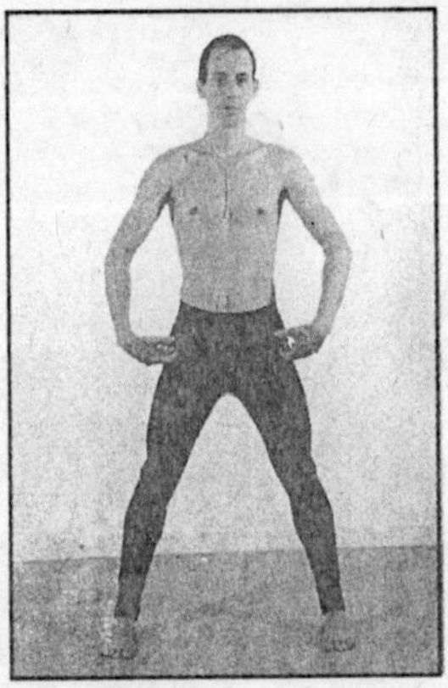
E-14

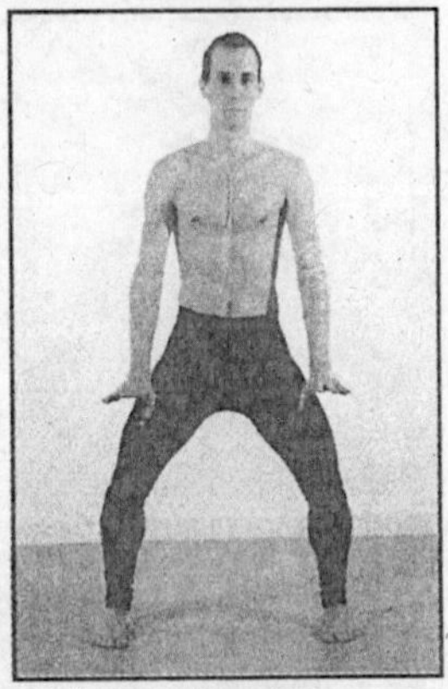
E-15

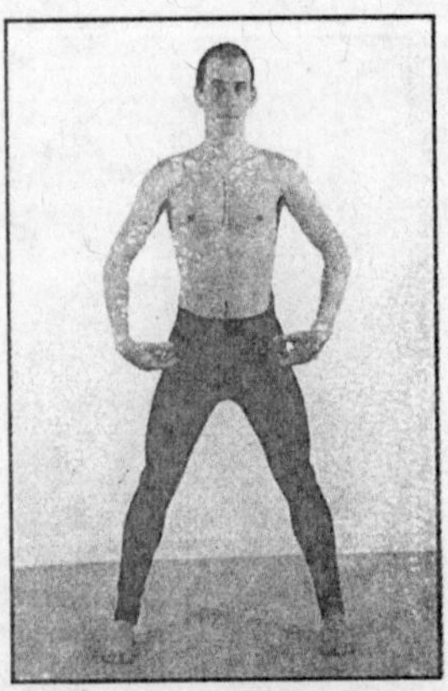
E-16

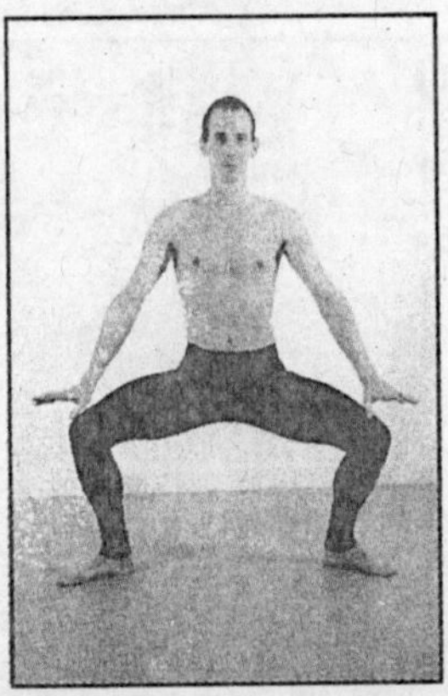
E-17

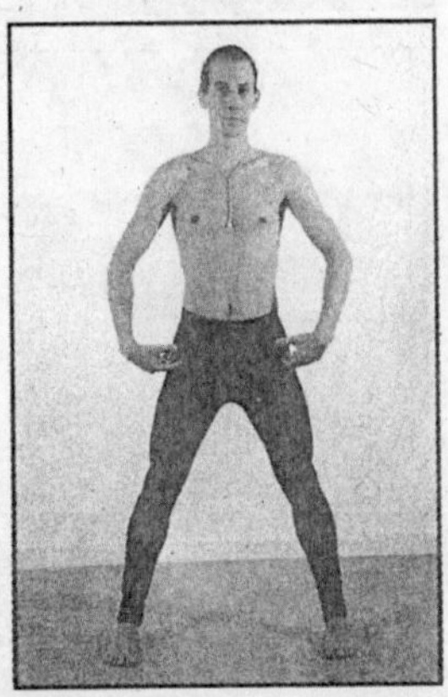
E-18

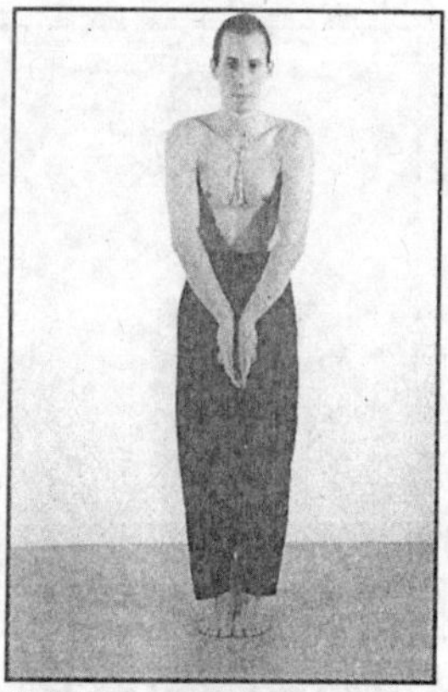
E-19

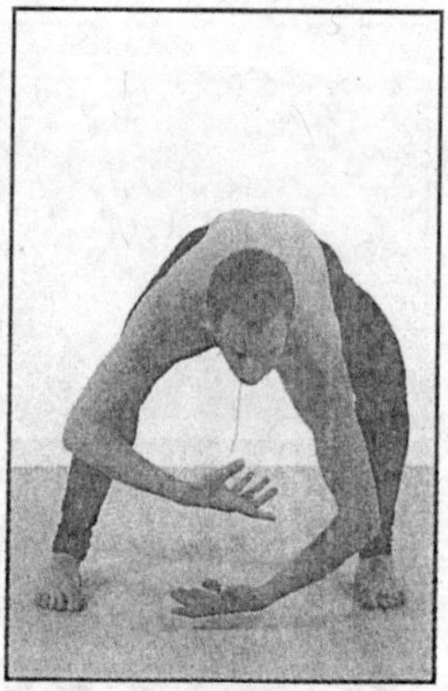
E-20

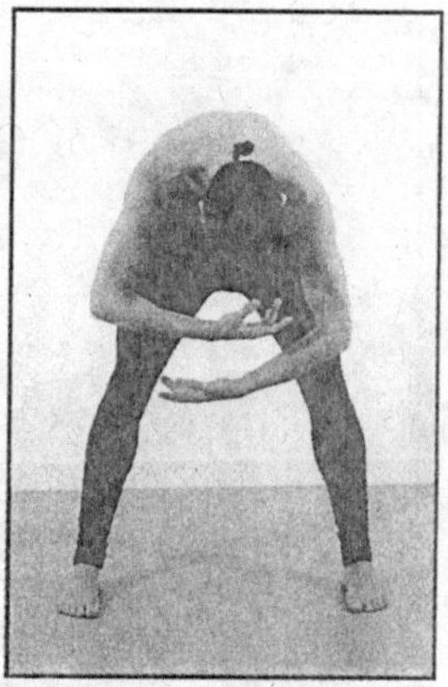
E-21

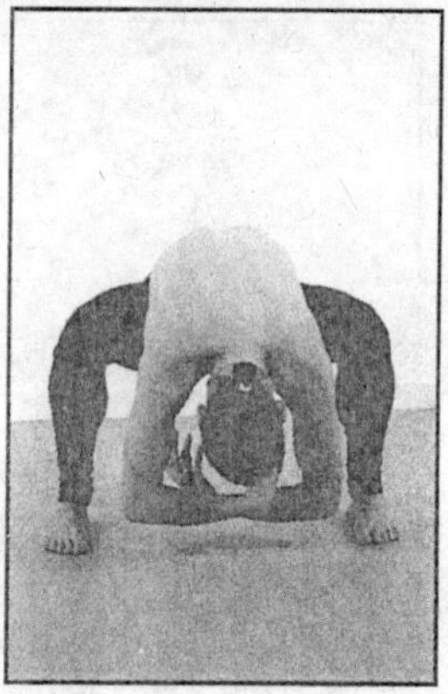
E-22

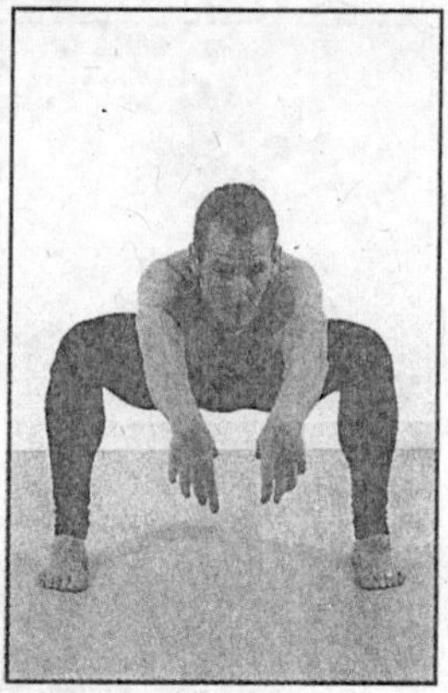
E-23

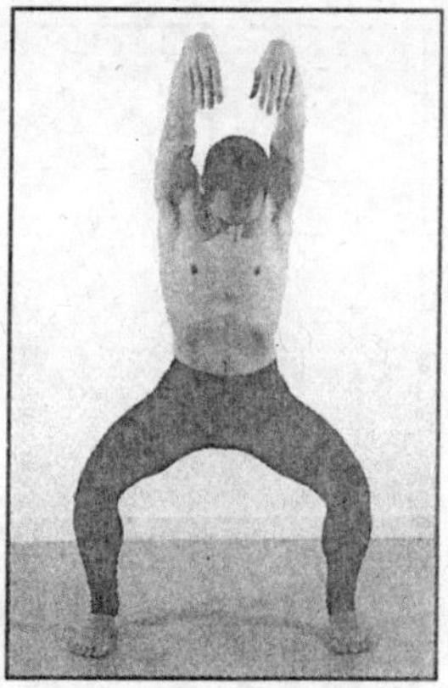
E-24

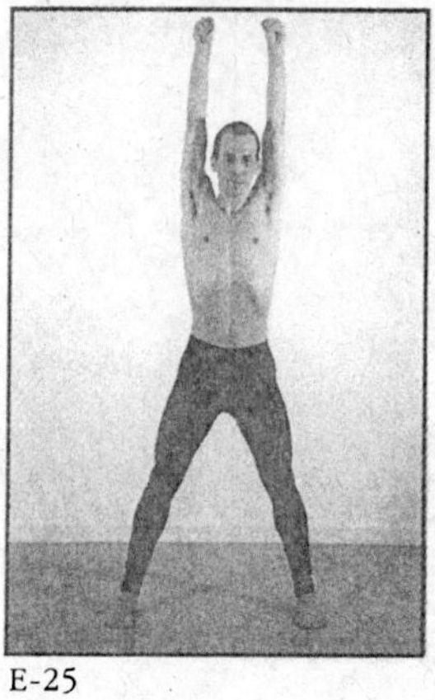
E-25

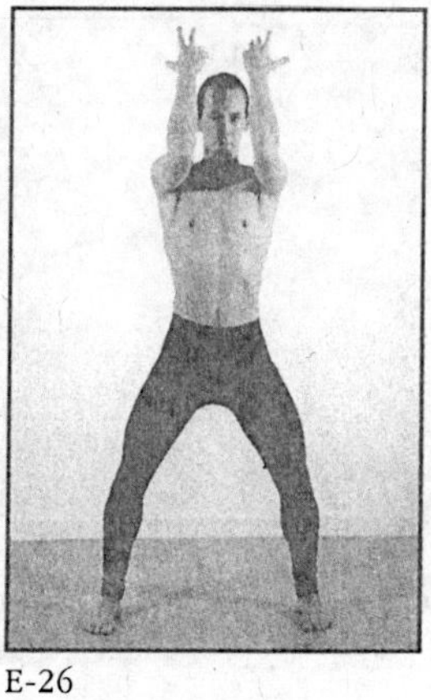
E-26

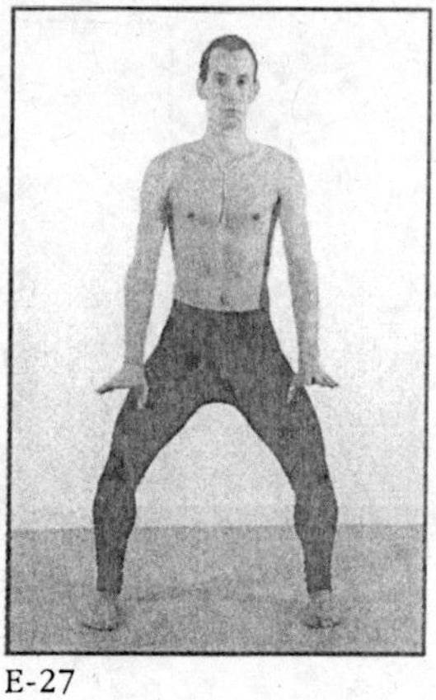
E-27

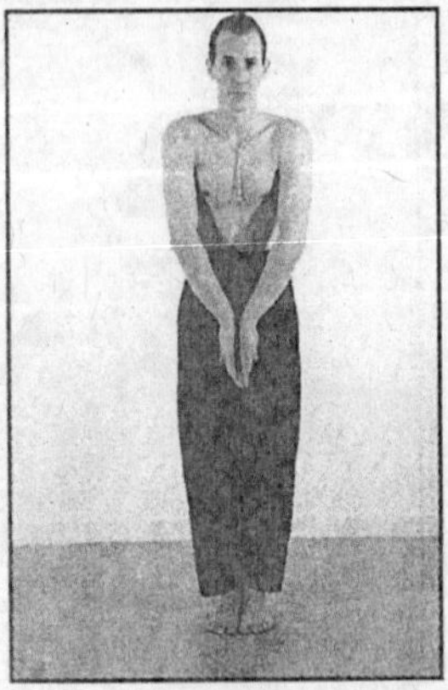
E-28

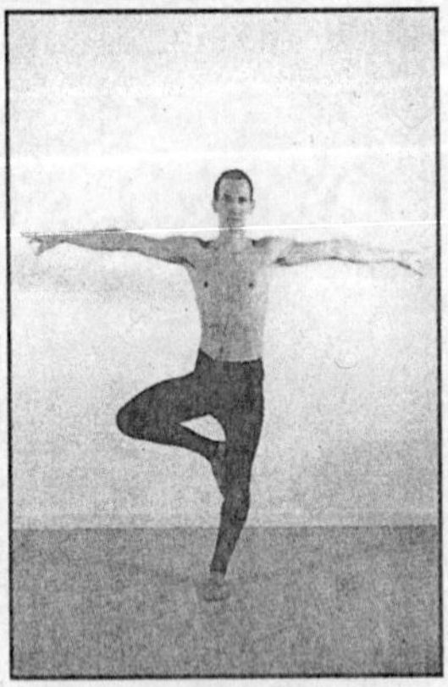
E-29

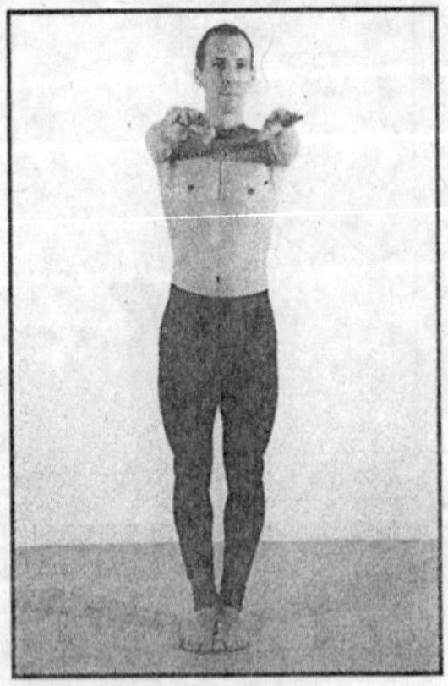
E-30

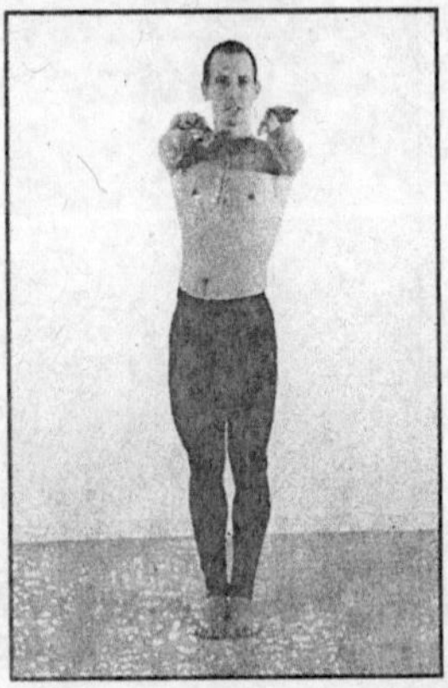
E-31

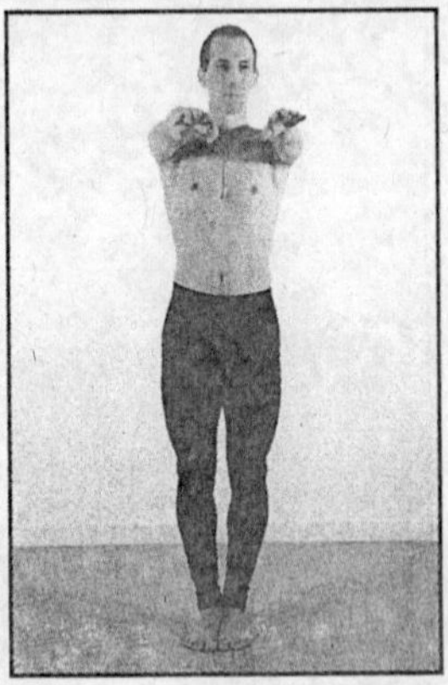
E-32

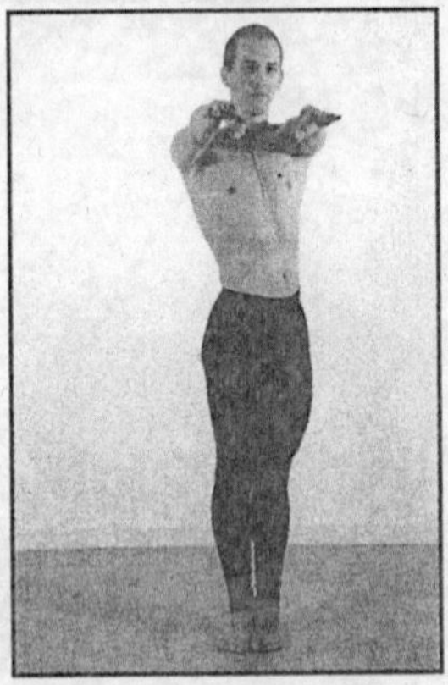
E-33

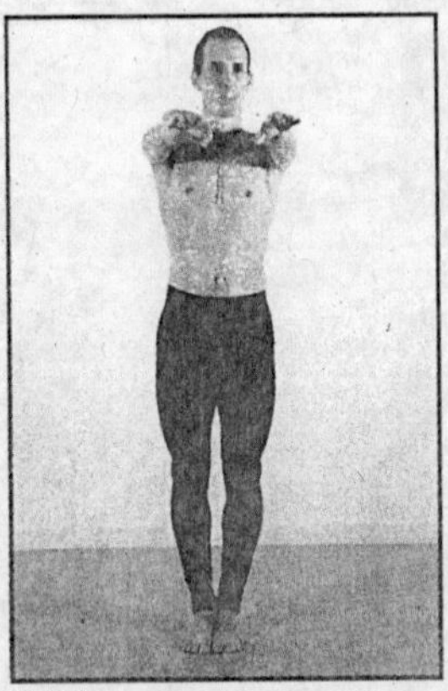
E-34

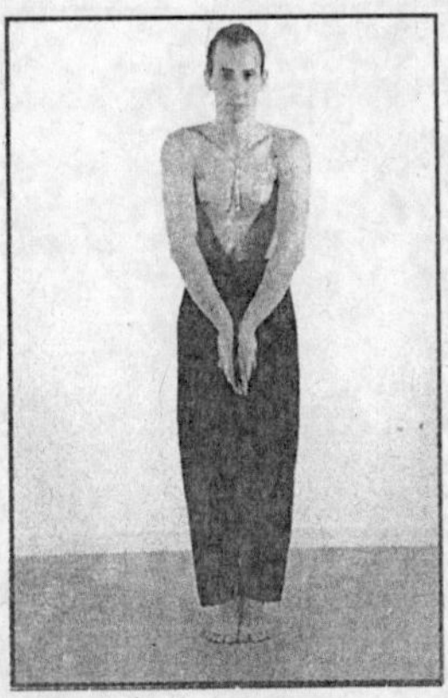
E-35

SALUTATION SERIES

Maṅgalam

Maṅgalam is a salutation to the gods in the form of prayer. Maṅgalam is happiness, prosperity, wealth, everything that is promising, and a solemn ceremony that is carried out on important occasions. The salutation itself does not form a series in the practice of Vyāyāma; however it is executed as an appendix to any of the series. In it, the essence of the practice of this discipline is found; so its execution at the end of each series, sets the objectives of Vyāyāma in the mind.

FIRST SALUTATION. Namaskāra
Vyaṅga pictures: F-1-2-3-4-5-6-7

I salute your true being

The adversary is saluted, seeking to communicate the need for improvement through the acknowledgement of faults and virtues that are observed in oneself. The opponent is the mirror of the practising persons, and their incentive for improvement.

It predisposes the fight by following the premise: "I will not unsheath my sword without courage, I will always do it with honour, and although you are my adversary, I will salute you."

We should keep in mind that the mystical origin of Vyāyāma Yoga comes from warriors and doesn't refer to fighting someone else's battle, but our own internal battle. Is there any war bigger than the one we fight within ourselves?

In this salutation we put both hands together looking into the eyes of the adversary signalling alertness and preparation for the unexpected.

SECOND SALUTATION. Praṇāma
Vyaṅga pictures: F-8-9

Salutation to the master

In order to establish the struggle for self-improvement, the person who practises needs to have a guide that knows how to lead and help him in difficult times and who inspires confidence, a master. Masters of the Yoga and Vyāyāma tradition tell us about our need to practise faith, or trust in the scriptures, in the words and wise advice of the master, and in our own potential.

In this salutation both hands are joined together over the head and the body is bent forward in the direction of the master without looking at him.

THIRD SALUTATION. Arpaṇam
Vyaṅga pictures: F-10-11-12-13-14

Salutation to the gods

We offer the gods our actions and thoughts in order to obtain their grace. They dwell inside us just as they do in the Universe, as the forces and powers that sustain everything. To please the gods is to collaborate in the maintenance of the balance of life. Otherwise, if we think that we are the epicentres of the Universe, this will lead to destruction because there is not enough strength in our interior to enable us to sustain everything and to be the dynamic force which moves it.

To perform this salute both hands are raised together above the head while looking up towards the sky.

FOURTH SALUTE. Śaraṇam
Vyaṅga pictures: F-15-16-17-18-19-20-21

Salutation to Gaṇeśa

Gaṇeśa is the god who protects Vyāyāma, dance and yoga. He is the one who removes obstacles which appear during the process of realization. To surrender to Gaṇeśa is to invoke the necessary strength to overcome difficulties.

Continuous practice and impartiality are the two indispensable factors necessary to obtain success. Along the way, numerous difficulties emerge, numerous forces which tend to draw us away from our objectives. Gaṇeśa is the strength which is capable of removing such difficulties.

To perform this salute, the arms and hands are placed above the head, while moving the torso to imitate the movement of an elephant's trunk.

FIFTH SALUTE. Arghya
Vyaṅga pictures: F-22-23-24-25

Salute to the Sun and the Moon

The sun is the force which creates outer life and the moon is our internal energy. This salute deals with the necessity of finding a balance between both in order for strength to be obtained and to achieve the objective of our practice. Without strength, there is no possibility of success.

To perform this salute, the arms trace a circle of the sun and the fingers of both hands come together at the level of the tan, symbolizing the moon.

SIXTH SALUTE.

Vyaṅga pictures: F-26-27-28-29-30-31-32-33-34-35-36-37-38-39

The steps of wisdom (3)

(1-1) Compassion, Karuṇā, to help those who have been left behind along the way and those who have yet to arrive, by showing them the way.

(1-2) Ability, Kauśala, to learn; who asks the right questions will learn well; who learns well will teach well.

(2) Harmony, Samatva, provides us with the necessary mental balance so that we do lose our way, helping us to be conscious of our weaknesses and to remember our past so that we are more tolerant with the difficulties of others.

(3) The force which drives your destiny, Hara.

Something has to die for something new to come to life. It is the resulting force of the practice that shall completely transform life, enabling everything to flourish again, so other destinies can enter our lives and expand it.

To perform this salute we take two steps back, while turning the torso and our gaze and projecting the body and the arms forwards, in an act that symbolizes that we are pushing our destiny.

SEVENTH SALUTE. Namaste

Vyaṅga pictures: F-40-41

To all, to our fellow members, searching for harmony

With our legs crossed, knees bent and hands together, we salute our fellow members one by one by looking into their eyes.

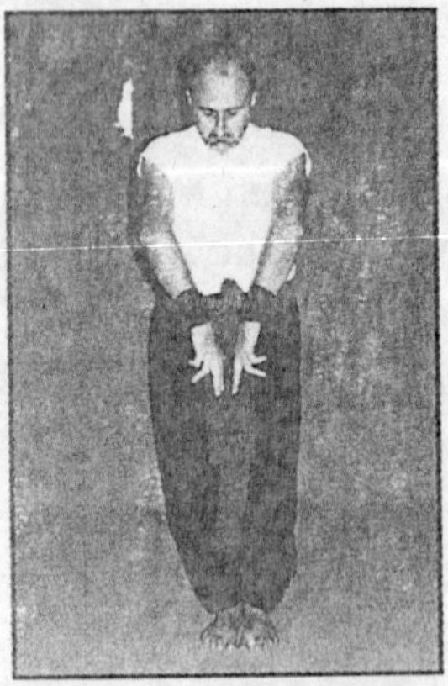
F-1

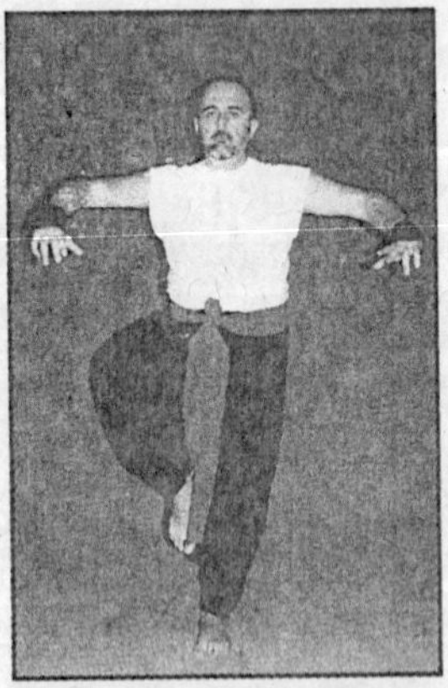
F-2

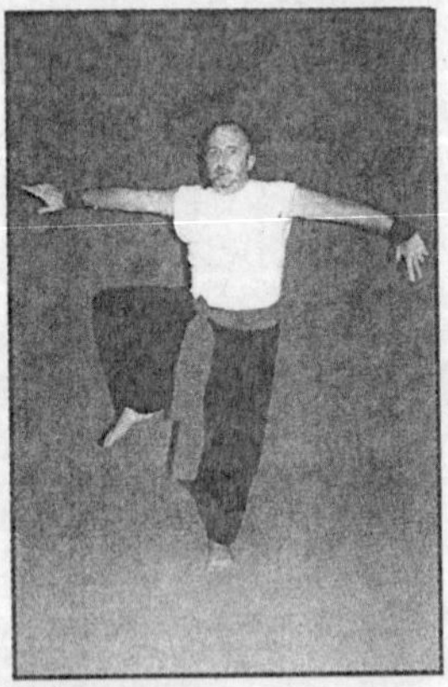
F-3

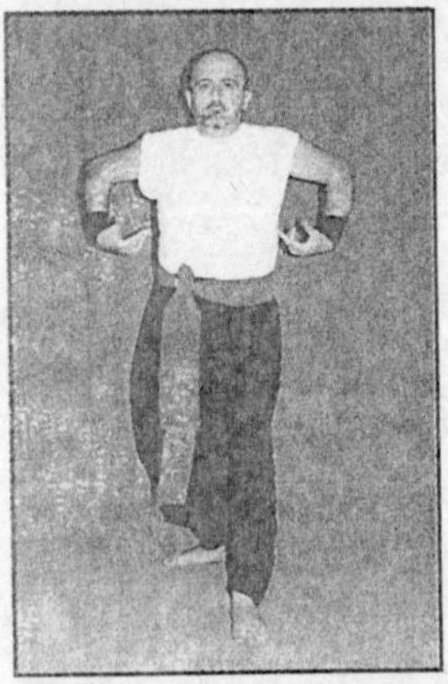
F-4

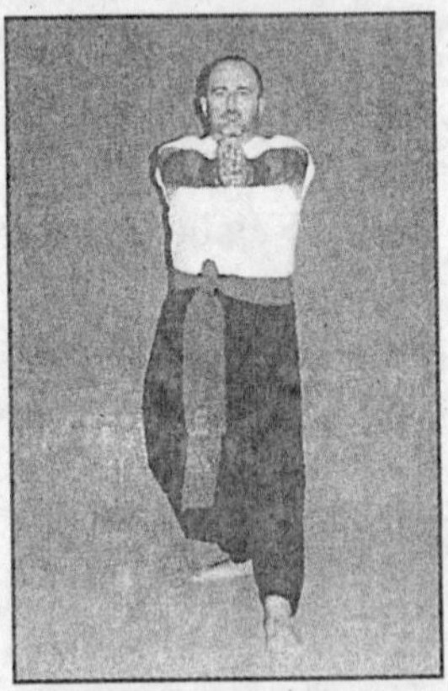
F-5

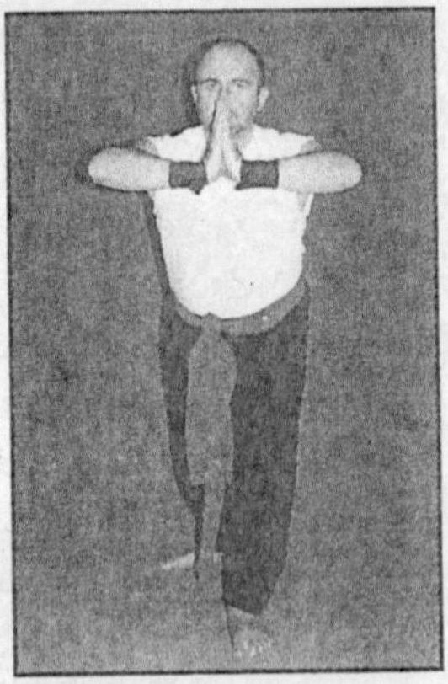
F-6

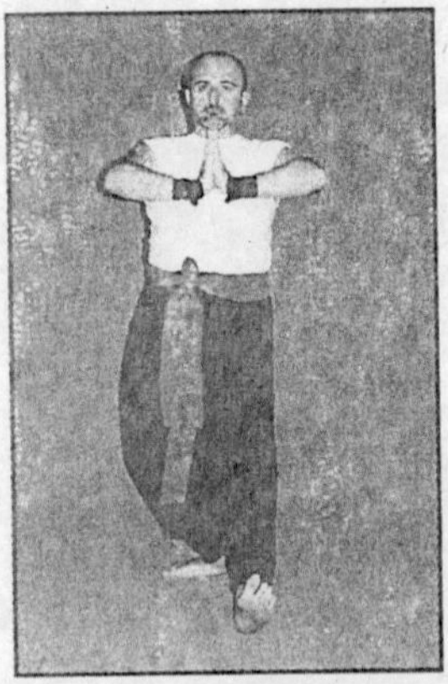
F-7

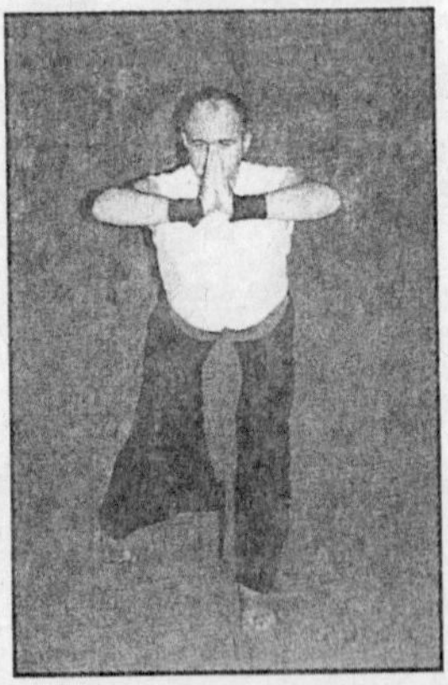
F-8

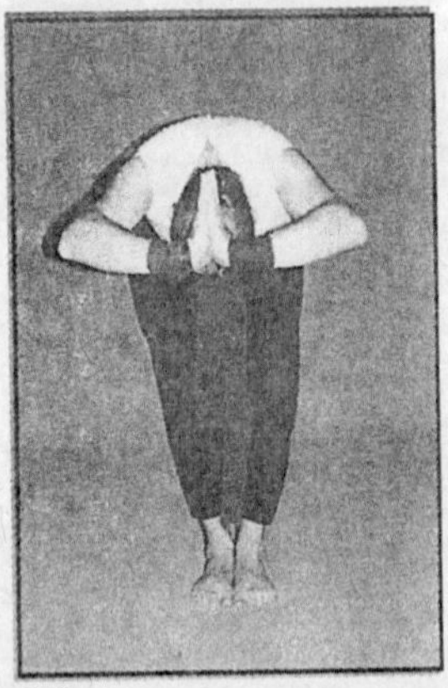
F-9

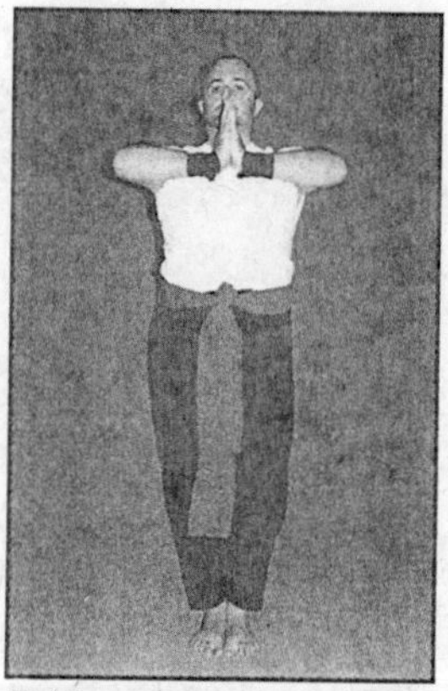
F-10

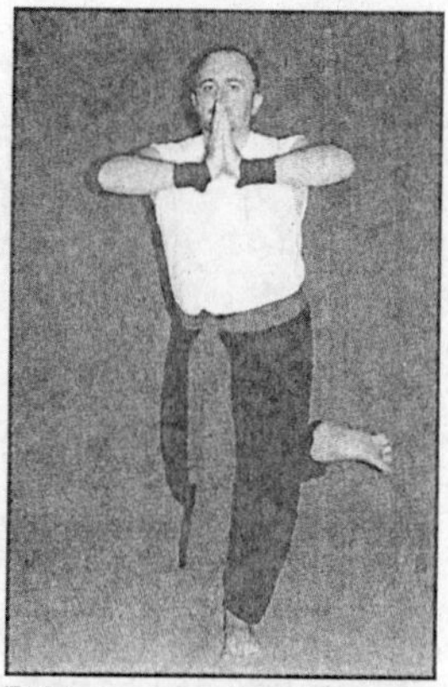
F-11

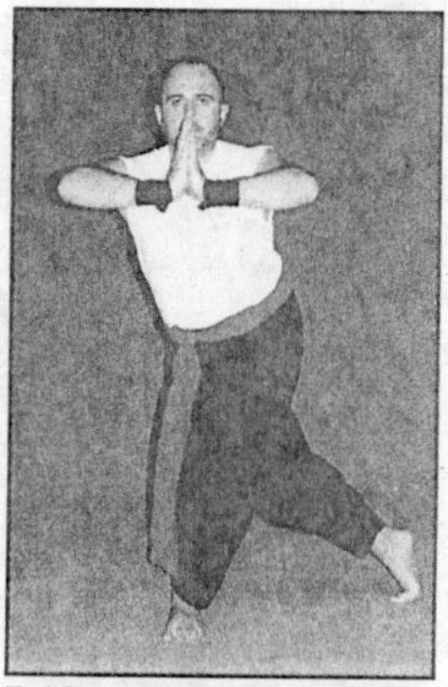
F-12

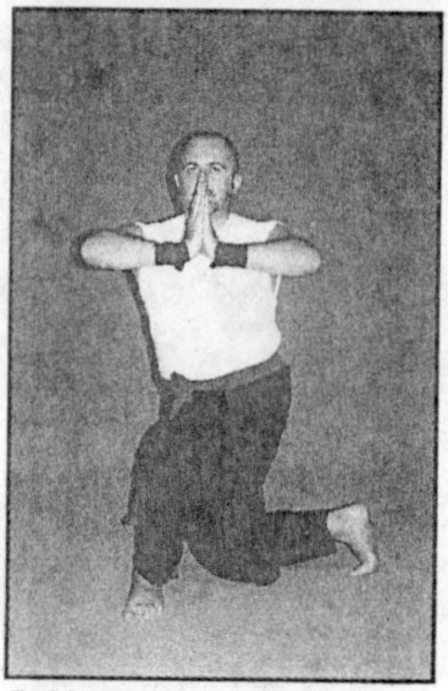
F-13

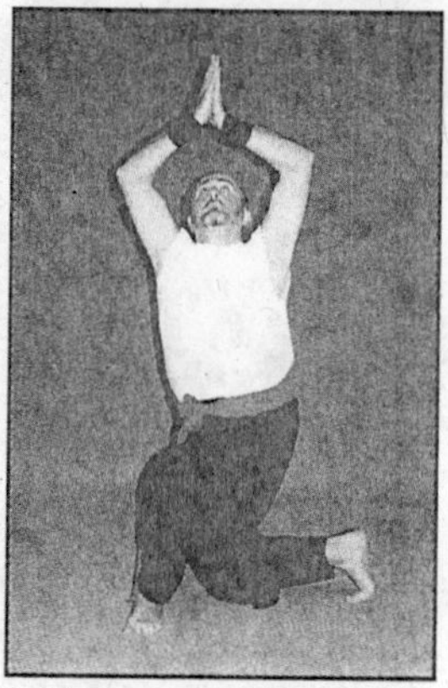
F-14

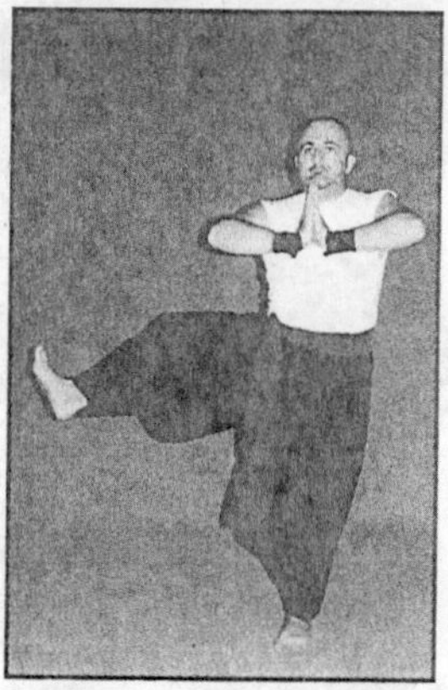
F-15

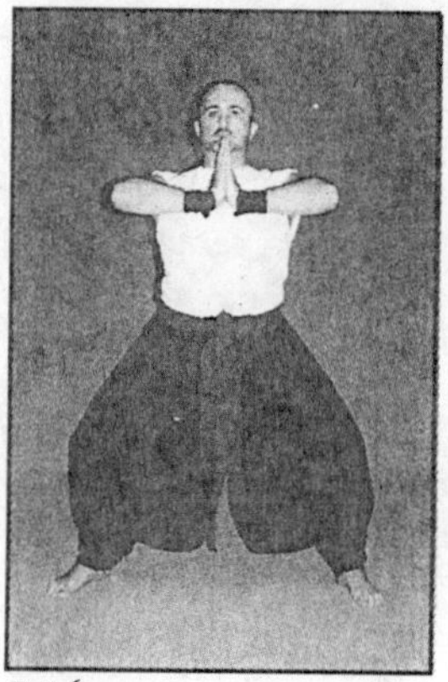
F-16

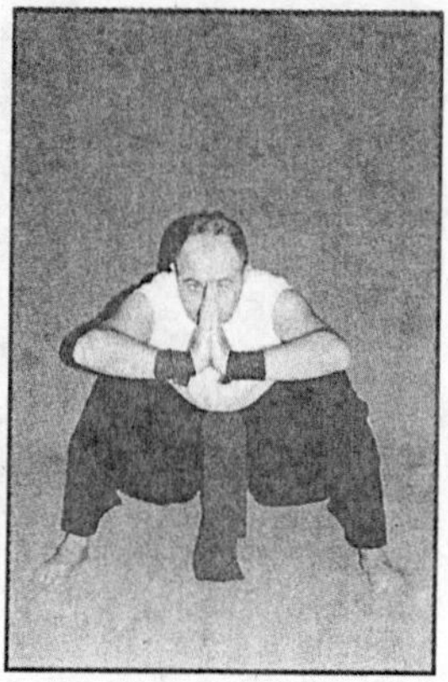
F-17

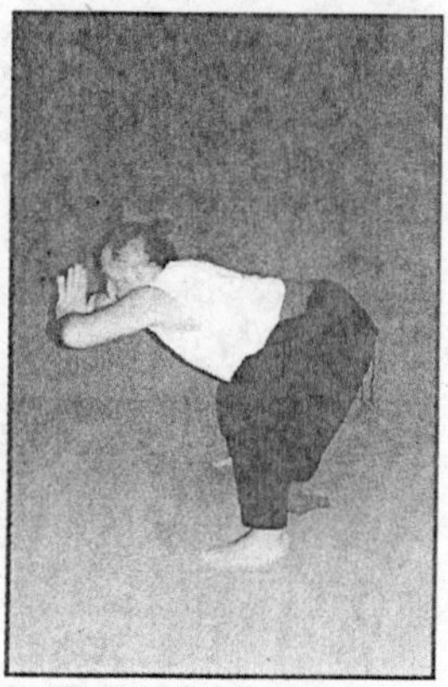
F-18 *Side view of previous movement*

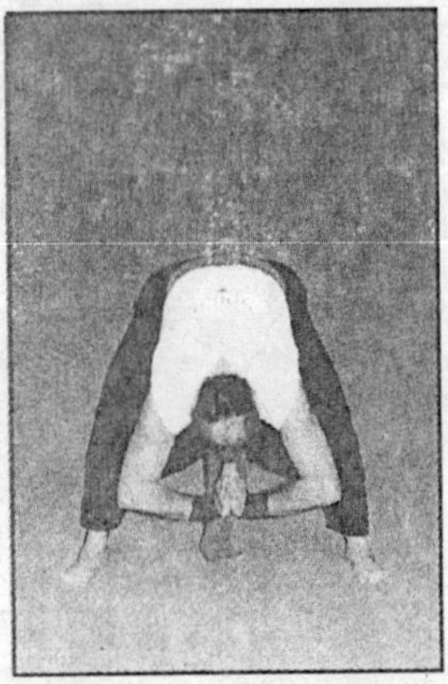

F-19

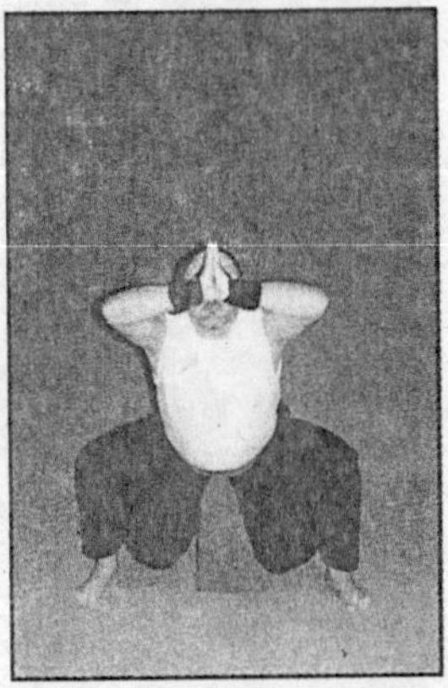

F-20

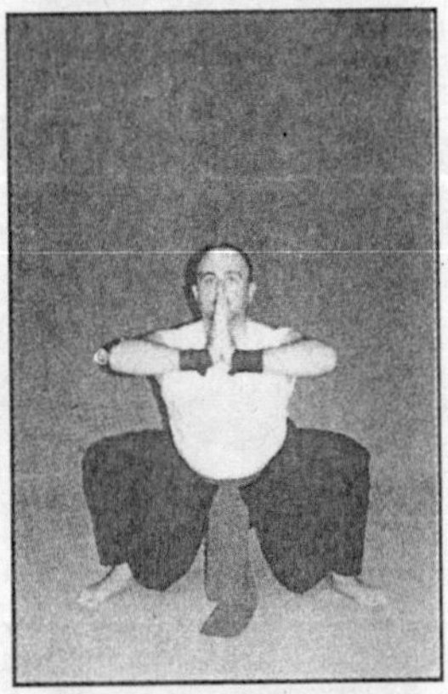

F-21

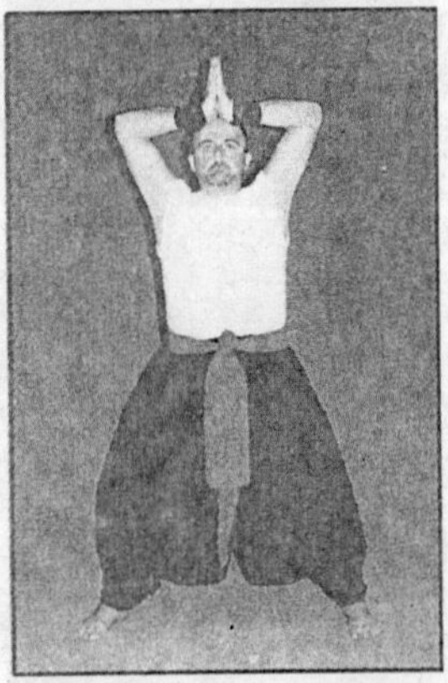

F-22

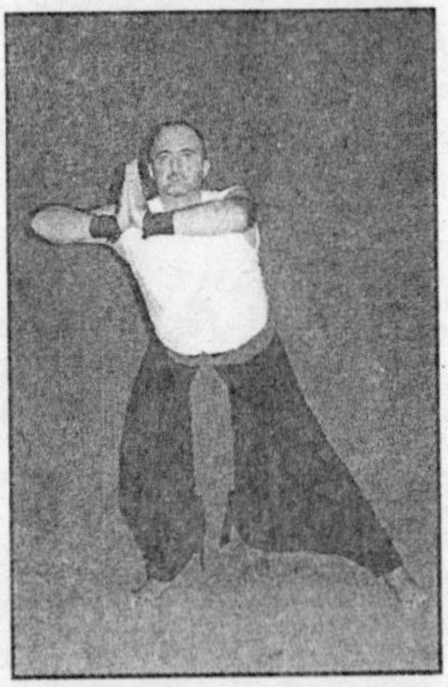

F-23

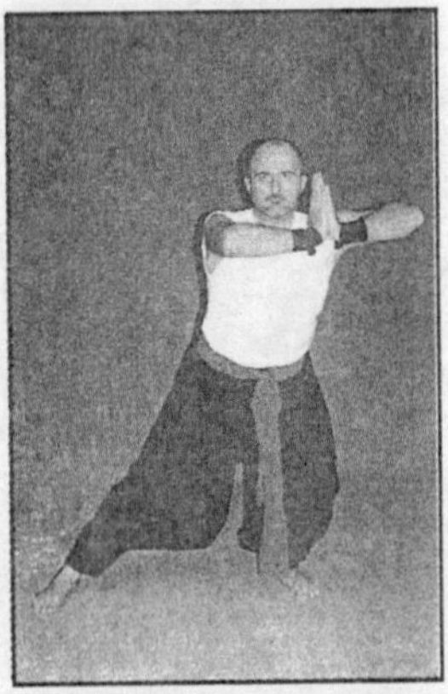

F-24

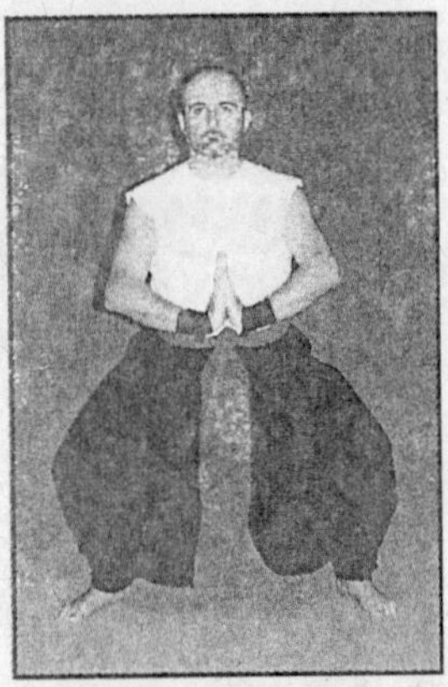

F-25

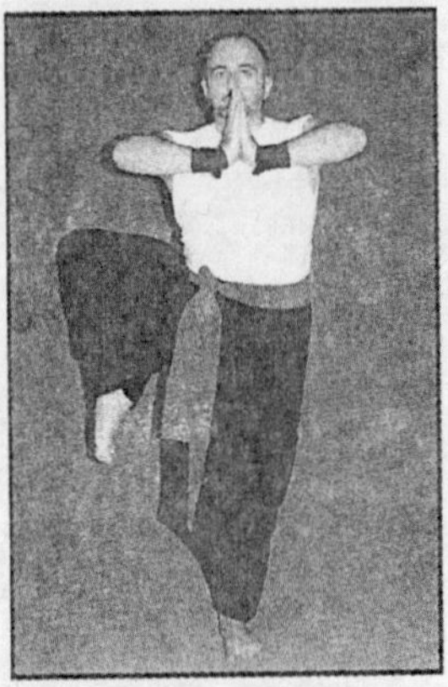

F-26

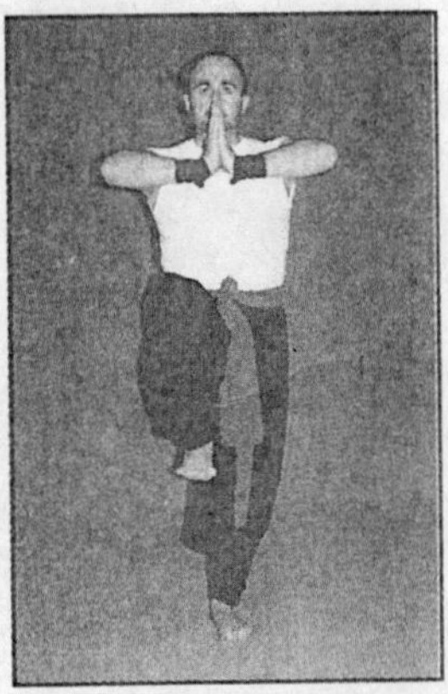

F-27

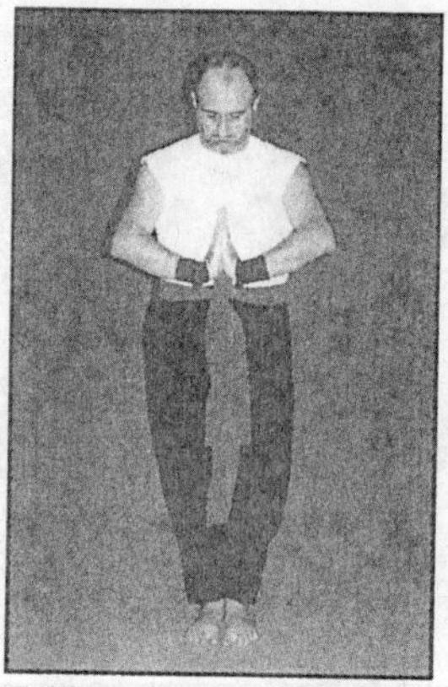

F-28

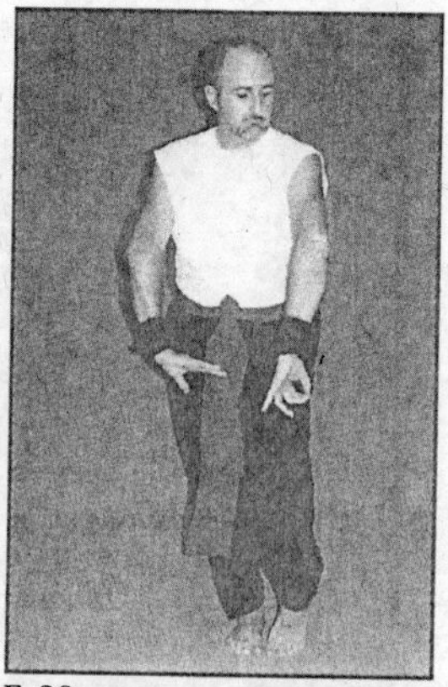

F-29

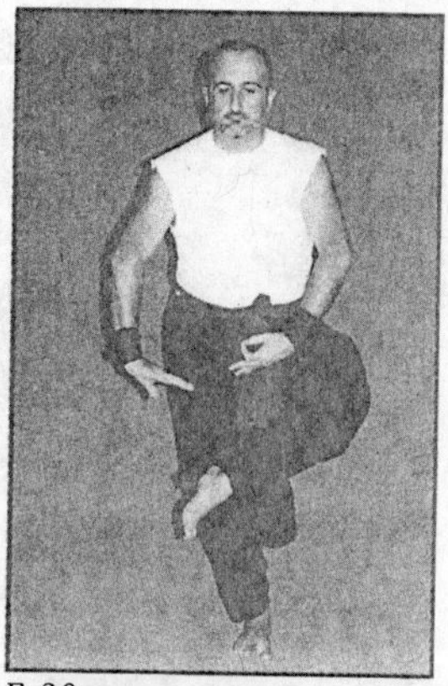

F-30

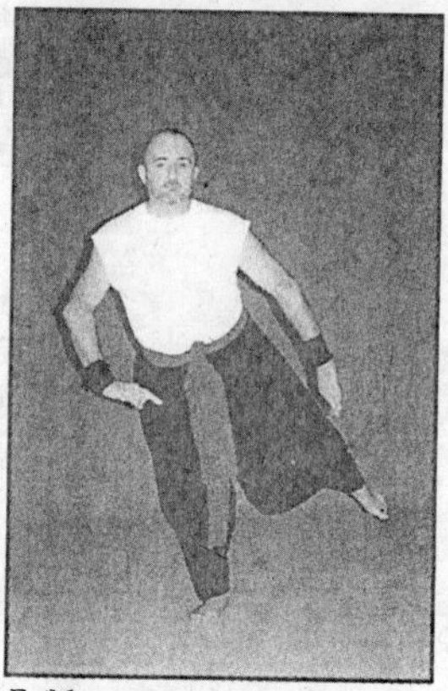

F-31

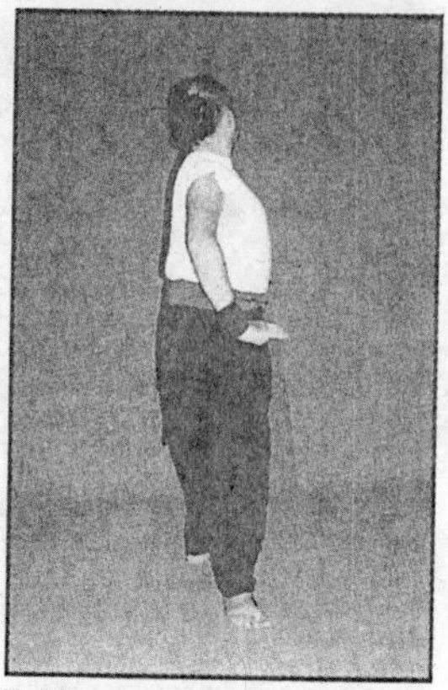

F-32a

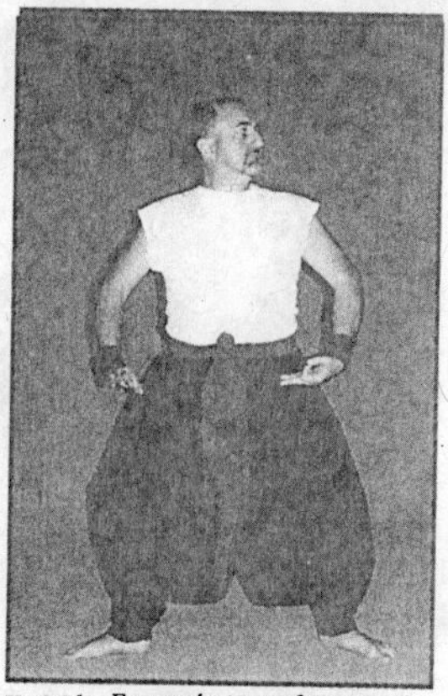

F-32b *Frontal view of previous movement.*

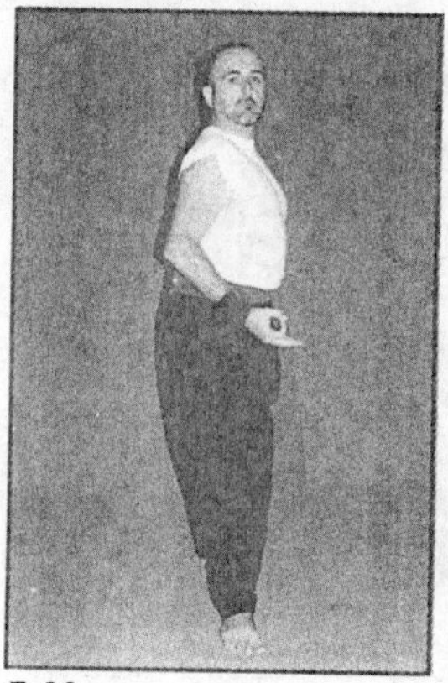

F-33

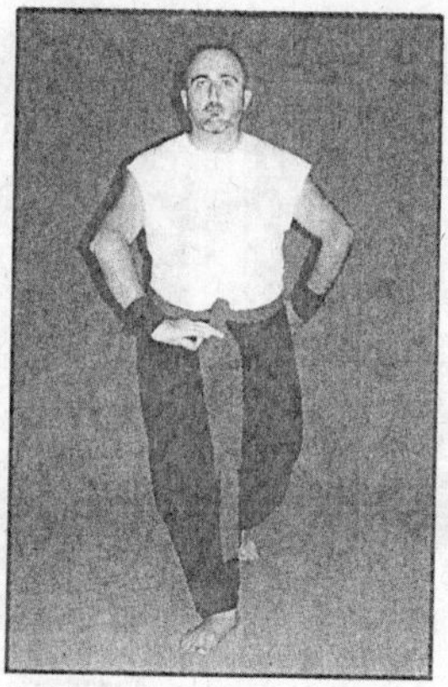

F-34

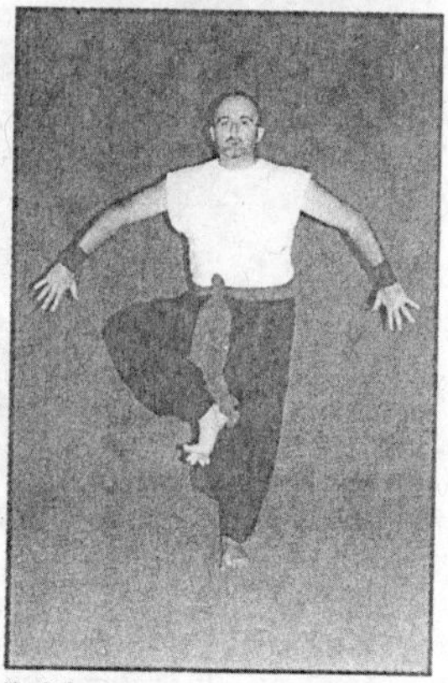

F-35

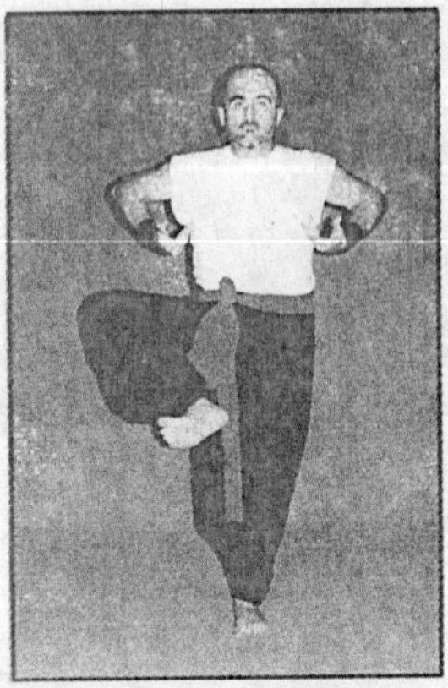
F-36

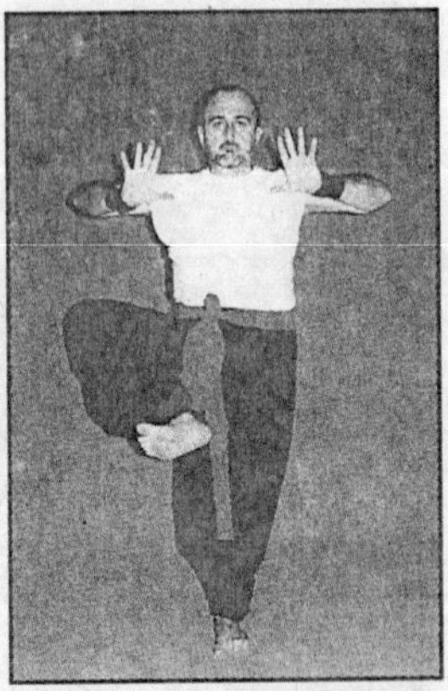
F-37

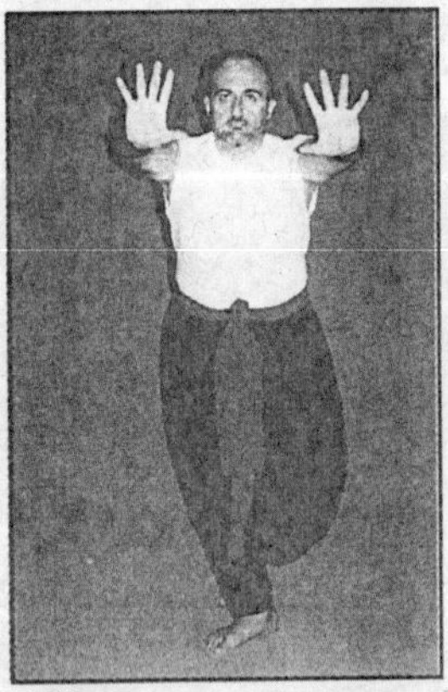
F-38

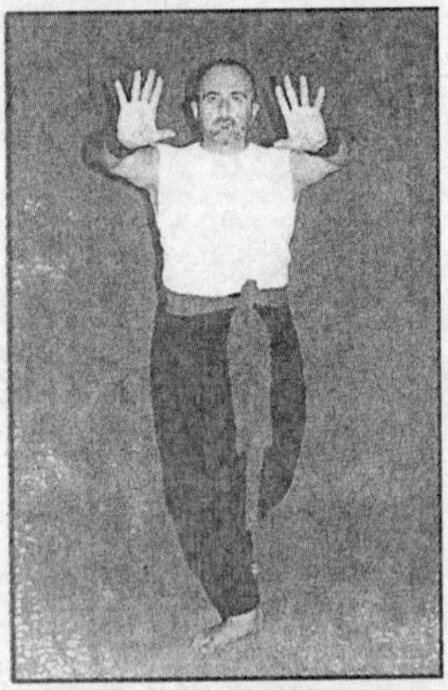
F-39

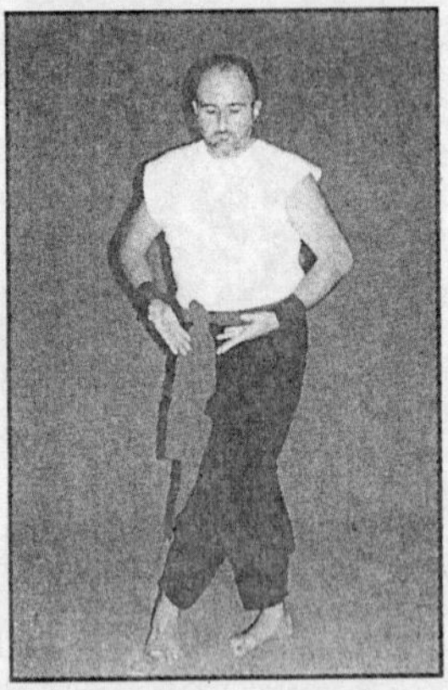
F-40

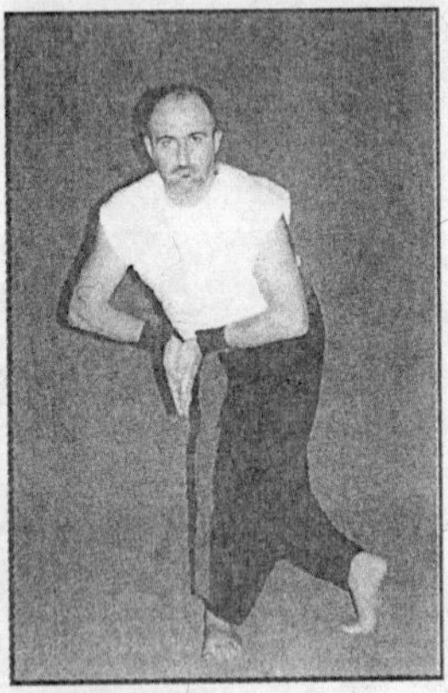
F-41

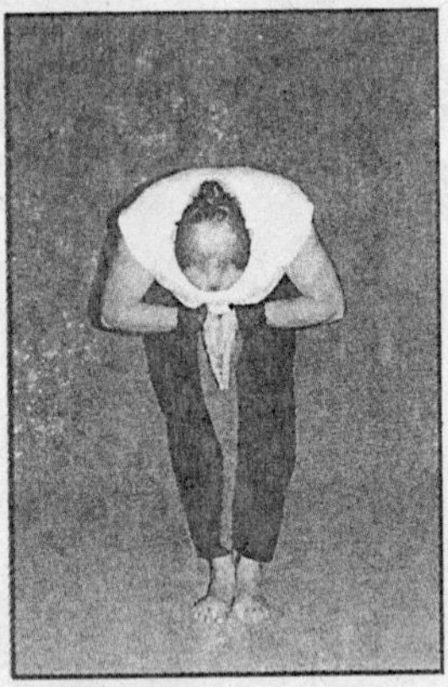
F-42

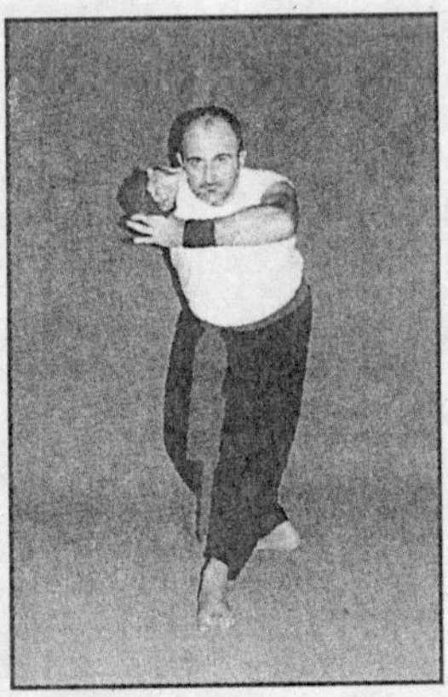
F-43

The Traditional School of Vyāyāma Yoga

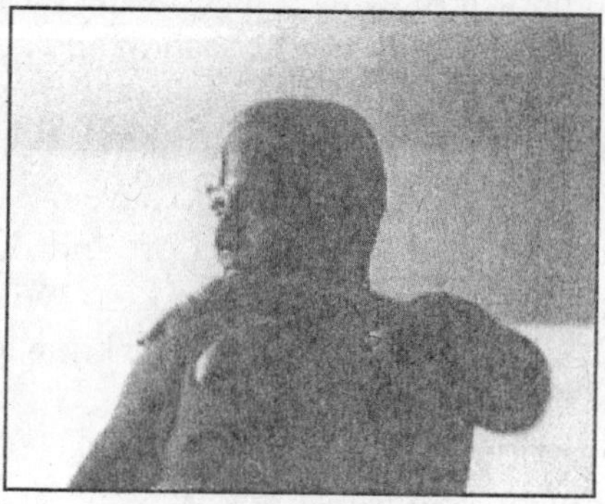

Swami Tilak

The Traditional School of Vyāyāma Yoga was inspired by the venerable Master Swami Tilak Paramahansa and subsequently founded and developed by Gurukul Master Javier Plazas who gives the opportunity to wishing to learn the teachings and profoundly understand this almost extinct discipline and art of immeasurable value for total health and well being.

For this and many other reasons, Javier Plazas has always kept this teaching closely guarded, protecting it against popularization by transmitting it in the same way he received it from his Master, with the same care and value.

This is why the school is called "Traditional School of Vyāyāma Yoga", as its teachings originated in a remote past and faithfully carry out orthodox standards even though it is being effectively adapted to use in our daily lives today. Javier Plazas is a non-conventional master who teaches in a personal, direct and serious way, with humor, severity and fondness.

The motto of the Traditional School of Vyāyāma Yoga is, "The mind is where the breath is", a saying that encompasses a great potential power; the training of the breath, its immense energy, and magical thought in order to make the impossible possible.

The purpose of the Traditional School of Vyāyāma is to diffuse an appropriate and updated method of the ancient techniques of Vyāyāma Yoga, which would otherwise not have been possible to learn in the modern world because of the difficulties and requirements it demands.

To avoid the fraud of opportunists, of the phoney's who are eager for notoriety and riches, and of the impatient who do not take time to learn but then immediately want to teach what they do not know, and to minimize the impact of the popularization and corruption that every such diffusion implies, the copyright, name and concept of Vyāyāma has been registered. This means that the use of the term and the technique is prohibited to all people who have not received the proper training to teach it. In this way, the effort and dedication of all the students receiving formal training is respected. With their enthusiasm, they are the official receivers of this great knowledge, guaranteeing its continuity for future generations.

With the publication of this book, Javier Plazas sets the beginning of the written diffusion of this marvellous technique around the world, in addition to the labour already begun in India by the ancient spiritual warriors.

MY MASTER SHRI SWAMI TILAK PARAMAHAMSA

When Swami Tilak was 30 years old, in approximately 1960, he undertook a Yātrā, (pilgrimage) with the aim of finally putting an end to a stage of his life dedicated to social work. Instead he looked for spiritual values that would park the way toward the Being.

Three years had passed from when he took the life of a Sannyāsī. In the beginning he left his work as an editor of a magazine to go in search of his Guru, travelling on foot in the strictest tradition of the renounced monks and living only on charity. It was his first experience as a young Sannyāsī and he would follow this way of life while travelling to more than fifty-six countries.

In this period he had many experiences in which he saw that god protected those who dedicated themselves to a spiritual life. His journey served to increase even more his motivation to dedicate himself completely to this life, but in spite of everything, he could not find his Guru to guide him in this journey. Disappointed with the lack of profundity of the spiritual organisations he returned to his previous job as an editor.

Three years later he unexpectedly disappeared. Nobody knew where he went and he was never heard of again. The fact is that Swami Tilak had taken the firm decision to search for his spiritual master, even if it took his entire life.

His first journey had demonstrated that he was not able to find the truth of the "Being" in the big and famous religious organisations nor in famous Gurus, so he avoided any contact with these important people. Instead, his footsteps directed him to the sacred River Narmada, where Śrī Adi Śaṅkarācārya, the founder of the ten orders of Swamis advaitas and a great exponent of Vedānta philosophy had realised a great part of his Sādhanā (spiritual practice).

Swami Tilak commented that in that stage of his life he had almost lost hope of finding the truth in this world, but finally his search led him to find his master, Bābā Bajaraṅga Dāsji Mahārāja.

About his meeting with his master Babaji, Swami Tilak said the following:

"It was afternoon, and the sun was about to set. I was tired so I sat on a rock. Some shepherds returning to their homes approached me and asked me to accompany them to their small village.

"Why must I go, perhaps there is something special in your little village?" I asked.

Finally on seeing their innocent looks and their sincere expressions I went with them.

That night the villagers told me that nearby lived a great Saint known for his austerity, knowledge and devotion. He was also the incarnation of love.

The following morning I resumed my journey along the river. I had scarcely walked a mile when I saw on the right a small cabin on the top of some white rocks and standing at the side of the cabin a young saint. Not wanting to stop, I continued on for some metres. I turned my head and I saw that the young saint was still there. A voice inside me said "Now that you have seen him what can you lose by going to pay your respects?"

I turned around and climbed up to the cabin. I found that the young saint was not alone. There was another saint, older, sitting surrounded by some devotees. I positioned myself in front of them and waited for a reaction.

I asked some customary questions and then he said:

"Are you going on a pilgrimage to the Narmadā?"

Not wanting to reveal myself, I said:

"No sir."

"What then is the aim of your journey?"

"None, sir."

"My son" he answered with a smile, "not even a blade of grass can leave its place without some aim, so how can you?"

His words penetrated deep within me and put me on guard. I had to acknowledge that I had been wrong.

"Sorry sir, I am looking for 'knowledge."

Without saying anything more, the saint stood up and started to water the plants. I felt offended to think that he had not paid any attention to me, so I decided to leave. When I asked to excuse myself he looked at me from head to toe and said laughingly, "Nobody comes here to leave, so how can you, my son?" With these words he completely deflated my ego and I noticed an unknown sensation all over my body. I had listened to many talks and religious statements but no one impressed me more than these first words of my master, so simple but so profound."

From that moment started years of pure happiness with Gurudeva, serving at the feet of his master Baba Bajaranga Dasji Maharaja. The cabin where they lived was very simple, without any comforts. It was an austere life. In the hermitage, together with Gurudeva and Babaji, lived some devotees, but never more than 5 or 6 people.

What was the teaching that Babaji imparted to his disciples? Gurudeva possessed a brilliant intellect and had a lot of knowledge of philosophical books (Upanishads) and of other sacred scriptures of the Vedic Culture.

He knew perfectly all the teachings of all the different schools within Hinduism, the philosophical statements of the great masters, and the doctrines of other religions. He also knew the different techniques of meditation and prāṇāyāmas, together with other yoga disciplines. He knew and loved the culture and history of his country. In his youth he had actively participated in some political parties fighting for the independence of India, including spending some months in prison for his patriotic ideology. He had a great talent for speaking and wrote easily.

There was no cultural or academic instruction, not even of the yoga method, and there was no need for monastic education: Gurudeva knew his path very clearly. Babaji taught Gurudeva to live in truth and recognise it wherever it was. Babaji was Gurudeva's Brahmavidyā Guru, the master who directly instructs in the knowledge of the nature of Brahman, "The Absolute." The teaching of Babaji can be summarized in a few words:

"My son, there are many saints and learned men in the world; first you must become a man!".

Babaji taught that a man was not envied for his ostentation, but respected for his simplicity. Humility does not signify gentleness but the disposition to recognise the greatness of others. At the end of all his journeys, Gurudeva carried with him two mantras that his Guru taught him. They summarise in great part the teachings he received. The first was the mantra of Assimilation.

"First free yourself of ego and then use words that give the same happiness to others as they give to you."

The second mantra was of Modesty.

"Modesty grants glory, while the anxiety for glory takes God away. Because of his reduced size, the ant can collect particles of sugar that enter in the dust, while the elephant can only dirty himself with them".

The formation of his character was the most important teaching that Gurudeva received during the time he stayed in the company of his master. He always considered that the profound love and compassion that Babaji felt towards all creatures manifested itself in a curious behaviour when someone met him. As soon as he saw a friend, on many occasions he cried. He was also terribly affected when someone left the Kuti.

Some, amongst them Gurudeva, did not understand this behaviour, confusing it with excessive sentimentality. Gurudeva reproached him for his tears.

"Who is grieving! Grief cannot come near to me. These are tears of love and they have nothing to do with grief." answered Babaji.

Soon Gurudeva could understand for himself the truth of Babaji words.

Although Babaji profoundly loved his disciple, and the time they spent together was for both of them the highest happiness of love and understanding, he did not delay in sending him away from Kutira for the first of his preaching journeys, knowing that it was this service that Gurudeva must give to humanity.

He said, "My son, the world is suffering terribly. The rich like the poor are living in miserable conditions. Man cannot live on bread alone. He needs divine grace and the light of spiritualism. You have to take on this task. It is urgent and important".

"But, Maharajaji" said Gurudeva, "I do not have the ability or the resources to do this."

"Do not worry. All will come to you without asking for anything. Have faith in me."

In this way, thanks to Babaji's vision, the whole world was able to benefit from the true spiritual message transmitted in the learned teachings of Gurudeva.

When he said goodbye to his master, he lovingly kissed him saying:

"Always remember that all houses, all denominations, all countries and all Gurus are yours. Share the happiness and grief of others. Be as clear as water and do not place any limits. Continue flowing, filling ditches and wells."

If Gurudeva had any doubts about the true indifference of his master, it was cleared up on an occasion when after an absence of eight years, he returned to the feet of his master. The order to take his message out of India soon came in the form of a journey that took him to the western world. In the pure atmosphere and spirit of the Kutira, Gurudeva felt very happy serving at the feet of his master again. He knew that Babaji felt proud of him. Didn't he say time and time again, showing his photograph to everyone "Look, this is my disciple. Now he is spreading dharma (the religion) all over the world."

Gurudeva knew the necessity of leaving and each day he said "I'm leaving, I'm leaving," but each day he thought, "Why the rush?" Eight years have passed, I'm going to stay here a while longer, "Where am I going to find as much peace?" "Where am I going to find anyone that loves me as much as Babaji?" Soon Babaji gave the reason.

One night, while talking to some devotees, he said:

"Some speak of leaving, however, they do not go. If you do not think of going, why speak about it?"

The following day Guruveda said goodbye to his master and started his great journey abroad.

During his padayātrā (pilgrimage on foot) of eight years throughout India, Gurudeva lost the few clothes he had. One day, his shoes broke. From that moment he never returned to wearing shoes. Another day his "kurtā" (shirt) tore, so he never wore another "kurtā" either. This continued until he was only left with a lunghi (a piece of cloth that covers from the waist to the feet) and a wool blanket.

During the last 20 years of his life, these were his only clothes. For the person who met Gurudeva for the first time, knowing that his life was spent travelling, it was a big surprise to see his luggage. He carried a lungi as a change of clothing, his toiletries and two books, the Rāmāyaṇa and the Mahābhārata.

On one occasion, during a radio interview, the presenter asked Guruveda:

"Swami, have you come to establish a sect of barefoot monks?"

"My friend" answered Gurudeva, "I havn't come to establish anything new. My only hope is that if I see a rich man surrounded by his possessions, comfortably seated in his house, but despite this fact he says to himself, 'Why am I not happy?' he could remember that monk who travels without money, dressed in two pieces of cloth and who did not even have shoes on his feet, but was totally happy. Maybe then he would see that happiness is in the realisation of the Internal Being and does not depend on material objects."

The standard custom was to treat all authorised religious men with pomp and ceremony, looking after them and not introducing political themes, other sects, privileged groups, authorities or rival schools into the conversation. It was also customary to wait several days before being received by him. The people were disconcerted at first but later happy with the free spirit of Gurudeva.

He rejected categorically any type of ostentation with regard to himself. His Guru had sent him to show himself as a pilgrim monk and to lighten the hearts of his devotees with his example and even more with his words. To show humility, he used a brush to clean his quarters. To show self-control, he never accepted a sweater, even though in Russia it was less than–10 degrees. To show modesty, he was always open to show his respect to any person of authority, even though he knew they were inferior to him. To show compassion, he personally answered all the letters he received, never less than 30 a week and personally attended to everyone who came looking for help. If he was in a city where someone he knew lived, he went to greet him even if he had to walk 10 kilometres.

To exhibit simplicity he never accepted money other than what he needed to travel to his next destination and when he travelled he always took the most economical form of transport. To show his power of faith in God, he travelled without money or help from any organisation. Many times he arrived in countries or cities where he knew no one and did not speak the language. He was not bothered by sleeping in the street or spending days without eating, waiting for the hand of God to protect him. These circumstances, instead of testing his faith, confirmed it, because in spite of the extremely risky manner in which he travelled, there was always someone to help him.

In all the houses he visited, Gurudeva cooked delicious meals for his hosts. In this way, through Prasad (food offered to God, cooked by a religious person), he purified the bodies and minds of all who ate his food. This was his silent blessing to everyone who gave him hospitality.

One day, a Pandit (a scholar) of the privileged group of Brāhmaṇas (the highest privileged group of priests, masters, etc.), wanted to determine if Gurudeva was a Brāhmaṇa Sannyāsī (of the privileged Brāhmaṇa group) to know if he must pay his respects or not. When Gurudeva found this out, he laughed to himself and prostrated himself before the Brāhmaṇa, saying that he was a caṇḍāla (member of the lowest group, the untouchables).

Gurudeva commented: "Thanks to the teaching that I received from my Guru, I feel comfortable in any place. Thanks to having an equal attitude towards others, I can penetrate the forces of different sects and schools of philosophy. Dualists and non-dualists have all opened their doors with happiness. The Brāhmaṇas and the pariahs have all offered me hospitality in their houses. Many times they have asked me "Swamiji, who are you?". "Are you Advaitin (non-dualist) or Dvaitin (dualist)?". "Are you Brāhamaṇa or Kṣatriya?"

"Vaiśya or Śūdra?" (Brāhmaṇa, Kṣatriya, Vaiśya and Śūdra are the four Hindu groups). "We are very surprised to see all types of people delighted to attend your conferences."

"AIR EATERS"

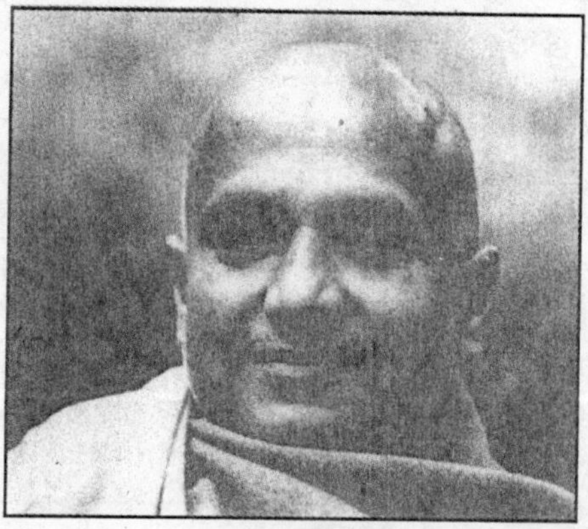

Swami Tilak

As Air Eaters we have been able to see through this book, the Vyāyāma Yoga practice is rooted in the most intimate nature of the person, seeking to instruct how to use the resources that are inside ourselves in order to achieve what would otherwise be impossible. A person who practises Vyāyāma Yoga gradually becomes an "air eater," a vyahaṛka, without noticing. Before ever having practised Vyāyāma yoga, breathing may have been an insignificant everyday activity, but as we bring Vyāyāma yoga into our lives, air ingestion becomes an indispensable way to obtain the best resources from any type of activity.

The "air eater," vyahaṛka, understands that the quality of his life is based on using internal resources in an appropriate way and that this continues by using the external resources in the same way. He understands and experiences that the source of pleasure comes from a correct use of breathing and that its control may provide a higher level of pleasure.

GUIDANCE DURING PRACTICE

Vyāyāma yoga was originally practised by warriors. Today, it can be practised by anyone of any age and allows the development of different techniques which can help to improve the practitioner's quality of life.

Practising Vyāyāma yoga provides physical well-being and strength, enhances the capacity to enjoy and allows the realization of happiness. It has been transmitted from master to disciple in a continuous succession to the present day. Because of this, although we are lucky to have this book, practising under the guidance of a qualified instructor will prevent possible mistakes while allowing the student to advance at a faster pace.

It is often observed in beginners and in those who are not no longer beginners, how a number of defects develop, which might later cause injury, should a qualified person not correct them.

You can learn Vyāyāma through the following activities developed by the Traditional School of Vyāyāma yoga: classes, seminars, conferences, workshops and especially the teachers' training course which consists of three levels:

I. Preparatory level, 100 hours.
II. Instructor's level, 100 hours.
III. Professor's level, 200 hours.

Someone attending these activities may have the purpose of becoming a teacher or just the objective of learning and practising in a deeper way.

Teachers' training course

This course is specifically structured for those interested in the deep knowledge of its teachings.

This course prepares the students to:

1. Practice Vyāyāma yoga in a more precise way.
2. Understand its philosophy and therapeutics.
3. Work individually in order to obtain enough resources to take care of our physical, emotional and spiritual health.
4. Teaching Vyāyāma yoga in the future, after completing the teachers' training course.

The teachings throughout the training period are based on the combination of three disciplines known as the TRIKA triad: Haṭha-Yoga, Vyāyāma and Dance. They are complemented by basic Āyurveda, basic Tantra philosophy, psychosomatic therapy and an introduction to Sanskrit and the philosophy of language.

The study of the topics described in the following list is accompanied by the practice of one or more of the Vyāyāma blocks of exercises and is developed during the three levels.

Programme contents

1. Initiation to the Vyāyāma yoga master programme

1.1. The meaning of Vyāyāma yoga.
1.2. The strength of the breath and a healthy body.
1.3. Basic principles of Vyāyāma yoga.
1.4. Energetic anatomy.
1.5. Āyurveda.
1.5.1. Origins of Āyurveda.
1.5.2. Foundations and principles of Āyurveda: the five elements and the three energies.
1.5.3. Doṣas and Guṇas: their characteristics
1.5.4. The seven dhātus, their formation and maintenance
1.5.5. The six flavours and their influence on health
1.6. The five harmony and health principles
1.7. Physiology and anatomy: bones, muscles, joints, circulation, breathing, digestion, excretion
1.8. Energetic anatomy and its relation to physiological anatomy

2. **Training programme**

2.1 Learning contemplation.
Setting the foundations for a meditative and introspective life that empowers the innate capacities and awakens creative and self-healing potential.

2.2 Learning body purification.
Purification of the essential elements: earth, water, fire, air and ether.

2.3 Learning breathing.
Introduction to the science of breathing, Svarodaya and the study of the five prāṇas and nāḍi (energetic channel) draining

2.4 Learning relaxation.
Through the stillness of the body, we learn to install in our interior the capacity to project this stillness on a day-to-day basis. We obtain serenity when we give the mind the appropriate and necessary activity.

2.5 Learning the ignition of the six powers.
The connection and disconnection of the physical and subtle body. Cakras, their composition and influence on the body, mind and spirit. How to purify and activate them.

2.6 Learning positive thought.
By thinking positively, we are providing the body with optimum health and harmony, we fight disease effectively and our lives are filled with light. We learn how to transform our negative thoughts into positive ones instead of repressing them.

2.7 Learning healing energy.
Health is what integrates a person with himself. We have an inner strength that we can use to heal ourselves and to heal others, or to be more receptive to treatments. The five basic principles of self-healing are studied.

2.8 Learning awareness of the three bodies.
Every human being, no matter what his level of evolution is, has the potential to reach the highest powers. The eight steps to achieve these powers are studied.

2.9 Learning Saṁyama meditation.
Saṁyama gives the guidelines for the acquisition of qualities of the mind, providing power over the nature of things, animals and persons. It is the dominance over the profound nature of anything, to unite subject and object. In tantric terms, this means to unite the person who meditates with the object of his meditation.

2.10 Learning to invoke the power of the three Gods.
Happiness comes from the spirit and life is full of happiness that transforms itself into vital energy. The three divine life-regulating forces are studied: The Power of the Creator, the Power of the Preserver and the Power of the Destructor.

2.11 Learning to invoke the power of the three Goddesses.
All beings carry inside them the duality of the masculine and feminine forces, the positive and the negative. Through their invocation we acquire the energetic knowledge of the deep duality that manifests itself in us as breath. The three divine forces, which are consort to the Creative, Preserver and Destructive powers are studied.

3. Global vision of the delivered knowledge.
Magisterial closing and a projection of the delivered knowledge in our everyday life is contemplated.

Where to Learn Vyāyāma

The Traditional School of Vyāyāma has two websites where you can find all the information you need: www.vyayama.org / www.saberser.org

If you have any questions about this book you can write to: escuelavedica@yahoo.es

Glossary of Sanskrit terms

Adhama kala	:	In the practice of Vyāyāma, this refers to a low impact exercise.
Ādi Tala	:	The different physical points in which a tala is projected.
Ājñā cakra	:	Energetic centre which has its physical projection in the space between the eyebrows.
Ahaṁkāra	:	False self, associated with a form in a physical body.
Ajapā-japa	:	The spontaneous repetition of a mantra caused by the inertia of conscious repetition.
Anāhata cakra	:	Energetic centre which has its physical projection at the level of the heart, in the centre of the chest.
Annamaya kośa	:	First substantial form of the physical body, Sthūla Śarīra, which is made of energy extracted from food.
Antaḥkaraṇa	:	Internal investigation organ used by the Ātman, the being itself, to know and to be projected in the outer world.
Anusvāra	:	The final vibration of the OM sound. Its chart representation corresponds to the dot placed over the letter M, indicating that in its pronunciation, it vibrates at the top of the head.
Apāna	:	Energy that controls the excreting processes of the body.
Artha	:	The principles of life transactions
Asidhara Vāda	:	One of the disciplines of the art of sword "to clutch the sharp sword"
Aśvattha	:	Sacred tree whose roots seem to grow to the sky and its branches go inside the earth
Ātman	:	Being. My self, that which determines my existence.
Āyurveda	:	The knowledge of life and of all that is necessary to improve our health and avoid disease. Vedic medicine
Bhairava	:	Fierce aspect of the God Śiva
Bodhidharma	:	Buddhist master of Indian origin who took the knowledge of Vyāyāma to China and afterwards to Japan
Bhārata Varṣa	:	The name given to India in ancient times, meaning Land of Light

Bhastrikā Svara : Type of breathing in which the movements are made with the thoracic area of the lungs, resembling the movement of a pair of bellows.

Bhūta Śuddhi Tantra : Classical scripture of Tantra knowledge

Bīja mantra : Seed or root sound from which other sounds originate. They contain great energetic power that is awakened when repeated.

Brahma : The power of the being that manifests in the Universe.

Brahman : The Absolute Being. He who determines all existence.

Brahma-dvāra : The gateway located at the end of the subtle energy channel known as Suṣumṇā, from which the state of realization is obtained.

Bhrāmarī svara : Type of breathing which resembles the sound of a bumble bee.

Buddhi : Intellect

Cakra : Centre where energy is generated and regenerated.

Caraka Saṁhitā : One of the most important classical texts where the basis of āyurvedic medicine is collected

Chiku Vāda : One of the disciplines of the art of the sword. "To take up the dagger".

Citta : Subconscious mind where all past experiences are stored.

Daṇḍa Vāda : One of the disciplines of the art of sword. "To brandish the stick".

Dhanur Vidyā : Vedic military art/science.

Dhanur Veda : The knowledge of archery.

Dharma : From the Sanskrit root "dhṛ": that which supports. It is the law which allows everything to be; the natural law, the social law, the spiritual law and the law of morality.

Durlabhasāra Tantra : One of the scriptures of Tantra knowledge.

Jñāna mudrā : Hand gesture that symbolizes knowledge.

Jñāna śakti : The power that gives the capacity for knowledge.

Guṇa : Quality or matter vibration state.

Guru : He who gives light in the darkness. A spiritual master.

Hasta Vāda : One of the martial art disciplines. "To expand the fists".

Haṭha : The force manifested through both the poles, positive and negative.

Icchā śakti : The power that gives the capacity for will power.
Iḍā : Subtle energy channel through which negative energy flows.
Jala : Water.
Janakarājā : Famous wise king.
Kālī : Goddess of death. The power that destroys everything.
Kālikā Purāṇa : Ancient Vedic text that describes the natures of Kālī.
Karma : From the Sanskrit root "kṛ", doing. All action entails a reaction.
Kanda : The place where Kuṇḍalinī dwells, the power of the serpent, situated at the base of the spinal column in its physical projection.
Kaṅga Mārga : The use of a sword.
Kāpālaka svara : Type of breathing in which the use of the diaphragm predominates with fast contraction movements.
Kāraṇa Śarīra : The third body, known as astral body and origin of the other two bodies.
Kāraṇa Vyāyāma : A magical form of practising Vyāyāma which is mainly performed with mantras, a special class of sounds which modifies mental states, and with saṁyama meditation, which allows the acquisition of a number of qualities.
Karnatak : Articulated way of producing sounds.
Kaṭha Upaniṣad : One of the scriptures belonging to the philosophy of the Absolute, Brahman.
Kauśala : Ability, capacity.
Krama Abhyāsa : Progression of linked movements.
Kriyā śakti : The power that gives the capacity for action.
Kudhan Vāda : One of the disciplines of the art of the sword. "To take up the wooden sword."
Kumbhaka antar : Breath retention with the lungs full of air.
Kumbhaka bahir : Breath retention with no air in the lungs.
Kuṇḍalinī : The latent and individualised Śakti Power.
Lakṣmī : Goddess of prosperity. The power that brings prosperity in its multiple forms.
Lakṣmī Tantra : One of the scriptures of Tantra knowledge.
Liṅga : Male sexual organ.
Madhyama kala : Moderate-impact Vyāyāma exercise.
Mahā Deva : Great god, the name of the God Śiva.
Mahā Devī : Great goddess, the name of the Goddess Pārvatī, consort of Śiva.

Mahā Nirvāṇa Tantra : One of the scriptures of Tantra knowledge.

Manas : Conscious mind. The faculty that allows for thought.

Maṇipūra Cakra : Energetic centre which has its physical projection in the solar plexus.

Mārga : Path.

Marmas : Energy connection cores.

Moda : State of happiness experienced when possessing what is desired.

Mokṣa : State of liberation.

Mudrā : Gesture performed primarily with the hands, with the objective of channelling energy in a determined way.

Mūlādhāra cakra : Energy centre which has its physical projection at the base of the spinal column.

Mumukṣutva : Intense desire for liberation.

Nāḍī : From the root "nad" which means movement. Among other meanings we can also find: river, current or flow.

Naṭya Śāstra : Scriptures where the knowledge of dance and music is collected.

Nyāsas : Special touches performed on different parts of the body pronouncing special sounds, with the objective of estblishing energy in the body part.

Om : The original vibration from which the whole Universe originated. The three letters that compose it, AUM, in their original vibration are the three basic states of the **Universe**: manifestation, preservation and destruction. It is the origin of the phonemes of the Sanskrit alphabet.

Pañcaprāṇas : The five essential vital energies.

Pañca Tantra : One of the scriptures of Tantra knowledge.

Paramaithuna : Sacred sexual act performed between a yogi and a yogini.

Piṅgalā : Subtle channel through which the positive energy flows.

Prakṛti : That to which everything returns. Matter in its essential state of manifestation.

Pramoda : State of happiness resulting from enjoying the object of desire.

Prāṇa : Vital energy

Prāṇamaya kośa : Vital form contained in the subtle body, formed by

		vital energy in its different manifestations. It is intimately linked to the physical body.
Pratyāhāra	:	Abstraction.
Āhāra	:	to eat, gobble up.
Pratyakṣa	:	Perception.
Priya	:	State of happiness resulting from seeing.
Pūraka	:	Inhalation.
Rajas	:	Excited energy vibration state.
Rājarṣis	:	Ancient wise men of royal origin.
Rāma	:	Incarnation of the God Viṣṇu. The source of pleasure.
Recaka	:	Exhalation.
Ṛddhi	:	Material power obtained by yoga practice.
Rudra	:	The God of destruction. The power that encompasses all, allowing all to return to its origin.
Rudrayāmala Tantra	:	One of the scriptures of Tantra knowledge.
Sahaja krama abhyāsa	:	Spontaneous practice of Vyāyāma. The original practice.
Sahasrāra Cakra	:	Energy centre which has its physical projection at the top of the head. It is the lotus of a thousand petals. When the energy rises to this point, the ultimate state of realization of yoga is achieved.
Samāna	:	Vital energy that controls the digestive processes.
Samatva	:	Harmony.
Samskāras	:	Latent impression. Seed.
Saṁyama	:	Meditation practice that seeks to acquire the qualities of the object of meditation.
Sanskrit	:	Original language of the Vedas. Perfect.
Sattva	:	Harmonic energy vibration state.
Śakti	:	From the root "śak" which means power, doing. It indicates activity and capacity. Śakti is power in general and any particular form of power.
Śakti gatis	:	Vyāyāma exercises that mobilize the śakti.
Śakti puṣṭis	:	Vyāyāma exercises that cover the śakti.
Śakti Śuddhis	:	Vyāyāma exercises that purify the śakti.
Śakti Urdanas	:	Vyāyāma exercises that regulate the pulsation of the śakti.
Śakti Vardhakas	:	Vyāyāma exercises that rejuvenate the śakti.
Śakti Vikāsakas	:	Vyāyāma exercises that strengthen the śakti.
Śiva Saṁhitā	:	One of the three most important classical texts of Haṭha yoga, the yoga of strength.
Śūnya	:	Vacuum, zero.

Siddhi : Spiritual power obtained through yoga practice.

Sthūla Vyāyāma : Vyāyāma practice in which most exercises are static and dense.

Śūkṣma śarīra : Subtle body.

Śūkṣma Vyāyāma : Vyāyāma practice in which most exercises are energetic.

Suṣruta Saṁhitā : Classical text of Āyurvedic medicine.

Svādhiṣṭhāna Cakra : Energy centre which has its physical projection at the level of the genital organs.

Svaras : Dynamic ventilations.

Svarodaya : The act of breathing is known as svara and changing from one nostril to the other is known as udaya, therefore the whole process is known as svarodaya. It is the science or knowledge of breathing and the states produced or reflected by it.

Taittirīya Upaniṣad : One of the scriptures of the philosophy or knowledge of the Absolute, Brahman.

Talas : Energy distribution centres.

Tamas : State in which matter vibrates at a low and dense frequency.

Tan : Energetic centre that determines the characteristics of a personality.

Tan hara Śakti : The tan is the neurological point of the 'area of strength', tan hara śakti and is divided in a frontal region known as tan Śakti and a rear region known as tan tala. The tan hara Śakti is where the balance of the body is concentrated and where the mind descends in order to achieve serenity and rest.

Tantra : That which expands the mind and frees consciousness. The knowledge that seeks the liberation of man through the use of energy in its diverse states.

Tridoṣa : The humours that control the activity of the body and mind.

Tripurasundarī : Goddess who dwells in the three cities. It refers to the three vibration states of matter. It is the power of the three goddesses together: Durgā, Lakṣmī and Sarasvatī.

Triśūla : Trident.

Udāna : Vital energy that controls the process of swallowing food.

Ujjayika svara : Breathing performed by emitting a whistling sound. It concentrates and fixes the mind.

Umā : Goddess consort of the God Śiva. The power that controls the activity of material nature.

Utta kala : High impact exercise in Vyāyāma practice.

Varṇaṭak : Non-articulated way of pronouncing sounds.

Vāta : One of the three humours that constitutes the nature of the human being according to āyurvedic medicine, in which the wind element predominates.

Vāyu : Wind. The God of wind. The power that drives everything.

Vāyuka : To have the presence of the God Vāyu. Breaths produced by sharply expelling air with a sound.

Vāyu kanda : Place where the breath resides.

Vicāra : Analysis.

Vikṣepa : State of mind agitation which leads to constant errors.

Vīravrata : Warrior. The one who preserves his virile energy.

Vīra Vrata Vidyā : The science of the strong ones. Vedic military art/ science.

Viṣṇu : The God who preserves the universe.

Viṣṇu Purāṇa : Ancient Vedic text that explains the nature of Viṣṇu.

Viśuddha cakra : Pure. Energy centre which has its physical projection at the level of the throat.

Vyāna : Vital energy that controls all the fluids and currents of the body.

Vyāyāma : The oldest energetic and curative gymnastics in the world. To tame the inner breathe. This Sanskrit term is comprised of two words: yama, which means 'to tame', and vyu, which means 'to stimulate, to incite', 'to push the air or internal and external breath'. Vyāyāma is the discipline that teaches you to tame the energy that comes from the air through breathing. Its different meanings demonstrate the depth of the technique:

1 Drag and brake down any solid, subtle or mental structure.
2 Separate essential elements filling the core.
3 Healthy sport or physical activity.
4 Fight between bodies.
5 Struggle to achieve a goal.

6 Warrior combat.
7 That which enables you to successfully challenging yourself.
8 Effort to overcome one's limitations.

Vyaṅgas	:	Each one of the Vyāyāma exercises. Movement.
Yantra	:	Geometrical diagram of occult powers.
Yoga Sūtras	:	Yoga aphorisms. Attributed to Patañjali Maharṣi.
Yoni	:	Female sexual organ.

BOOKS OF RELATED INTEREST FROM NAB

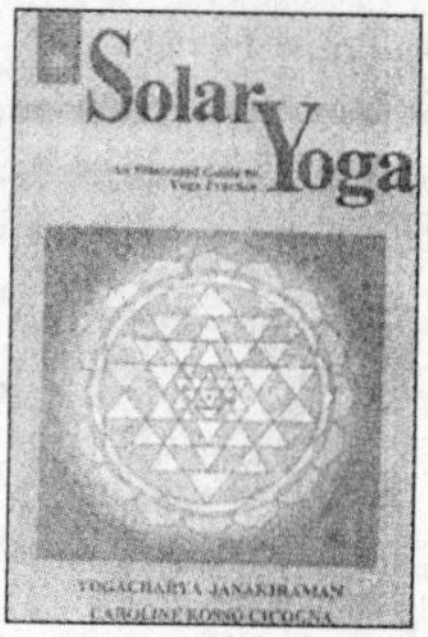

SOLAR YOGA

All Illustrated Guide to Yoga Practice

—Yogacharya Janakiraman and Caroline Rosso Cicogna

This book offers new insights into the age-old discipline of Solar Yoga. It treats a carefully selected number of classical Yoga practices in a novel manner, integrating the use of sound vibrations with that of postures and breathing techniques at the physical, psychic and spiritual levels.

ISBN: 978-81-7822-247-9

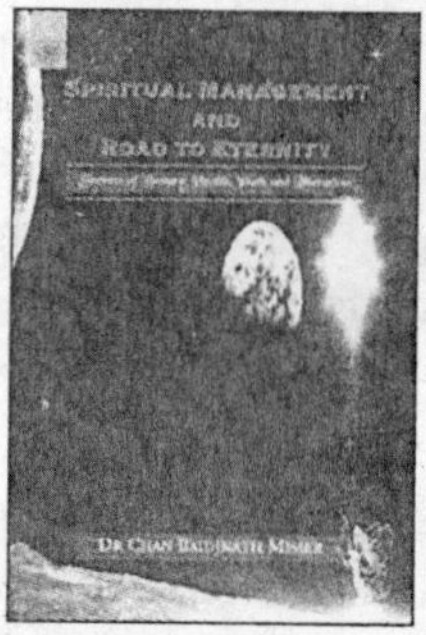

SPIRITUAL MANAGEMENT AND ROAD TO ETERNITY

Secrets of Beauty, Health, Youth and Liberation

—Dr. Chan Baidjnath Misier

This book integrates the various aspects of yoga and shows how to find inner strength, to establish a way of living that brings you inner peace, health, energy and happiness throughout your life. Self-realization and union with God are the threads through all the subjects in this paper, with an explanation of proper breathing, meditation and puja with easy practices.

ISBN: 978-81-7822-278-3

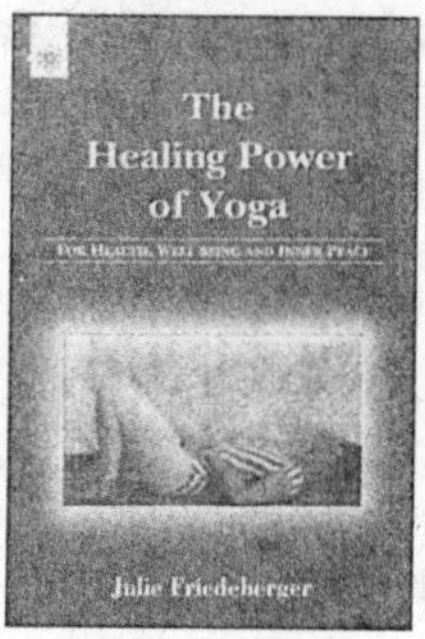

THE HEALING POWER OF YOGA

For Health, Well-Being and Inner Peace

—Julie Friedeberger

This is a book about yoga, a holistic system for creating and sustaining balance and harmony on all the levels of our being : body, mind, emotions and spirit.

ISBN: 978-81-7822-181-6

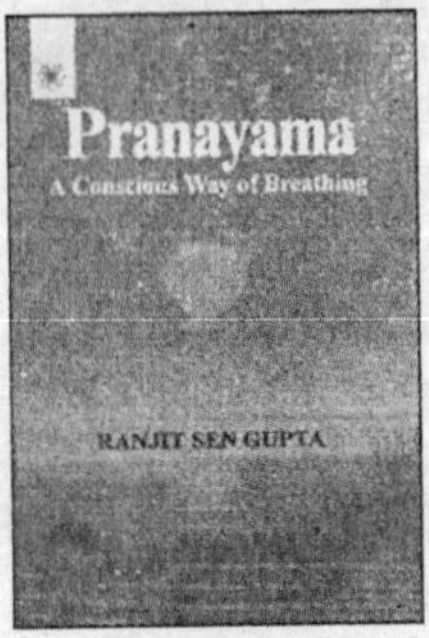

PRANAYAMA
A Conscious Way of Breathing
—Ranjit Sen Gupta

Pranayama is the conscious perception and guidance of life energies which unfold self in complex form in the psychophysical system of all living beings.

ISBN: 978-81-7822-083-3

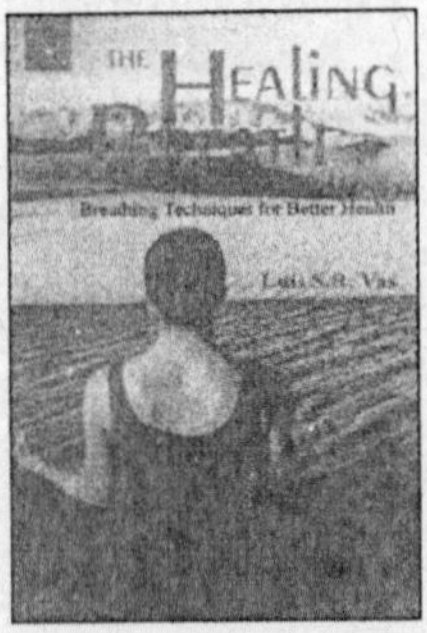

THE HEALING BREATH
Breathing Techniques for Better Health
—Luis S.R. Vas

This book covers the numberous benefits that simple breathing techniques, which are described here, can bring us. Of all these things, from coffee to ginseng to artificial stimulants to working out, they found that just 15 minutes of deep breathing can give us all the energy we need for the day.

ISBN: 978-81-7822-164-9

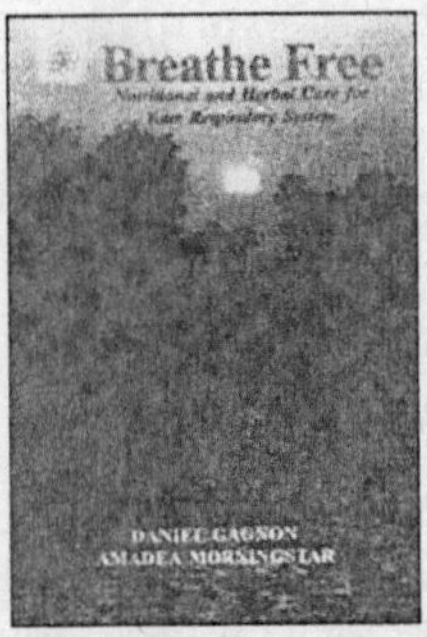

BREATHE FREE
Nutritional and Herbal Care for Your Respiratory System
—Daniel Gagnon and Amadea Morningstar

For the first time here is a self help book that tells it all. An expose on respiratory diseases and their natural treatment learn how you can heal and/or manage: Common Cold/Flu, Allergies/Hay Fever, Cough/Sore Throat, Aids and Related Respiration Infection, Earache/ Asthma, Pleurisy/Pneumonia, Bronchitis/ Emphysema.

ISBN: 978-81-7822-018-5